Oral Lichen Planus and Lichenoid Lesions

Gaetano Isola • Simona Santonocito
Rosalia Leonardi • Alessandro Polizzi

Oral Lichen Planus and Lichenoid Lesions

Etiopathogenesis, Diagnosis and Treatment

Springer

Gaetano Isola
Department of General Surgery and Surgical-Medical Specialties
School of Dentistry
University of Catania
Catania, Italy

Simona Santonocito
Department of General Surgery and Surgical-Medical Specialties
School of Dentistry
University of Catania
Catania, Italy

Rosalia Leonardi
Department of General Surgery and Surgical-Medical Specialties
School of Dentistry
University of Catania
Catania, Italy

Alessandro Polizzi
Department of General Surgery and Surgical-Medical Specialties
School of Dentistry
University of Catania
Catania, Italy

ISBN 978-3-031-29764-9 ISBN 978-3-031-29765-6 (eBook)
https://doi.org/10.1007/978-3-031-29765-6

This Springer imprint is published by the registered company Springer Nature Switzerland AG
The registered company address is: Gewerbestrasse 11, 6330 Cham, Switzerland

Foreword

My thoughts and thanks go to my colleagues at the University of Catania (Catania, Italy) who designed and published this valuable volume entitled *Oral Lichen Planus and Lichenoid Lesions*.

The authors, in six chapters, provide complete clinical and laboratory pathways, enhanced by a comprehensive update of the literature about these diseases. All this allows the reader both to follow and to deepen certain aspects, under the stimulus of the controversies that the topics of Oral Lichen Planus and Lichenoid Lesions have offered in recent decades; it is the case of the differential diagnoses among these lesions, and their malignant transformation.

The current lack of clarity and standardization in diagnosis and treatment seems to contribute to the unimproved prevalence of oral squamous cell carcinoma and its high mortality, and the general low awareness of potentially malignant oral disorders.

I am sure that it will help all young practitioners orient themselves in dealing with such a complex issue, both in the diagnostic and therapeutic steps, correlating these diseases with the systemic aspects related.

It will provide an excellent stimulus for older and more experienced readers for further study, research, and critical analysis.

In the face of such an important and strategic objective, this text constitutes a well-successful experiment that has been able to integrate, in a synergistic design, the authors' skills and knowledge, enriched by an important work of analysis and comparison of bibliographic sources, with a precious accuracy and iconographic richness.

Giuseppina Campisi
University of Palermo
Palermo, Italy

Contents

Introduction

1

The mouth can be regarded as the window of the body: it can reflect, even at an early stage, a systemic disease state. The oral mucosa, primarily, is derived embryologically from the invagination of the ectoderm, and, therefore, it is not surprising that it may be involved in disorders primarily associated with the skin.

Lichen planus (LP) is a chronic mucocutaneous disorder of stratified squamous epithelium that may affect the oral, esophageal, laryngeal, nasal, conjunctival, anal, and genital mucous membranes, skin, nails, and scalp (causing alopecia) [1–3]. OLP (oral lichen planus) is considered to be a chronic inflammatory clinical condition, of noninfective origin, affecting the stratified squamous epithelium of the oral cavity and the underlying lamina propria [4]—derived from the Greek word "leichen" meaning tree moss and from the Latin word "planus" meaning flat. The term "lichen" was applied to the disease because of the common presentation of the flat lesions that suggested a resemblance to lichens [1].

Ferdinand von Hebra (1816–1880), professor at the Viennese school of dermatology and leader of modern dermatology, was the first to provide, in 1860, a scientific description of certain chronic inflammatory lesions of the skin, confluent with each other and characterized by papular eruptions, itchy eruptions, hence the name "lichen ruber" (from the Latin ruber meaning red) which was later referred to as "lichen planus" for the not particularly noticeable redness and the characteristic flatness of the lesions, which would better describe the pathognomonic nature of the lesion.

Significant contributions to the description of the disease were made by the famous British surgeon and British dermatologist Erasmus Wilson (1809–1884) who redefined in 1866 the "lichen ruber" of Hebra and called it "lichen planus" (LP). He described several clinical cases of lichen planus, in which he treated with an iron-arsenical mixture, Fowler's solution (1% solution of potassium arsenate biacid), and a mercury bichloride lotion, all substances used in the past as medicines for various ailments, now considered toxic and dangerous [5].

In 1895, the French pathologist Louis Frédéric Wickham (1861–1913) observed the characteristic hyperkeratotic striae, whitish and arborescent skin striae on the surface of papules, known today as "Wickham's striae" [6].

LP was therefore mainly diagnosed on the basis of objective and clinical-morphological aspects of the lesions until in 1906, when William Dubreuilh (1857–1935) and Ferdinand-Jean Darier (1856–1938), universally recognized as the father of French dermatology, described the histopathological changes [7].

Despite the first description of LP dating back to the second half of the nineteenth century, thanks to the studies of Erasmus Wilson, the pathogenic mechanisms that cause LP are still not fully clarified.

G. Isola et al., *Oral Lichen Planus and Lichenoid Lesions*,
https://doi.org/10.1007/978-3-031-29765-6_1

The diagnostic aspects also remain controversial, differential histological and nosological aspects that guide the formulation of the diagnosis, as well as the actual potential for malignant transformation of OLP. All these factors constitute the aspects that describe the complexity of this pathology.

References

1. Gupta S, Jawanda MK. Oral lichen planus: an update on etiology, pathogenesis, clinical presentation, diagnosis and management. Indian J Dermatol. 2015;60(3):222.
2. Mutafchieva MZ, et al. Oral lichen planus–known and unknown: a review. Folia Med (Plovdiv). 2018;60(4):528–35.
3. Crincoli V, et al. Oral lichen planus: update on etiopathogenesis, diagnosis and treatment. Immunopharmacol Immunotoxicol. 2011;33(1):11–20.
4. Bermejo-Fenoll A, López-Jornet P. Familial oral lichen planus: presentation of six families. Oral Surg Oral Med Oral Pathol Oral Radiol Endod. 2006;102(2):e12–5.
5. Wilson E. Addresses and papers read at the thirty-fourth annual meeting of the British medical association: on lichen planus: the lichen ruber of Hebra. Br Med J. 1866;2(302):399.
6. Keller Rivers J, Jackson R, Orizaga M. Who was Wickham and what are his striae? Int J Dermatol. 1986;25(9):611–3.
7. Shklar G. Lichen planus as an oral ulcerative disease. Oral Surg Oral Med Oral Pathol. 1972;33(3):376–88.

Epidemiology

2

Oral lichen planus (OLP) is one of the most common dermatological diseases occurring in the oral cavity [1], but the exact incidence and prevalence are unknown [2]. It is estimated that the prevalence in the world population of OLP could range from 0.22 to 5% [3]. The incidence, on the other hand, has been identified as 2.2% [4] and the female-to-male ratio is 2:1. The disease begins on average between the ages of 30 and 60 [very rare cases have been reported in young and even in pediatric subjects (Table 2.1)] and is often reported in familial cases or in conjunction with other immune-reactive diseases [5, 6]. Twenty percent of females and 15% of males with OLP also manifest cutaneous and genital LP lesions. Furthermore, it is estimated that 70–77% of cutaneous LP patients concomitantly manifest OLP lesions [5–8]. However, further well-designed studies, with standardized methods, and criteria in different populations are needed to obtain more reliable data [9].

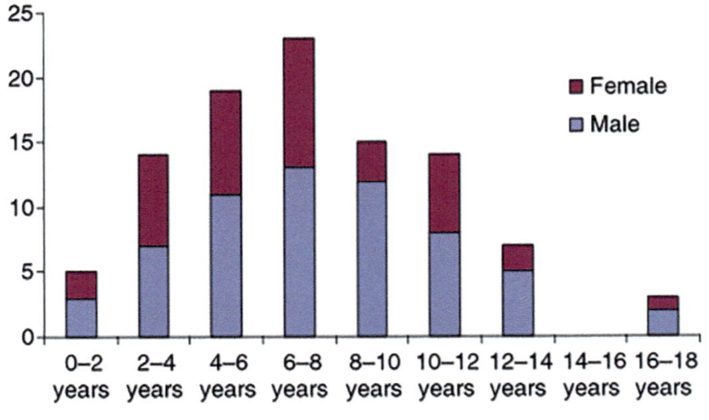

Graph associated with Table 2.1

G. Isola et al., *Oral Lichen Planus and Lichenoid Lesions*,
https://doi.org/10.1007/978-3-031-29765-6_2

Table 2.1 Subgroups of patients according to gender and age of onset

Epidemiology of LP in a child population of 100 individuals	
No of patients	100
M/F	61/39
Age in years (range)	8.76 (2–18)
Age of onset in years (range)	7.6
No of positive cases due to family history	2
Oral involvement (OLP)	17%

(With associated graph)—taken from Kanwar A.J. and De D. (2009)

References

1. Elenbaas, Andrea, Reyes Enciso, and Kamal Al-Eryani. "Oral lichen planus: a review of clinical features, etiologies, and treatments." Dentistry Review 2.1 (2022):100007.
2. Gupta S, Jawanda MK. Oral lichen planus: an update on etiology, pathogenesis, clinical presentation, diagnosis and management. Indian J Dermatol. 2015;60(3):222.
3. Gorouhi F, Davari P, Fazel N. Cutaneous and mucosal lichen planus: a comprehensive review of clinical subtypes, risk factors, diagnosis, and prognosis. Sci World J. 2014;2014:742826.
4. De Rossi SS, Ciarrocca K. Oral lichen planus and lichenoid mucositis. Dent Clin. 2014;58(2):299–313.
5. Farhi D, Dupin N. Pathophysiology, etiologic factors, and clinical management of oral lichen planus, part I: facts and controversies. Clin Dermatol. 2010;28(1):100–8.
6. Kanwar A, De D. Lichen planus in childhood: report of 100 cases. Clin Exp Dermatol. 2010;35(3):257–62.
7. Stoopler ET, Sollecito TP. Oral lichen planus. CMAJ. 2012;184(14):E774.
8. Scully C, Carrozzo M. Oral mucosal disease: lichen planus. Br J Oral Maxillofac Surg. 2008;46(1):15–21.
9. Carrozzo M. How common is oral lichen planus? Evid Based Dent. 2008;9(4):112–3.

3 Aetiology

OLP is considered a chronic mucocutaneous inflammatory disorder of unknown etiology. The most relevant hypotheses explain the disease as a T lymphocyte-mediated immune reaction, probably induced/favored by factors of exogenous and/or endogenous origin [1].

3.1 Factors of Exogenous Origin

3.1.1 Infectious Agents

CD8+ T lymphocytes, active in OLP and localized with apoptotic keratinocytes, are known for their role in inducing programmed cell death in virally infected cells [2].

Therefore, viral infections of the oral mucosa could be involved in the development of OLP lesions [3]. There are numerous associations between OLP and viral infections that have been studied, cytomegalovirus (CMV), herpes simplex virus-1 (HSV-1), Epstein-Barr virus (EBV) [4], human herpesvirus-6 (HHV-6) [5], human papillomavirus (HPV) [6–8], and human immunodeficiency virus (HIV) [9], but no significant correlations have been found [10].

Recently, however, some research seems to reevaluate the role of HPV in OLP (see Sect. 4.5.1).

With regard to hepatitis B virus (HBV), it appears that the risk of developing LP in hepatitis B surface antigen (HBsAg)-positive patients is twice as high as in HBsAg-negative patients [11]. Furthermore, anti-HBV antibodies have been observed in the lichenoid eruptions of OLP patients after the administration of several anti-HBV vaccines [12].

There is currently relevant evidence that, at least in some geographic areas, especially in the Mediterranean area, OLP may be associated with hepatitis C virus (HCV) infection, probably due to concomitant extrahepatic effects of HCV, such as cryoglobulinemia and other autoimmune and immune-reactive disorders in general [13–15]. The pathogenetic mechanism linking OLP and HCV is based on the discovery of circulating antibodies against the oral epithelium identified in OLP patients with concomitant HCV infection and the fact that the cytokine mediating OLP is triggered by HCV infection [16]. Furthermore, HCV replication, by polymerase chain reaction/reverse transcription or in situ hybridization, was detected in the epithelial cells of the oral mucosa involved in the OLP. In addition, HCV-specific CD4+ and CD8+ lymphocytes have been detected in the subepithelial band of the oral mucosa. This suggests that possibly HCV-specific T lymphocytes may play a role in the development of OLP; however the OLP-HCV etiopathogenetic connection still remains controversial and requires further prospective and interventional studies for a better understanding [17]. The geographical variability in the OLP-HCV association could be attributable to a specific genetic haplotype in the

G. Isola et al., *Oral Lichen Planus and Lichenoid Lesions*,
https://doi.org/10.1007/978-3-031-29765-6_3

population (such as HLA-DR6) [18], to environmental factors, or even to the viral genotype of HCV itself. However, answers to these hypotheses have not yet been found [14, 15]. One study also evaluates a polymorphism on the gene encoding for interleukin-8 (IL-8) as possibly involved in the development and progression of PLO in HCV-positive patients [19]. From a clinical point of view, one study shows that HCV infection and toxic hepatitis status alone does not appear to cause clinical exacerbations of OLP. The alteration of hepatic hematological liver markers can induce such exacerbations, independent of the underlying pathology. Therefore in hepatopathic patients with OLP, especially in cases of elevated transaminases, collaboration between hepatologist and oral pathologist is vital in order to achieve better control of the clinical course of the disease [20].

Finally, as specified by a systematic review and meta-analysis of the literature, the association between the two diseases underlines the importance of hepatitis C virus screening in patients with oral lichen planus [21].

Studies on the correlation between OLP and bacterial infections are still at an early stage. Such microorganisms could cause, support, or exacerbate the course of the disease [22]. Studies on *Helicobacter pylori* have not shown an association with OLP [10]. Recent observations show significant increases in *Fusobacterium* and *Campylobacter* colonies and decreases of *Porphyromonas* in the saliva of patients with erosive OLP. The increase in these bacterial forms could cause or sustain lesion exacerbations [23]. Analyses of a recent study found high concentrations of *Fusobacterium*, *Leptotrichia*, and *Lautropia* in patients with OLP compared to healthy controls, in which streptococci were present, suggesting that OLP may be associated with dysbiosis of the oral cavity microbiome [24]. About the relationship between bacterial colonization and OLP, studies are relevant on toll-like receptors (TLRs), a subset of receptors that recognize microbial molecules. Indeed, the expression of these receptors in saliva and biopsies of oral lichen planus patients was different compared to healthy controls [25–28]. In addition, one study identifies a polymorphism in the TLR-3 gene that could play a significant role in the etiology of OLP [29]. Therefore, careful removal of oral microbial biofilm is recommended during the clinical course and management of OLP gingival and mucosal lesions [10].

3.1.2 Factors Causing Lichenoid Reactions

Certain dental restorative materials, drugs, and foods may be potential exogenous factors capable of triggering clinically and histologically similar exogenous factors capable of triggering lesions that are clinically and histologically similar to those observed in OLP: in this case, we speak of oral lichenoid reactions or lesions (OLR or OLLs) [30], in which it is possible to identify a specific causative factor, the removal of which usually leads to regression of the lesions [31], although some studies suggest that this may also not be the case [32]. Furthermore, these substances may also amplify the extent of pre-existing OLP lesions, generating complications in the management and clinical course of the disease [33]. We can distinguish contact OLL (OLCHR (oral lichenoid contact hypersensitivity reaction)), drug-induced OLL (OLDRs (oral lichenoid drug reactions)), and OLL associated with graft-versus-host disease (GvHD) [31].

Antigenic contact reactions (together with granulomatous reactions and reactions to tuberculin) constitute a type of delayed cell-mediated hypersensitivity reactions, or type IV reactions according to the Gell and Coombs classification, also known as DTH (delayed-type hypersensitivity). These reactions are mediated by cellular elements and not by antibodies, especially by Th1 CD4+ T helper (Th) lymphocytes (which act by activating phagocytosis and direct cytotoxicity mechanisms) and, in some cases, also by CD8+ cytotoxic T lymphocytes (which act mainly on macrophages and B lymphocytes). Antigenic contact reactions are triggered by the uptake of an external antigen by Langerhans cells, which, migrating through the epithelium and various tissues, present the processed antigen to CD4+ helper T lymphocytes in the lymph node. In reality, some substances do not have an antigenic character, unlike some metals, but, by penetrating the skin/mucosa, they can bind to specific surface proteins and thus acquire an allergenic character [34] (in this case we speak of "haptens"). There are many dental materials capable of triggering contact OLL, such as silver amalgam restorations that trigger low-level mercury exposures. Several studies have reported the presence of OLL in the mucosa adjacent to such types of restorations, and it was identified, from a histopathological point of view, the presence of spongiosis at such sites, suggesting that this histopathological alteration may be a helpful marker to suspect association with the restorative material [35, 36]. But, in addition to amalgam, there are also other materials that have been identified as possible cause of contact OLL: gold, cobalt, palladium, chromium, glass ionomer cements, and even nonmetallic materials such as epoxy resins (composite) and ceramics [37–41]. It has been found that food, toothpaste flavorings, and some food additives such as cinnamic aldehyde (cinnamates) could constitute contact allergens and produce lichenoid reactions (see Table 3.1) [40].

Drug-induced OLL also constitutes a type of delayed cellulomediated hypersensitivity reaction [34]. Drugs that can induce lichenoid reactions include antihypertensive drugs (including methyldopa, some ACE inhibitors), β-blockers, NSAIDs, some antimalarial drugs, oral hypoglycemic drugs (sulfonylureas such as chlorpropamide), allopurinol, antiretroviral drugs, and gold salts and penicillamine (used to treat rheumatoid arthritis) (see Table 3.2) [30, 38, 39, 44–47]. These drugs may exacerbate a latent pathology or a previous disorder rather than cause the pathology [48].Within the group of symptoms of graft-versus-host disease (GvHD) are also OLLs which may therefore occur in patients undergoing stem cell transplantation or bone marrow transplantation. In these patients, concomitant immunosuppressive therapy increases the risk of developing neoplasms, defining these types of lichenoid reactions as lesions with high malignant potential [38].

Table 3.1 Substances associated with oral lichenoid contact reactions

Contact OLL (OLCHR)	
Metallic dental materials	*Non-metallic dental materials*
– Silver, beryllium, bismuth	– Ceramics
– Mercury chloride 0.1%	– Acrylic compounds
– Cobalt, chromium	– Composites
– Mercury ammoniate 1%	– Glass ionomers
– Mercury metal	*Flavoring agents*
– Nickel	– Balsam of Peru
– Gold	– Cinnamates (cinnamic aldehyde)
– Palladium	– Eugenol
– Copper	– Menthol
– Tin	– Mint (peppermint)
	– Anti-tartar toothpastes

Taken and modified from Müller S. et al. (2017)

3.1.3 Habits and Trauma Factors

An etiological correlation between cigarette smoking and OLP has been suggested in some Indian communities [49]; however in most patients with OLP, there is no increase in the prevalence of this habit [50]. Betel nut chewing is also more prevalent in Indian patients with OLP than those without [51–53]. Studies have shown that spoiled abutidins potentially damaging oral tissues such as smoking and alcohol intake could promote a neoplastic degeneration of OLP lesions (see Sect. 4.5.1).

Theoretically also chronic mucosal trauma such as bruxism, malpositioned teeth, or incongruous dentures could also increase the risk of cancer of concomitant OLP lesions, but there are as yet no data in the literature that elaborate on these aspects. It is therefore recommended that dentists pay particular attention to possible traumatic factors on mucous membranes with OLP lesions, which are already more prone to neoplastic transformation than healthy oral mucosae (see Sect. 4.5). Finally, the Koebner phenomenon could partially explain the localization of lesions in the sites most subjected to trauma.

Table 3.2 Drugs associated with oral lichenoid reactions

Drug-induced OLL (OLDR)	
Antihypertensive drugs, diuretics, antiarrhythmics, and antianginal drugs – β-blockers (*atenolol, metoprolol, propanolol*) – Diuretics (*chlorothiazide, hydrochlorothiazide, furosemide*) – α2-agonists (*methyldopa*) – ACE inhibitors (*enalapril, captopril*) NSAIDS – Salicylates (*acetylsalicylic acid, mesalazine*) – Heteroaryl acetic acids (*diclofenac*) – Arylpropionic acids (*ibuprofen, naproxen*) – Indole and indene acetic acids (*indomethacin*) Antidiabetic drugs – Insulin – Sulfonylureas (*chlorpropamide, glipizide, glibenclamide* [42], *tolbutamide*) Anti-dyslipidemic drugs – Statins (*fluvastatin, lovastatin, pravastatin, simvastatin*) Antigout medications – Inhibitors of uric acid synthesis (*allopurinol*) Psychopharmaceuticals and CNS drugs – Sedative-hypnotics: *benzodiazepines* – Antidepressants: *tricyclic antidepressants* – Antimaniacals (*lithium*) – Anticonvulsants: hydantoins (*phenytoin*); carboxylic acids (*valproic acid*); iminostilbenes (*carbamazepine*)	Antibiotics – Antituberculars (*isoniazid, rifampicin*) – Aminoglycosides (*streptomycin*) – Tetracyclines Antivirals – Antiretrovirals (*zidovudine* [43]) Antifungals – Azole derivatives (ketoconazole) – Polyene macrolides (amphotericin B) Antiprotozoal drugs – Antimalarials (*chloroquine, hydroxychloroquine, quinacrine, quinidine*) Biological drugs – Anti-CD20 (*obinutuzumab, rituximab*) – Anti-CD80/86 (*abatacept*) – Anti-TNF-α (*infliximab, adalimumab, certolizumab, etanercept*) Other drugs – Dapsone (*antibiotic, immunomodulator*) – Bismuth (*anti-ulcer (peptic ulcer)*) – Gold salts (*antirheumatic*) – Penicillamine (*antirheumatic, treatment for Wilson's disease*) – Sulfasalazine (*MICI treatment*) – Levamisole (*anthelmintic*)

Excerpted and modified from Müller S. et al. (2017)
CNS central nervous system, *GERD* gastroesophageal reflux disease, *IBD* chronic inflammatory bowel disease

3.2 Factors of Endogenous Origin

3.2.1 Genetic Factors

Research has also focused on a possible genetic predisposition, and in particular many authors have evaluated the association between OLP and various genetic polymorphisms. The presence of these polymorphisms, although the cause is unclear, supports the autoantigenic hypothesis [54]. There is a demonstrated association between most idiopathic forms of cutaneous LP and HLA-DR1 [55] (HLA (human leukocyte antigen), the major histocompatibility complex; see Sect. 4.1.2). HCV-related OLP appears to be particularly associated with the HLA class II allele HLA-DR6 [18, 49]. A significant association between erosive OLP and the HLA-DR3 allele has also been observed [53]. HLA-Aw19 and HLA-28 also appear to be associated with OLP, whereas HLA-A11 and HLA-A26 appear to be more associated with erosive forms [56]. Other possible associations have also been observed with HLA-A3, B3, B5, B7, B8, and DRw9 [57]. Increased HLA-DR9 and HLA-te22 antigens have also been reported in Chinese OLP patients [58]. It is possible that HLA-DQ1 may be a resistance factor for the disease [59]. It has also been reported in a Chinese family with five members affected by OLP, and a hereditary predisposition caused by a mutation in chromosome 3p14-3q13 has been suggested [60]. Polymorphisms of several cytokines have also been studied (see Sect. 4.3.1). However, the current evidence in the literature does not allow the conclusion that the disease is genetically determined [31].

3.2.2 Autoimmunity

One possible explanation for OLP could be an autoimmune response to epithelial autoantigens [22]. A single study reports evidence in favor of an autoimmune process through the in vitro expansion of T lymphocytes isolated from the skin of two patients with chronic cutaneous LP. And it was observed that such laboratory-cultured T cells are able to destroy autologous keratinocytes through a direct cytotoxicity mechanism [61]. A further study, in which the prevalence of autoantibodies was assessed in 82 Indian patients suffering from OLP, shows the presence of AMA (anti-mitochondrial antibodies) in 45 patients, AKA (anti-keratinocyte antibodies) in 27 patients, and Dsg3 (anti-desmoglein 3 antibodies) in 24 patients [62]. It was also observed that normalizing vitamin D levels in OLP patients improves the clinical course of the disease, as it does in other autoimmune diseases [63]. However, although OLP is characterized by a dysregulation of the immune response, none of the studies reported so far have provided definitive evidence for autoimmunity, i.e., a response to self-antigens [22].

3.2.3 Heat Shock Proteins (HSPs)

Possible self-antigens in OLP could be heat shock proteins (HSPs), which are expressed by all cell types and essentially function for cell communication, differentiation, and growth, signal transduction, and apoptosis [64]. The high levels of expression of HSPs found in OLP lesions determine their potential role as autoantigens in disease pathogenesis [65]. It is assumed that dysregulation of the gene responsible for the expression of these proteins in epithelial cells and its inability to suppress the immune response results in the recognition of the body's own HSPs as non-self-antigens [44]. On the other hand, the increased expression of these proteins can be caused also by factors of exogenous origin such as temperature changes, UV light, drugs, viruses, etc. The question then arises whether HSPs are the main etiological factor of the disease or whether their increase is a consequence of another factor of exogenous origin [31].

3.2.4 Psychological Disorders' Correlation with OLP

Several authors argue that psychological disorders such as stress, anxiety, and depression may play a role in the etiology of OLP. Anxiety and depression would in fact be more common conditions in patients with cutaneous/oral lichen planus than in healthy controls, and patients with the disease report a development or exacerbation of lesions during periods of increased emotional tension [66–72]. Other studies have also found a positive association between OLP and psychological disorders [73–75]. Two more recent studies have also shown this correlation using the DASS (Depression Anxiety Stress Scale), which is a questionnaire consisting of a series of symptoms divided into three subscales for depression, anxiety, and stress [76, 77]. The fact that acute and chronic psychological stresses can influence the development of the disease could be explained by the fact that stressful situations are able to promote a dysregulation of immune functions leading to an alteration of the Th1/Th2 cytokine balance with an increase in the Th2 response (which is associated with a risk of developing autoimmune diseases) [78–82]. These changes in the immune response are induced mainly via neuroendocrine mediators of the hypothalamic-pituitary-adrenal axis and the sympathetic noradrenergic system [83]. In fact, one study found higher levels of anxiety, depression, stress, and cortisol in the saliva of OLP patients compared to healthy subjects [84]. In contrast, another study found that these parameters did not differ between patients with OLP and the control group [78]. In fact, it should be pointed out that several authors have not found an association between OLP and psychological disorders [67, 69, 78]. Probably, the lack of a methodological standardization of the studies is responsible for the controversial results. Furthermore, the etiology of OLP is complex and presumably depends on the interaction of several factors [44]. The same chronic distress caused by OLP may, in itself, constitute an additional stressor and partially explain the association [85]. To date, it can therefore be concluded that a definitive cause-effect relationship has not yet been proved. However, it cannot be ruled out that psychological disorders may play a secondary, rather than primary, role in the development of OLP, as well as other inflammatory conditions [22].

3.2.5 Correlation with Other Systemic Diseases

In addition to liver disease and certain infectious conditions (already analyzed in Sect. 3.1.1), lichen planus of the oral cavity has been associated with numerous systemic diseases, although the scientific debate still remains open on the subject.

For several years, authors have been studying the possible relationship between OLP and diabetes mellitus [86, 87]. An increased incidence of diabetes has been shown in patients with OLP compared to the general population [88], and an altered response to oral glucose administration has also been found in the former [88, 89]. Varying proportions of diabetes incidence between the two diseases were found in OLP patients (2.4–11.5%) [90], whereas in the population with diabetes mellitus, the incidence of OLP would be 1.6% of cases [91]. However, other studies revealed that there was no positive correlation between the two diseases [92, 93]. Another study performed on 50 patients, in which fasting blood glucose and HbA1C levels were compared, showed no significant differences between patients with OLP and healthy subjects [11]. A recent meta-analysis, which analyzed 831 studies from the literature between 1973 and 2016, shows instead a substantial association between OLP and diabetes and that the risk of developing lesions from OLP is higher than in control subjects. The authors conclude that the non-significant in previous studies was probably due to the different selection of age, gender, type of diabetes mellitus, medication, and criteria [94].

Hypertension has also been correlated in the etiology of OLP [57]. One study found an incidence of hypertension in 19.2% of cases in a sample of 130 patients with OLP [95], whereas other authors exclude a possible relationship between the two conditions [92].

The association between lichen planus and heart disease could be related to chronic systemic inflammation [90]. A state of dyslipidemia has been found in OLP patients [96–99], which, together with hypertension, diabetes, and smoking, constitutes a risk factor for cardiovascular episodes. It appears that particularly atrophic-erosive lesions from lichen planus may favor an increased risk of developing acute coronary syndrome. But further investigation is needed to better investigate this possible correlation [100]. Some authors have also found occasional associations between oral/cutaneous LP and certain autoimmune diseases such as primary biliary cirrhosis, chronic active hepatitis, ulcerative colitis, myasthenia gravis, thymoma [101], systemic lupus erythematosus, Sjögren's syndrome, and others, but there is a lack of documentation of the criteria used to diagnose OLP. Unfortunately, many studies of the association between OLP and other systemic conditions do not apply uniform diagnostic criteria, and the use of both clinical and histopathological evaluations is rare [22].

Certain thyroid disorders may also correlate with OLP. In particular, a report of 15 Italian cases shows that Hashimoto's thyroiditis in patients with OLP is much more common (14.3%) than in the general population (1%), and it was found that Hashimoto's thyroiditis preceded the onset of OLP in 93.3% of those patients. The authors claim that in Hashimoto's thyroiditis patients, circulating thyroid antibodies could trigger an organ-specific autoimmune response also at the oral level, leading to the development of lesions by LP. Therefore, given the high number of asymptomatic cases of chronic autoimmune thyroiditis, thyroid screening (especially for Hashimoto's thyroiditis) is recommended in women over 40 years of age with OLP [102]. Another study performed on a sample of 152 patients with OLP shows an association with hypothyroidism. Thyroxine treatment does not appear to have influenced the course of oral lesions [103]. In both studies, the diagnosis of OLP in all patients was based on defined clinical and histopathological criteria [104] (see Sect. 5.3). The pathophysiological mechanisms that could explain these associations are not yet known [22].

Another possible association between OLP and Good's syndrome has been studied. Good's syndrome is a rare condition consisting of thymoma (tumor of the thymic epithelial cells) with adult-onset immunodeficiency characterized by hypogammaglobulinemia, low levels or absence of B cells, and variable alterations in cell-mediated immunity involving CD4+ T cells [105]. Good's syndrome is associated with a predisposition to infections and also with several autoimmune diseases such as myasthenia gravis, pure erythrocyte aplasia, systemic lupus erythematosus, and polymyositis [106]. Most studies evaluating the association between Good's syndrome and OLP are based on the free application of clinical criteria alone [107–109]. Maehara et al. described two cases of oral mucositis in patients with Good's syndrome, and, through the investigation of immunohistochemistry, they compared the lesions immunologically with those of 15 patients with OLP; from the results obtained the authors concluded that the two diseases have different pathogenesis [110]. The real limitation of this study is that clinical and histopathological criteria used for diagnosis are not provided. Therefore, to date, there is no evidence of correlation with OLP, and it is possible that the oral lesions that could be found in patients with Good's syndrome are due to the coexistence of this pathology with multiple infectious and autoimmune conditions that can cause oral mucositis from causes other than OLP [22].

Chronic inflammatory bowel diseases (IBD) such as Crohn's disease and ulcerative rectocolitis have also occasionally been described concomitant with OLP [111]. Furthermore, a 1998 study advanced the hypothesis of a possible correlation between OLP and celiac disease where 22 out of 39 patients with OLP had antibody positivity to celiac disease [112]. In contrast, Scully et al. did not diagnose celiac disease in the 103 patients studied, concluding that the association could be accidental [113]. Some patients with LP or lichenoid reactions showed allergic reactions to certain foods and additives such as cinnamic aldehyde [40]. Lichen planus lesions have also been observed on the skin or mucous membranes of patients with various neoplasms such as breast cancer, metastatic adenocarcinoma, retroperitoneal sarcoma, gastric carcinoma, thymoma, Castleman's disease, pituitary adenoma, and non-Hodgkin's lymphoma [40]. Finally, OLP has occasionally been associated with varied conditions as psoriasis, lichen sclerosus, urolithiasis, Turner syndrome, etc. and agents used for the treatment of gallstones [40].

Although many factors have been studied in relation to OLP, to date, it can be inferred that the etiology of this pathology is complex and remains partly mysterious, presumably depending on the interaction of several factors of exogenous and/or endogenous origin.

References

1. Shklar G. Lichen planus as an oral ulcerative disease. Oral Surg Oral Med Oral Pathol. 1972;33(3):376–88.
2. Edwards KM, et al. Anti-viral strategies of cytotoxic T lymphocytes are manifested through a variety of granule-bound pathways of apoptosis induction. Immunol Cell Biol. 1999;77(1):76–89.
3. Sugerman PB, Sabage N. Oral lichen planus: causes, diagnosis and management. Aust Dent J. 2002;47(4):290–7.
4. Sand LP, et al. Prevalence of Epstein-Barr virus in oral squamous cell carcinoma, oral lichen planus, and normal oral mucosa. Oral Surg Oral Med Oral Pathol Oral Radiol Endodontol. 2002;93(5):586–92.
5. Yildirim B, Sengüven B, Demir C. Prevalence of herpes simplex, Epstein Barr and human papilloma viruses in oral lichen planus. Med Oral Patol Oral Cir Bucal. 2011;16(2):e170–4.
6. Campisi G, et al. HPV DNA in clinically different variants of oral leukoplakia and lichen planus. Oral Surg Oral Med Oral Pathol Oral Radiol Endodontol. 2004;98(6):705–11.

7. Gorsky M, Epstein JB. Oral lichen planus: malignant transformation and human papilloma virus: a review of potential clinical implications. Oral Surg Oral Med Oral Pathol Oral Radiol Endodontol. 2011;111(4):461–4.
8. Wen S, et al. Detection and analysis of human papillomavirus 16 and 18 homologous DNA sequences in oral lesions. Anticancer Res. 1997;17(1A):307–11.
9. Kumari R, Singh N, Thappa DM. Hypertrophic lichen planus as a presenting feature of human immunodeficiency virus infection. Indian J Dermatol. 2009;54(5):8.
10. Lodi G, et al. Current controversies in oral lichen planus: report of an international consensus meeting. Part 1. Viral infections and etiopathogenesis. Oral Surg Oral Med Oral Pathol Oral Radiol Endodontol. 2005;100(1):40–51.
11. Nosratzehi T. Oral lichen planus: an overview of potential risk factors, biomarkers and treatments. Asian Pac J Cancer Prev. 2018;19(5):1161.
12. Patrk I, et al. Cutaneous reactions in patients with chronic hepatitis C treated with peginterferon and ribavirin. Dermatology. 2014;228(1):42–6.
13. Younossi ZM. Hepatitis C infection: a systemic disease. Clin Liver Dis. 2017;21(3):449–53.
14. Lodi G, Pellicano R, Carrozzo M. Hepatitis C virus infection and lichen planus: a systematic review with meta-analysis. Oral Dis. 2010;16(7):601–12.
15. Carrozzo M, et al. Hepatitis C virus-associated oral lichen planus: is the geographical heterogeneity related to HLA-DR6? J Oral Pathol Med. 2005;34(4):204–8.
16. Lavanya N, et al. Oral lichen planus: an update on pathogenesis and treatment. J Oral Maxillofac Pathol. 2011;15(2):127.
17. Patil S, et al. Epidemiological relationship of oral lichen planus to hepatitis C virus in an Indian population. Oral Health Dental Manag. 2012;11(4):199–205.
18. Carrozzo M, et al. Increased frequency of HLA-DR6 allele in Italian patients with hepatitis C virus-associated oral lichen planus. Br J Dermatol. 2001;144(4):803–8.
19. Azab NA, et al. Interferon gamma and interleukin 8 gene polymorphisms in patients with hepatitis C virus related oral lichen planus. Arch Oral Biol. 2018;96:189–94.
20. Bombeccari GP, et al. Ruolo delle epatopatie nella fase acuta del lichen planus orale. Dental Cadmos. 2012;80(4):171–81.
21. Alaizari N, et al. Hepatitis C virus infections in oral lichen planus: a systematic review and meta-analysis. Aust Dent J. 2016;61(3):282–7.
22. Kurago ZB. Etiology and pathogenesis of oral lichen planus: an overview. Oral Surg Oral Med Oral Pathol Oral Radiol. 2016;122(1):72–80.
23. Wang K, et al. Analysis of oral microbial community and Th17-associated cytokines in saliva of patients with oral lichen planus. Microbiol Immunol. 2015;59(3):105–13.
24. He Y, et al. Dysbiosis of oral buccal mucosa microbiota in patients with oral lichen planus. Oral Dis. 2017;23(5):674–82.
25. Srinivasan M, Kodumudi KN, Zunt SL. Soluble CD14 and toll-like receptor-2 are potential salivary biomarkers for oral lichen planus and burning mouth syndrome. Clin Immunol. 2008;126(1):31–7.
26. Zunt S, et al. Soluble forms of Toll-like receptor 4 are present in human saliva and modulate tumour necrosis factor-α secretion by macrophage-like cells. Clin Exp Immunol. 2009;156(2):285–93.
27. Janardhanam SB, et al. Differential expression of TLR-2 and TLR-4 in the epithelial cells in oral lichen planus. Arch Oral Biol. 2012;57(5):495–502.
28. Kho H-S, et al. MUC1 and Toll-like receptor-2 expression in burning mouth syndrome and oral lichen planus. Arch Oral Biol. 2013;58(7):837–42.
29. Stanimirovic D, et al. TLR 2, TLR 3, TLR 4 and CD 14 gene polymorphisms associated with oral lichen planus risk. Eur J Oral Sci. 2013;121(5):421–6.
30. Bagan J-V, Eisen D, Scully C. The diagnosis and management of oral lichen planus: a consensus approach. Oral Biosci Med. 2004;1:21–7.
31. Mutafchieva MZ, et al. Oral lichen planus–known and unknown: a review. Folia Med (Plovdiv). 2018;60(4):528–35.
32. Müller S. The lichenoid tissue reactions of the oral mucosa: oral lichen planus and other lichenoid lesions. Surg Pathol Clin. 2011;4(4):1005–26.
33. Weedon D. The lichenoid reaction pattern (interface dermatitis). Skin Pathol. 2002;2:42–3.
34. Spadari F, et al. Lichen planus orale: revisione della letteratura. Doctor Os • aprile 2017 • XXVIII 04.
35. McParland H, Warnakulasuriya S. Oral lichenoid contact lesions to mercury and dental amalgam—a review. J Biomed Biotechnol. 2012;2012:589569.
36. Katsura T, et al. Allergic reaction to metal restrations associates with oral lichen planus and oral lichenoid lesions. J Japanese Society for Oral Mucous Membrane. 2007;13(1):1–7.
37. Scully C, Carrozzo M. Oral mucosal disease: lichen planus. Br J Oral Maxillofac Surg. 2008;46(1):15–21.
38. Al-Hashimi I, et al. Oral lichen planus and oral lichenoid lesions: diagnostic and therapeutic considerations. Oral Surg Oral Med Oral Pathol Oral Radiol Endodontol. 2007;103:S25.e1–S25.e12.
39. Serrano Sánchez P, et al. Drug-induced oral lichenoid reactions: a literature review. Eur J Clin Pharm. 2010;73:1523–37.
40. Scully C, et al. Update on oral lichen planus: etiopathogenesis and management. Crit Rev Oral Biol Med. 1998;9(1):86–122.
41. Issa Y, et al. Healing of oral lichenoid lesions after replacing amalgam restorations: a systematic review. Oral Surg Oral Med Oral Pathol Oral Radiol Endod. 2004;98(5):553–65.
42. Zhou G, et al. Increased B7-H1 expression on peripheral blood T cells in oral lichen planus correlated with disease severity. J Clin Immunol. 2012;32(4):794–801.

43. Ohno S, et al. Enhanced expression of Toll-like receptor 2 in lesional tissues and peripheral blood monocytes of patients with oral lichen planus. J Dermatol. 2011;38(4):335–44.
44. Payeras MR, et al. Oral lichen planus: focus on etiopathogenesis. Arch Oral Biol. 2013;58(9):1057–69.
45. Arora SK, et al. Lichen planus: a clinical and immuno-histological analysis. Indian J Dermatol. 2014;59(3):257.
46. Wenzel J, et al. Type I interferon-associated cytotoxic inflammation in lichen planus. J Cutan Pathol. 2006;33(10):672–8.
47. Rice PJ, Hamburger J. Oral lichenoid drug eruptions: their recognition and management. Dent Update. 2002;29(9):442–7.
48. Crincoli V, et al. Oral lichen planus: update on etiopathogenesis, diagnosis and treatment. Immunopharmacol Immunotoxicol. 2011;33(1):11–20.
49. Gorsky M, et al. Smoking habits among patients diagnosed with oral lichen planus. Tob Induc Dis. 2004;2(2):1–6.
50. Rajendran R. Oral lichen planus. J Oral Maxillof Pathol. 2005;9(1):3.
51. Trivedy C, Craig G, Warnakulasuriya S. The oral health consequences of chewing areca nut. Addict Biol. 2002;7(1):115–25.
52. Stoopler ET, Parisi E, Sollecito TP. Betel quid-induced oral lichen planus: a case report. Cutis. 2003;71(4):307–11.
53. Reichart PA, Warnakulasuriya S. Oral lichenoid contact lesions induced by areca nut and betel quid chewing: a mini review. J Investig Clin Dent. 2012;3(3):163–6.
54. Gorouhi F, Davari P, Fazel N. Cutaneous and mucosal lichen planus: a comprehensive review of clinical subtypes, risk factors, diagnosis, and prognosis. Sci World J. 2014;2014:742826.
55. Nasa GL, et al. HLA antigen distribution in different clinical subgroups demonstrates genetic heterogeneity in lichen planus. Br J Dermatol. 1995;132(6):897–900.
56. Ognjenović M, et al. Oral lichen planus and HLA A. Coll Antropol. 1998;22:89–92.
57. Gupta S, Jawanda MK. Oral lichen planus: An update on etiology, pathogenesis, clinical presentation, diagnosis and management. Indian J Dermatol. 2015;60(3):222.
58. Sun A, et al. Association of HLA-te22 antigen with anti-nuclear antibodies in Chinese patients with erosive oral lichen planus. Proc Natl Sci Council Repub China Part B Life Sci. 2000;24(2):63–9.
59. Porter K, et al. Class I and II HLA antigens in British patients with oral lichen planus. Oral Surg Oral Med Oral Pathol. 1993;75(2):176–80.
60. Wang Z, et al. Genetic linkage analysis of oral lichen planus in a Chinese family. Genet Mol Res. 2011;10(3):1427–33.
61. Sugerman P, Satterwhite K, Bigby M. Autocytotoxic T-cell clones in lichen planus. Br J Dermatol. 2000;142(3):449–56.
62. Nikam BP, et al. Prevalence of autoantibodies and the clinical spectrum of disease in an Indian patient subpopulation with lichen planus. Indian J Public Health Res Dev. 2019;10(10)
63. Gupta J, et al. Vitamin D in the treatment of oral lichen planus: a pilot clinical study. J Indian Acad Oral Med Radiol. 2019;31(3):222.
64. Tavassol F, et al. Heat-shock protein expression and topical treatment with tacrolimus in oral lichen planus: an immunohistochemical study. Int J Oral Maxillofac Surg. 2008;37(1):66–9.
65. Pearl LH, Prodromou C. Structure and mechanism of the Hsp90 molecular chaperone machinery. Annu Rev Biochem. 2006;75:271–94.
66. Rojo-Moreno J, et al. Psychologic factors and oral lichen planus: a psychometric evaluation of 100 cases. Oral Surg Oral Med Oral Pathol Oral Radiol Endod. 1998;86(6):687–91.
67. McCartan B. Psychological factors associated with oral lichen planus. J Oral Pathol Med. 1995;24(6):273–5.
68. Eisen D. The clinical features, malignant potential, and systemic associations of oral lichen planus: a study of 723 patients. J Am Acad Dermatol. 2002;46(2):207–14.
69. Rödström PO, et al. Erosive oral lichen planus and salivary cortisol. J Oral Pathol Med. 2001;30(5):257–63.
70. Vallejo MG-P, et al. Anxiety and depression as risk factors for oral lichen planus. Dermatology. 2001;203(4):303–7.
71. Manolache L, Seceleanu-Petrescu D, Benea V. Lichen planus patients and stressful events. J Eur Acad Dermatol Venereol. 2008;22(4):437–41.
72. Garcia-Pola MJ, Huerta G. Anxiety as an etiologic factor in oral lichen planus. Med Oral. 2000;5(1):7–13.
73. Koray M, et al. The evaluation of anxiety and salivary cortisol levels in patients with oral lichen planus. Oral Dis. 2003;9(6):298–301.
74. Chaudhary S. Psychosocial stressors in oral lichen planus. Aust Dent J. 2004;49(4):192–5.
75. Ivanovski K, et al. Psychological profile in oral lichen planus. J Clin Periodontol. 2005;32(10):1034–40.
76. Kalkur C, Sattur AP, Guttal KS. Role of depression, anxiety and stress in patients with oral lichen planus: a pilot study. Indian J Dermatol. 2015;60(5):445.
77. Manczyk B, et al. Evaluation of depression, anxiety and stress levels in patients with oral lichen planus. J Oral Sci. 2019;61(3):391–7.
78. Girardi C, et al. Salivary cortisol and dehydroepiandrosterone (DHEA) levels, psychological factors in patients with oral lichen planus. Arch Oral Biol. 2011;56(9):864–8.
79. Marshall GD Jr, et al. Cytokine dysregulation associated with exam stress in healthy medical students. Brain Behav Immun. 1998;12(4):297–307.
80. Andersson I, Lorentzen J, Ericsson-Dahlstrand A. Analysis of adrenocortical secretory responses during acute and prolonged immune stimulation in

inflammation-susceptible and-resistant rat strains. J Neuroendocrinol. 2000;12(11):1096–104.
81. Windle R, et al. Increased corticosterone pulse frequency during adjuvant-induced arthritis and its relationship to alterations in stress responsiveness. J Neuroendocrinol. 2001;13(10):905–11.
82. Bosch JA, et al. Acute stress evokes selective mobilization of T cells that differ in chemokine receptor expression: a potential pathway linking immunologic reactivity to cardiovascular disease. Brain Behav Immun. 2003;17(4):251–9.
83. Kemeny ME, Schedlowski M. Understanding the interaction between psychosocial stress and immune-related diseases: a stepwise progression. Brain Behav Immun. 2007;21(8):1009–18.
84. Shah B, Ashok L, Sujatha G. Evaluation of salivary cortisol and psychological factors in patients with oral lichen planus. Indian J Dent Res. 2009;20(3):288.
85. Carrozzo M, Thorpe R. Oral lichen planus: a review. Minerva Stomatol. 2009;58(10):519–37.
86. Albrecht M, et al. Occurrence of oral leukoplakia and lichen planus in diabetes mellitus. J Oral Pathol Med. 1992;21(8):364–6.
87. Lundström IM. Incidence of diabetes mellitus in patients with oral lichen planus. Int J Oral Surg. 1983;12(3):147–52.
88. Lowe N, et al. Carbohydrate metabolism in lichen planus. Br J Dermatol. 1976;95(1):9–12.
89. Powell SM, et al. Glucose tolerance in lichen planus. Br J Dermatol. 1974;91(1):73–5.
90. Cassol-Spanemberg J, et al. Oral lichen planus and its relationship with systemic diseases. A review of evidence. J Clin Exp Dent. 2018;10(9):e938.
91. Jelinek JE. Cutaneous manifestations of diabetes mellitus. Int J Dermatol. 1994;33(9):605–17.
92. Ansar A, Farshchian M, Ghasemzadeh Seyed M. Comparison of the frequency of diabetes mellitus in the patients with lichen planus and normal controls: a case-control study. Dermatol Cosmet. 2011;2:78.
93. Saini R, et al. Oral mucosal lesions in non oral habit diabetic patients and association of diabetes mellitus with oral precancerous lesions. Diabetes Res Clin Pract. 2010;89(3):320–6.
94. Mozaffari HR, Sharifi R, Sadeghi M. Prevalence of oral lichen planus in diabetes mellitus: a meta-analysis study. Acta Inform Med. 2016;24(6):390–3.
95. López-Jornet P, Parra-Perez F, Pons-Fuster A. Association of autoimmune diseases with oral lichen planus: a cross-sectional, clinical study. J Eur Acad Dermatol Venereol. 2014;28(7):895–9.
96. Dreiher J, Shapiro J, Cohen A. Lichen planus and dyslipidaemia: a case–control study. Br J Dermatol. 2009;161(3):626–9.
97. Arias-Santiago S, et al. Cardiovascular risk factors in patients with lichen planus. Am J Med. 2011;124(6):543–8.
98. Arias-Santiago S, et al. Lipid levels in patients with lichen planus: a case–control study. J Eur Acad Dermatol Venereol. 2011;25(12):1398–401.
99. López-Jornet P, Camacho-Alonso F, Rodríguez-Martínes M. Alterations in serum lipid profile patterns in oral lichen planus. Am J Clin Dermatol. 2012;13(6):399–404.
100. Conrotto D, et al. Can atrophic-erosive oral lichen planus promote cardiovascular diseases? A population-based study. Oral Dis. 2018;24(1–2):215–8.
101. Abbate G, et al. Neoplastic transformation of oral lichen: case report and review of the literature. Acta Otorhinolaryngol Ital. 2006;26(1):47.
102. Lo Muzio L, et al. Possible link between Hashimoto's thyroiditis and oral lichen planus: a novel association found. Clin Oral Investig. 2013;17(1):333–6.
103. Siponen M, et al. Association of oral lichen planus with thyroid disease in a Finnish population: a retrospective case-control study. Oral Surg Oral Med Oral Pathol Oral Radiol Endod. 2010;110(3):319–24.
104. van der Meij EH, van der Waal I. Lack of clinicopathologic correlation in the diagnosis of oral lichen planus based on the presently available diagnostic criteria and suggestions for modifications. J Oral Pathol Med. 2003;32(9):507–12.
105. Kelesidis T, Yang O. Good's syndrome remains a mystery after 55 years: a systematic review of the scientific evidence. Clin Immunol. 2010;135(3):347–63.
106. Bernard C, et al. Thymoma associated with autoimmune diseases: 85 cases and literature review. Autoimmun Rev. 2016;15(1):82–92.
107. Arnold S, et al. Three difficult cases: the challenge of autoimmunity, immunodeficiency and recurrent infections in patients with Good syndrome. Br J Dermatol. 2015;172(3):774–7.
108. Macdonald J, Mangold A, Connolly S. Good syndrome and lichen planus: case and review. J Eur Acad Dermatol Venereol. 2014;28(12):1828–30.
109. Malphettes M, et al. Good syndrome: an adult-onset immunodeficiency remarkable for its high incidence of invasive infections and autoimmune complications. Clin Infect Dis. 2015;61(2):e13–9.
110. Maehara T, et al. Cytokine profiles contribute to understanding the pathogenic difference between Good syndrome and oral lichen planus: two case reports and literature review. Medicine. 2015;94(14):e704.
111. Georgakopoulou EA, et al. Oral lichen planus as a preneoplastic inflammatory model. J Biomed Biotechnol. 2012;2012:759626.
112. Jokinen J, et al. Celiac sprue in patients with chronic oral mucosal symptoms. J Clin Gastroenterol. 1998;26(1):23–6.
113. Scully C, Porter S, Eveson J. Oral lichen planus and coeliac disease. Lancet. 1993;341(8861):1660.

4 Pathogenesis

OLP is a disorder with a complex pathogenesis, which has not yet been fully clarified and is the subject of various hypotheses. It is a chronic inflammatory disease characterized by apoptosis of basal keratinocytes of the oral epithelium induced by activation of cytotoxic CD8+ T lymphocytes [1].

An early event in the disease mechanism involves the expression of a keratinocyte or the exposure of an antigen that can be an auto-peptide or a heat shock protein [2]. Indeed, in OLP, cell-mediated immune processes can be induced by exogenous factors or even directly by endogenous conditions, although the immune mechanisms generated are often maintained by both conditions [3].

T lymphocytes (mainly CD8+ but also some CD4+ or T helper (Th) cells), migrating into the epithelium during normal surveillance or because they are attracted by chemokines, come into contact with the antigen at the level of basal keratinocytes: this mechanism therefore occurs either by chance or by chemotactic attraction [4]. The migrated CD8+ T lymphocytes are activated either directly through antigen binding to the major histocompatibility complex (MHC)-I on keratinocytes or indirectly through activated CD4+ T helper lymphocytes [5]. In fact, within the oral epithelium, there are antigen-presenting cells (or APCs), i.e., a group of cells specialized in recognizing an antigen and presenting it to the T lymphocytes: these include B lymphocytes, macrophages, and, in the OLP, especially dendritic cells (in the oral epithelium known as Langerhans cells). The Langerhans cell interacts with the antigen by internalizing and processing it. Once the maturation process is complete, migrates from the non-lymphoid tissue to the peripheral secondary lymphatic organs (lymph nodes, spleen) and the antigenic proteins obtained from the degradation of the pathogen are then exposed in order to present the antigen to lymphocytes through the expression of MHC-II. Thus, activated Langerhans cells will be able to stimulate T lymphocytes, which in turn will release a series of cytokines with a paracrine effect: the increased concentration of these cytokines produced by CD4+ cells is the key event in the pathogenesis of OLP [3]. Specifically, CD4+ cells are activated by APC cells through two mechanisms: the production of interleukin IL-12 (together with the co-expression of CD40 and CD80; see Sect. 4.1.3) and the antigen presentation to Th cells through the expression of MHC-II. Activated CD4+ T helper lymphocytes, in turn, activate CD8+ cytotoxic T lymphocytes through receptor interaction and the production of IL-2 and IFN-γ interferon. Finally, activated cytotoxic T lymphocytes kill basal keratinocytes through the action of tumor necrosis factor (TNF)-α, Fas-FasL interaction, and granzyme B-induced apoptosis [2, 6], all of which are involved in the activation of the caspase cascade (extrinsic pathway of apoptosis). Together, these

G. Isola et al., *Oral Lichen Planus and Lichenoid Lesions*,
https://doi.org/10.1007/978-3-031-29765-6_4

events represent the cell-mediated immunopathogenesis of OLP and are schematized in Fig. 4.1.

The immunopathogenesis of OLP also involves the non-specific immune response carried out by the action of matrix metalloproteinases (MMPs), chemokines, and mast cells [4, 7]. In contrast, the specific immune response involves CD4+ helper lymphocytes and CD8+ T-cytotoxic lymphocytes. Thus, both pathogenetic mechanisms of specific and non-specific immunity are active in the pathogenesis of oral lichen [3]. Finally, a role has also been suggested of humoral immunity in OLP due to the presence of circulating anti-desmoglein 1 and 3 autoantibodies [8] and the identification of IgA and IgM [9].

The activation of the non-specific immune response further exacerbates the accumulation of lymphocytes T cells, keratinocyte apoptosis, and mast cell protease-induced basement membrane destruction [10]. The integrity of the basement membrane is maintained by the secretion of fibers collagen type IV and laminin 5 by basal keratinocytes. In turn, to prevent apoptosis, they require a cell survival signal derived from the basement membrane. Apoptotic keratinocytes are no longer able to maintain the integrity of the basement membrane, and in turn, if the latter is not intact, it cannot send the cell survival signal. Thus, a vicious circle is established that favors the chronic course of the disease [4, 11].

The possible role of matrix metalloproteases (MMPs) and tissue inhibitors of metalloproteases (TIMPs) in the genesis and maintenance of OLP. Metalloproteases constitute a family of zinc-dependent enzymes of the protease group (endopeptidases). Their action consists of degradation of proteins in the extracellular matrix allowing the cells to pass through them: a process that allows, for example, leucocytes to invade tissues in inflammatory processes but which also occurs in carcinomas with marked metastatic spread [3]. In particular, high concentrations of MMP-9 and TIMP1 have been found in OLP

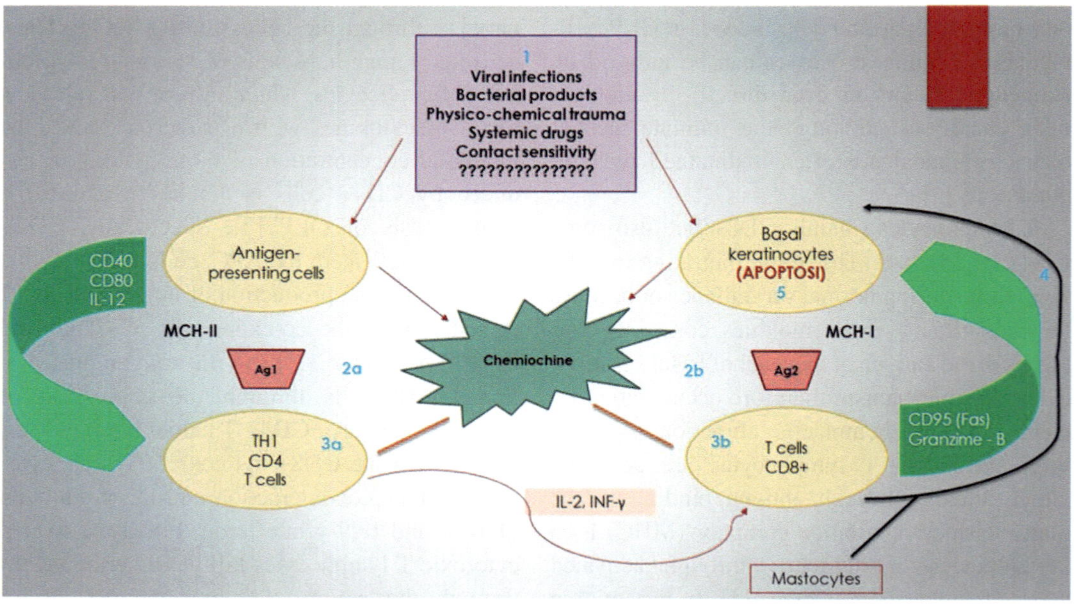

Fig. 4.1 Immunopathogenesis of OLP (modified from Spadari F. et al. 2017). (1) Exposure to the etiological factor of exogenous or endogenous origin. (2a) APC cells process antigen expressed through MHC-II. (2b) Basal keratinocytes expose antigen via MHC-I. (3a) Chemotactic recall and activation of CD4+ T lymphocytes through antigen presentation by APC cells and their production of IL-12 and expression of CD40 and CD80. (3b) Chemotactic recall and activation (direct and indirect, respectively) of CD8+ T lymphocytes through antigen presentation by keratinocytes and production of IL-2 and IFN-γ by Th lymphocytes. (4) Expression of cytotoxic action by CD8+ T lymphocytes. (5) Keratinocyte apoptosis

lesions. MMP-9, together with its activators released by T lymphocytes, cleaves type IV collagen fibers resulting in basement membrane degeneration [7, 12].

Chemokines constitute a large group of low-molecular-weight proteins in the family of cytokines. Their main function is the activation and recruitment (chemotaxis) of leukocytes to sites of inflammation [3]. A member of the chemokine family produced by various cells, including activated T lymphocytes, is called CCL5 or RANTES (Regulated on Activation, Normal T cells Expressed and Secreted) which plays a critical role in the recruitment of various inflammatory cells and especially lymphocytes and mast cells into the OLP [1]. Its main receptor is CCR5 [3], but other surface receptors for RANTES have also been identified in the OLP, such as CCR1, CCR3, CCR4, CCR9, and CCR10 [4, 13]. It has also been observed that these chemokines are associated with increased mast cell density in skin OLP and LP lesions [3]. RANTES is secreted by activated T lymphocytes, keratinocytes, and numerous other cells [14]. Its effect causes the recruitment and degranulation of mast cells which in turn release TNF-α and chymase which further upregulate the secretion of RANTES by T cells. Once again, a vicious circle is established that is responsible for the chronic course of the disease [12].

It has been shown that at least 60% of tissue mast cells are degranulated in the context of tissues with OLP, compared to the 20% mast cell degranulation observed in normal control mucosa [15]. TNF-α regulates the expression of vascular adhesion molecules such as CD62E (E-selectin), CD54 (ICAM-1) and CD106 (VCAM-1) by endothelial cells of the subepithelial vascular plexus: the expression of vascular adhesion molecules is required for the adhesion of lymphocytes to the luminal surfaces of blood vessels and their subsequent extravasation [5]; TNF-α also stimulates the secretion of RANTES from T cells [1]. Chymase is a protein that is able to activate and induce the production of MMP-9 by lymphocytes, thus demonstrating the indirect role of mast cells in basement membrane destruction [14]. Furthermore, it appears that the mast cell density is more pronounced at basement membrane colliquation sites, suggesting that mast cells may also play a direct role in the basal degenerative process, as well as in the intraepithelial migration of CD8+ T lymphocytes [13].

Macrophages may also promote lesion exacerbation through the production of pro-inflammatory cytokines such as TNF-α and IL-1b [16]. TNF-α produced by macrophages can trigger apoptotic processes in basal keratinocytes and, indirectly, may promote basement membrane degeneration by MMP-9 produced by the T lymphocytes themselves [17].

4.1 Cells Involved in the Pathogenesis of OLP

OLP is characterized by a complex immunopathogenesis involving different cell populations (Table 4.1). In the early stages of lesions, the levels of CD4+ T lymphocytes, macrophages, and dendritic cells are higher than in the advanced stages, which are characterized by high levels of CD8+ T lymphocytes [50]. This distribution suggests that in the early stages there is a predominance of APCs and cells that induce the inflammatory response, whereas in the advanced stages, the concentration of defense cells increases, which will lead to apoptosis of the keratinocytes [51].

4.1.1 Oral Keratinocytes

The oral cavity is lined by a multilayered squamous epithelium made up of 90% keratinocytes, with the remaining 10% consisting of keratinocytes, while the remaining 10% consists of Langerhans cells, melanocytes, Merkel cells, and cells of the immune system (mainly lymphocytes and macrophages) [18]. This epithelium rests on the lamina propria and submucosa and consists of a basal layer made up of cubic or cylindrical cells that anchor on the basement membrane by means of hemidesmosomes [19].

These cells undergo high proliferation allowing the continuous renewal of the oral epithe-

Table 4.1 Cells involved in OLP

Cells	Function	Role in the OLP	References
Oral keratinocytes	Main constituents of the oral squamous epithelium. They participate in metabolic and immune functions	Expression of the antigen that triggers the immune reaction. Expression of chemokines, TLR, VDR, miR, β-defensins, histamine, and thymic stromal lymphopoietin	[18–30]
Endothelial cells	Inner lining of blood vessels. They participate in metabolic and immune functions	Expression of vascular adhesion molecules and VEGFR. Production of chemerin, IL-1α, IL-6, and IL-8	[5, 31–36]
Myeloid DCs (including LC)	Antigen presentation by MHC-II	Production of several cytokines including IL-12 and expression of CD40 and CD80, with which it stimulates CD4+ T lymphocytes	[3, 37]
Plasmacytoid DCs	Antigen presentation by MHC-II	Stimulation of cytotoxic effects mediated by NK and CD8+ T cells by IFN-α production	[3, 31, 37]
Macrophages	Innate immunity expressed through intense phagocytic activity. They are divided into M1 (pro-inflammatory activity) and M2	Production of TNF-α and IL-1b which stimulate the production of keratinocyte RANTES and T lymphocyte MMP9	[16, 17, 38, 39]
B lymphocytes	Protagonists of humoral immunity. They express BCR and MHC-II for CD4+ activation. Can differentiate into plasma cells and memory lymphocytes	Low involvement. High expression of salivary IgA in OLP	[40–42]
CD4+ T lymphocytes	Once activated by APC cells, they can differentiate into Th1, Th2, and Th17 lymphocytes	Once activated, they release TNF-α, IL-2, and IFN-γ that allow stimulation of CD8+ and promote the chronic course of lesions	[3, 16, 40, 41]
CD8+ T lymphocytes	Once activated, they become cytotoxic effector lymphocytes	They induce keratinocyte death by means of TNF-α, perforin, protease, FasL, and granzyme B. They destroy the basement membrane by releasing MMP-9	[4, 14, 38]
Regulatory T lymphocytes	They allow the maintenance of immune tolerance toward the self. Suppress inflammation	Poorly expressed in OLP lesions	[13, 38, 43]
NK cells	They do not require MHC for activation, but IL-2 and IL-12. They induce cell death via perforins and certain serine proteases	NK cells have been identified in lesions, but their functions are not yet defined	[38, 40, 44, 45]
Mastocytes	Inflammatory and immunomodulatory tissue repair and remodeling function	They release numerous substances from their granules when stimulated	[14, 15, 40, 41, 46–49]

lium by compensating for the loss of cells through superficial desquamation [52]. Above the basal layer is the stratum spinosum where the cells, in histological sections, appear with cytoplasmic extensions of a spinous appearance. The upper layer is the granular layer where larger, flattened cells containing keratohyaline granules reside. Finally, the most superficial layer is the stratum corneum layer consisting of flattened cells containing keratin. Today the keratinocytes are no longer considered simple structural elements of the epithelium, but cells that participate in metabolic and immune functions [19].

As already mentioned, the basal keratinocytes, through the production of type IV collagen fibers and laminin 5, maintain the integrity of the basement membrane, which in turn is essential for preserving the viability and preventing apoptosis of keratinocytes. In OLP, keratinocytes are the target cells that undergo apoptosis, and, for this mechanism to occur, it is first necessary for these cells to express an antigen (as yet unknown) in the early stages of disease development.

Once active, these keratinocytes secrete chemokines attracting lymphocytes and other immune cells that initiate the inflammatory process culminating in keratinocyte apoptosis. The apoptotic keratinocytes are no longer able to maintain the integrity of the basement membrane, and in turn these, being no longer intact, can no longer send the cell survival signal. Thus the vicious circle is established that favors the chronic course of the disease [4, 11]. Recently it has also been demonstrated that oral keratinocytes possess a histamine transport and metabolization apparatus, and some authors have put forward the hypothesis that an imbalance in histamine metabolism and transport could partly contribute to the pathogenesis of OLP [20] (see Sect. 4.4.4).

4.1.2 Antigen-Presenting Cells (APCs) and Humoral Immunity

In the pathogenesis of oral lichen, an important role is played by antigen-presenting cells (APCs), i.e., a cell class capable of exposing antigens on their membrane surface via MHC-II (major histocompatibility complex) molecules and stimulating the activity of virgin CD4+ lymphocytes. They can also expose (as well like any nucleated cell) antigens also via MHC-I molecules through which CD8+ T lymphocytes are stimulated. Professional APC cells, i.e., those capable of presenting antigen to CD4+ T lymphocytes via MHC-II, are macrophages, B lymphocytes (these two expose antigen mainly to already activated T lymphocytes), and dendritic cells (the most effective in activating and virgin Th lymphocytes). In contrast, nonprofessional APC cells do not normally express MHC-II molecules but do so only under cytokine stimulation. The MHC class II allows the expression of antigens of extracellular origin, whereas MHC class I allows the expression of antigens of cytoplasmic origin [53]. The human MHC gene cluster (located in the short arm of chromosome 6) was later also referred to as the HLA (human leucocyte antigens) system because the molecules encoded by it were first recognized in leucocytes. This gene system is present in different loci (i.e., chromosome regions where a gene is present). The genes of the HLA system are grouped into three classes:

1. The class I region (HLA-1) includes the HLA-A, HLA-B, and HLA-C loci where the genes coding for the MHC class I (MHC-I) molecules expressed by all nucleated cells of the organism are located in the HLA-A, HLA-B, and HLA-C loci.
2. The class II region (HLA-2), also known as the D region, includes the HLA-DP loci, HLA-DQ, and HLA-DR loci where the genes coding for the MHC class II (MHC-II) molecules are expressed especially by cells of the immune system (APCs, lymphocytes, etc.).
3. The class III region (HLA-3) includes genes coding for other factors, including the cytokines TNF-α and TNF-β.

The nomenclature of histocompatibility molecules involves the use of a capital letter (A, B, or C for HLA-1 and P, Q, or R for HLA-2/HLA-D), preceded by the acronym HLA, indicating the locus, followed by an Arabic number indicating the allele: e.g., HLA-DR6 (the one found in the association between HCV and OLP) indicates allele 6 of the DR locus.

The genes of the MHC system are transmitted according to Mendelian laws and are all codominant.

Thus, offspring express both MHC genes located on chromosome 6 of paternal origin and those on chromosome 6 of maternal origin. These are highly polymorphic genes, and this means that for each of them there are many allelic variants: the allele indicates the single copy of a pair of genes occupying the same locus in the two homologous chromosomes.

The alleles of a gene usually differ from each other only in a few nucleotide sequences; therefore, the encoded proteins differ slightly from each other, and this difference is responsible for the biological individuality of everyone. The set of alleles, present on a single homologous chromosome, transmitted en bloc to offspring is called a haplotype. The combination of all the alleles present in an individual represents its genotype. Thus, with haplotype transmission en bloc, the offspring inherit three HLA-1 genes and three HLA-2 genes from their father and three HLA-2 genes from their mother, whereby the cells will express six HLA-1 and six HLA-2 molecules, almost always different from each other. For several years, it has been known that possession of certain genes of the MHC system is associated with an increased risk of developing certain diseases, especially autoimmune diseases [40]. As seen before, lichen of the oral cavity could be one of these (see Sect. 3.2.1).

Within the pathogenesis of OLP, the APC cells most involved are the dendritic cells (DCs), in epithelia known as Langerhans cells (LCs). These cells are capable of expressing both histocompatibility antigens (MHC-I and MHC-II). Dendritic cells are differentiated from hemopoietic stem precursors in the bone marrow. Before encountering with an antigen, DCs are referred to as "immature." In this form they are in non-lymphoid tissues, such as the skin and mucous membranes, where antigens can be encountered. Once an antigen through specific receptors (pattern recognition receptor, PRR; Toll-like receptor (TLR)) is internalized, DCs undergo a maturation process. The mature DCs migrate to peripheral secondary lymphatic organs (such as lymph nodes and the spleen) where they present the antigenic protein to T lymphocytes [3]. Different subsets of dendritic cells in OLP are mature and immature myeloid DCs (both Langerhans cells and stromal DCs) and plasmacytoid DCs [54]. Mature myeloid DCs produce Th1 cytokine IL-12, whereas plasmacytoid DCs are the main producers of IFN-α [37]. This cytokine in particular can induce cytotoxic effects by activating NK cells, CD8+ T lymphocytes, and FasL-mediated apoptosis, all of which are known to occur in OLP [31]. It has also been observed how the different subgroups of DCs (LC, myeloid, and plasmacytoid DCs) can also be recruited through expression of the chemotactic agonist chemerin by endothelial cells lining the blood vessels [31]. Among DCs, Langerhans cells (LCs) are the most studied. The LCs are mainly located in the suprabasal layer of the multilayered compound epithelium of the oral mucosa and epidermis [3]. High numbers of these cells have been observed on the basal layer of the epithelium with OLP lesions [55]. As explained above (see Chap. 4), the LC, having recognized the antigen, migrates to secondary lymphatic organs and presents it to lymphocytes through the expression of MHC-II, producing a primary immune response (initial sensitivity to the antigen).

When LCs then recapture the antigen, it will be recognized by the circulating memory of T lymphocytes which will induce a secondary immune response (release a series of cytokines with a paracrine effect) which will lead to the appearance of clinical signs of the disease [56–58]. Macrophages play a fundamental role in defense processes and are characterized by intense phagocytic activity. Their precursors, monocytes, are formed in the bone marrow and use the circulatory stream as a distribution route to all districts. In the peripheral tissues, macrophages (recruited especially in the presence of chemotactic signals) can divide producing new macrophages. Due to their motility and phagocytic activity, together with the neutrophil granulocytes, they constitute fundamental agents in defense processes. They are in fact cells capable of phagocytosing, bacteria, cell debris, tumor cells, foreign bodies, and various antigens: all ingested material undergoes the action of lysosomal enzymes. In chronic inflammatory granulomatous diseases, they cluster together to form polynucleated giant cells [38]. The macrophages are normally present in healthy oral mucosa and are present in greater numbers during pathological processes [17]. Macrophages are divided into M1 (with pro-inflammatory activity) and M2 (with anti-inflammatory activity) according to their effector functions [39]. M1 macrophages can cause an exacerbation of OLP lesions through the production of pro-inflammatory cytokines such as TNF-α and IL-1b [16].

These in turn have the function of regulating the presence of adhesion molecules on the surface of endothelial cells, inducing the production of chemokines (RANTES) by keratinocytes and leading to an increased recruitment of inflammatory cells at the site of injury. In addition, TNF-α produced by macrophages can initiate apoptotic processes in basal keratinocytes and, indirectly, can promote basement membrane degeneration by MMP-9 produced by T lymphocytes [17].

B lymphocytes, together with natural killer (NK) lymphocytes, unlike T lymphocytes, form and complete their maturation in the bone marrow. The mature B lymphocytes that enter the circulatory torrent mainly localize in the secondary lymphoid organs (only 15% are present in the circulatory torrent). These B lymphocytes are referred to as "virgin" or "naive" until the moment they encounter the antigen, an event that leads to the activation of these cells, protagonists of humoral specific immunity. B lymphocytes express several markers on the membrane surface, including the receptor for antigen, termed the "B-cell receptor" (BCR). This receptor is responsible for the direct recognition of the antigen and the formation of a bond with it. Recognition is defined as direct because the BCR-antigen interaction occurs without the simultaneous intervention of other molecules; otherwise it occurs with the "T-cell receptor" (TCR), the antigen receptor of T lymphocytes, which only recognizes protein antigens in association with MHC-I or MHC-II molecules. Furthermore, the BCR, unlike the TCR, can recognize, in addition to antigens of a protein nature, also those of a lipid or glycidic nature. The interaction of the B lymphocyte with the antigen leads to its activation, i.e., proliferation and differentiation into plasma cells (synthesis and secretion of immunoglobulins or antibodies specific for the stimulating antigen) and into a memory lymphocyte that will preside over the secondary response.

However, the response to protein antigens by B lymphocytes, unlike those of a lipid or glycidic nature lipid or glycidic nature, requires a second stimulation mediated by Th lymphocytes through the secretion of various cytokines (IL-2, IL-4, IL-5, IL-6). Therefore, protein antigens are considered T-dependent antigens, whereas glycidic and lipid antigens are called T-independent antigens. Protein antigens are therefore processed and complexed to MHC-II molecules on the surface of B lymphocytes: this will enable recognition by CD4+ T lymphocytes via their TCR. In this respect, the B lymphocytes performed the function of an APC cell.

The activated Th lymphocyte will stimulate, through cytokine secretion (IL-2 in particular), the differentiation of B lymphocytes into plasma cells and memory lymphocytes. The plasma cells are dedicated to the production of immunoglobulins of which five classes are identified: IgG, IgM, IgA, IgD, and IgE.

IgG constitutes the largest proportion (70–80%) of all circulating immunoglobulins: they are involved in the primary response (the first contact with the antigen), but the concentration of specific IgG gradually increases in the serum, thereafter constituting the main antibodies of the secondary response (given by further contact and penetration of the antigen into the body). The increased production of specific IgG, which is associated with an increase in their affinity for affinity for the antigen, is caused by the presence in the body of memory B lymphocytes, formed during the primary response and expressing an antigen-specific BCR. The specific IgG remains in the blood for several months to a few years. This mechanism is the basis of immunological memory:

- IgM is an emergency immunoglobulin as they are the first to be released after antigenic stimulation and constitute 10% of circulating Ig. The concentration of specific IgM in serum peaks 7–14 days after contact with the antigen and progressively decreases over the following days. IgM is therefore involved in the primary response to the antigen.
- IgA is predominantly present in secretions and is therefore referred to as secretory Ig. Once secreted by plasma cells, IgA is taken up on the basal side of the epithelial cells that line the mucous membranes. Part of this IgA will be released in the secretions, while the other aliquot will remain attached to the cell surface.
- IgD has a low concentration in biological fluids, most of it being expressed on the membrane of B lymphocytes in the form of BCR (BCR can be considered as an M- or D-class immunoglobulin that is not secreted but

remains attached to the plasma membrane of the plasma membrane of the B lymphocyte).

- IgE, compared to the other classes, is provided with an Fc fragment specific for receptors present on the surface of mast cells and basophil granulocytes. IgE concentrations normally increase in allergic or parasitic patients [40].

Regarding oral lichen, a study by Sugerman et al. in 2002, reported that B cells probably contribute little or nothing in pathogenesis. The authors noted that the literature did not provide a detailed analysis of the role of these cells in lichen and therefore ruled out a possible role of plasma cells and antibodies [4]. However, subsequent studies have reassessed the role of humoral immunity, for instance, a positivity for anti-desmoglein 1 and 3 antibodies in patients with erosive lichen (18 positive out of 22 tested) but not reticular form (3 positive out of 15) [8]. Another study identified elevated serum levels of IgA and IgM in patients with OLP, and slight nonsignificant increases in IgG levels [9]. A recent meta-analysis analyzed serum and salivary Ig levels reported in several studies that compared healthy and OLP patients. An absence of a proper elevation in serum levels, but rather an alteration in salivary levels of both IgG and IgA, had been found. Considering the few studies conducted on saliva, the results suggested that salivary IgA levels (the only ones with significant differences) have higher values than serum levels. Therefore, it is possible that salivary immunoglobulins may play a significant role in the pathogenesis of OLP [59].

4.1.3 T lymphocytes and Apoptosis

T lymphocytes, unlike B cells, leave the bone marrow still in an undifferentiated state to complete the maturation process in the thymus (which together with the marrow constitutes the primary lymphoid organs in humans). Within this gland the T lymphocytes come into contact with thymic stromal cells from which they receive a series of information that makes them capable of expressing the TCR (T-cell receptor) which, unlike the BCR, is able to exclusively recognize peptides derived from protein antigens exposed in association with MHC molecules (see Sect. 4.1.2). The maturation process of T lymphocytes in the thymus is much more complex than that of B lymphocytes in the bone marrow, as it involves the formation of two functionally different classes of T lymphocytes (CD4+ and CD8+). Moreover, these undergo a process of clonal selection that takes place in two stages: a positive selection in which all T lymphocytes equipped with a TCR that does not recognize any MHC-peptide complexes are eliminated (i.e., cells capable of recognizing MHC either presenting autologous or foreign peptides survive) and a negative selection that induces apoptosis of T lymphocytes that recognize MHC-peptide complexes as autologous peptides. Clonal selection induces the phenomenon of immune tolerance, as it leads to the elimination of self-reactive T lymphocytes and thus enables the immune system's ability to distinguish its own (self) from its non-self. Mature T lymphocytes leave the thymus (to reach secondary lymphoid organs such as the spleen, lymph nodes, appendix, tonsils, etc. and the various body districts via the blood and lymph) which are already divided into two populations:

- Some lymphocytes, during the thymic maturation process, acquire the membrane marker CD4 (CD4+ T lymphocytes) and are able to recognize with their TCR antigens presented in association with MCH-II expressed by APC cells. They assume the functions of T helper (Th) lymphocytes because they regulate all specific immune responses by means of synthesis and secretion cytokinesis.
- Other T lymphocytes, on the other hand, during the thymic maturation process, acquire the membrane marker CD8 (CD8+ T lymphocytes) and are able to recognize with their TCR antigens presented in association with MCH-I molecules, expressed with varying intensity by almost all cells of the organism. Once activated, they differentiate and take on the function of cytotoxic effector lymphocytes (CTLs) capable of causing cytotoxicity to target cells.

The immune system can respond to antigenic stimulation in different ways, namely, through the action of immunoglobulin-producing B lymphocytes or through T lymphocytes. The prevalence of the first or second type of response depends on the type of antigenic stimulation and the preferential release of certain cytokines rather than others [40]. Virgin CD4+ T lymphocytes, upon leaving the thymus, make contact with an antigen presented by APC cells; they are classified into three subgroups, Th1, Th2 (these two derive from the differentiation of Th0 lymphocytes characterized by a mixed cytokine profile [31]), and Th17, indistinguishable morphologically but characterized by different cytokine productions [16]. These cytokines will condition the type of immune response following to antigenic stimulation: that is, the immune response may be polarized in a Th1 or Th2 direction, also because cytokines of one type inhibit the production of those of the other type and block the proliferation of lymphocytes belonging to the other subpopulation, but also stimulate the proliferation and function of cells of the homologous class [40]:

1. Th1 polarization (i.e., the maturation of virgin CD4+ T lymphocytes into Th1 effector lymphocytes) is promoted by the release of IL-12 by mature myeloid dendritic cells and macrophages which are in turn stimulated by the release of IL-12, IL-18, and especially IFN-γ by NK cells (the latter also produced by the T lymphocytes themselves) [37]. This immune reaction is regulated by various transcription factors (STAT-1, STAT-4, T-bet) and is also favored by the release of co-stimulatory signals (together with IL-12) such as CD40 and CD80 by APC cells: IL-12 will bind to IL-12R (receptor), while CD40 and CD80 will bind to CD154 and CD28, all of which are expressed on the membrane of CD4+ T cells, thus promoting a Th1 response [40]. In this regard, CD (cluster of differentiation) denotes a large group of molecules on the cell surface, useful as cellular markers for the identification and isolation of leukocyte populations. This nomenclature has been universally adopted by the scientific community. CD molecules can act physiologically in different ways, as receptors or ligands, often playing a role in cell signaling or cell adhesion mechanisms. CD indicates a provisional CD designation, whereas capital letters that follow a CD number (e.g., CD45RO) indicate a junctional variant of the extracellular domain of a cell surface molecule. A lower-case letter following a CD number (e.g., CD1a, CD1b, CD1c, CD1d, or CD1e, which would be β2-microglobulin) indicates several molecules that share a common chain, or it may indicate a number of different members of the same gene family (e.g., CD66a, CD66b, CD66c, CD66d, CD66e, and CD66f). On the other hand, the use of L (ligand) has been removed, so, for example, CD154 should no longer be referred to as CD40L [60]. The main cytokines released by Th1 lymphocytes are IL-2, TNF-α, and IFN-γ [16]. The vast majority of studies performed on oral mucosa and peripheral blood shows a type 1 (Th1) cell-mediated immune response in patients with OLP [44]. This type of response includes cytotoxicity mediated by CD8+ T lymphocytes (often found at the epithelial-connective interface and sometimes adjacent to apoptotic keratinocytes) [61, 62] and is also confirmed by the presence of cytotoxicity-related molecules such as granzyme, perforin, and Tia-1, all molecules detected in the epithelium and connective tissue [63, 64]. Further evidence showing the prevalence of a Th1 profile in OLP is given by transcription of the T-bet factor (regulator of Th1 cells) which overrides transcription of the GATA-3 (Th2-related) factor in the peripheral blood of affected patients [65], detection of IFN-γ-positive cells (Th1 cells produce IFN-γ) [62], expression of CD45RO memory T cells that produce mainly Th1 cytokines [66], overexpression of IFN-γ and TNF-α [62, 67, 68], and absence of eosinophilic granulocytes in the inflammatory infiltrate which also confirms the prevalence of the Th1 profile [69]. However, it has been suggested that, in OLP lesions, some Th1 lymphocytes might actually be Th0 lymphocytes, as they appear to produce Th2 cyto-

kines (such as IL-4, IL-5, and IL-13) but also IFN-γ. From the data of the same study, it appears that there is a higher prevalence of Th0 and Th17 lymphocytes in erosive lesions and of Th2 lymphocytes in reticular lesions [70].

2. Polarization in the Th2 direction (i.e., maturation of virgin CD4+ T lymphocytes into Th2 effector lymphocytes) follows two main conditions: helminthic infestation and penetration into the body by allergens. This immune response is stimulated by the production of IL-4 (released by the T lymphocytes themselves at the beginning of their activation) and is regulated by the transcription factors GATA-3 and STAT-6, which favor the transcription of genes coding for the main Th2 cytokines: IL-4, IL-5, and IL-13. Other Th2 cytokines are IL-3, IL-6, and IL-10 [40]. All these cytokines are crucial for antibody production [16]. The Th2-type immune response involves the release of plasma cellular IgE and the activation of eosinophilic granulocytes and mast cells, the cells that play a key role in the defense against helminths and type I hypersensitivity reactions [40]. As mentioned earlier, the Th2 response does not appear to be prevalent in OLP compared to the Th1 response. Furthermore, it is important to specify that the Th1/Th2 response pattern is not always so clear-cut, as it is subject to numerous genetic and acquired variables [40].
3. This last concept is even more valid bearing in mind that more recent research has led to the discovery of a third type of polarization, called Th17, namely, the maturation of virgin CD4+ T lymphocytes into Th17 effector lymphocytes, so called because they produce large amounts of IL-17. They exhibit effector functions distinct from Th1 and Th2 lymphocytes and play an important role in the clearance of pathogens that are not adequately handled by the latter [71]. This immune response is stimulated by the action of IL-6, IL-21, TGF-β, and IL-23, which enable the expansion of Th17 lymphocytes through STAT-3, ROR-γ, and ROR-α factors [72]. These cytokines are produced by activated APC cells after contact with pathogens [73]. Differentiated Th17 cells, in addition to IL-17, can produce IL-26 [16], IL-21, IL-22, and GM-CSF (granulocyte macrophage colony-stimulating factor) which exert protective effects against extracellular parasites (bacteria and fungi) and participate in the immune barrier [74]. Th17 lymphocytes are potent tissue inflammatory inducers and have been identified as being primarily responsible for the pathogenesis of several autoimmune diseases [75–78] and allergic diseases [79, 80], and it is discussed their role in neoplastic diseases is also debated, as there are conflicting studies on the effects pro-/anti-tumor effects (according to one review, this discordance could be explained by the different cytokine profiles linked to the high degree of plasticity of these cells) [71]. As mentioned earlier, it is known that Th17 lymphocytes also play a role in the pathogenesis of OLP, especially in erosive forms [70]. For example, one study showed a significantly higher proportion of Th1 and Th17 cells and IL-17 serum levels significantly higher than that of controls, especially in the atrophic-erosive rather than reticular forms [81]. A strong increase was also observed in epithelial immunostaining for IL-17 and IL-23 in OLP lesions and a significantly higher number of IL-23+ lymphocytes (detection with cytoplasmic immunostaining) in erosive forms [82] (see Sect. 4.3.1 "IL-17").
4. In general, in oral lichen lesions, CD4+ T cells constitute the numerically predominant population numerically predominant and often occur in small clusters located deeper in the lymphocyte-rich subepithelial band—or in the lamina propria [83], but are not present in areas of basement membrane degeneration [84]. As explained above (see Chap. 4), CD4+ T lymphocytes are activated by APC cells through several mechanisms: the production of interleukin IL-12 (together with the co-expression of CD40 and CD80) and antigen presentation through the expression of MHC-II. CD4+ cells thus activated will in turn activate cytotoxic CD8+ T lymphocytes

through the release of a series of cytokines (such as TNFα [4], IL-2, IFN-γ) with a paracrine effect and through a receptor interaction [3], more precisely between RCAR (request to cytotoxic activity receptor) on the surface of CD4+ cells and RCA on the surface of CD8+ T lymphocytes [16]. Furthermore, local IFN-γ production promotes the maintenance of MHC-II molecule expression through keratinocytes, thus contributing to the chronic course of lesions [85].

The chronic course of OLP may also be due to:

- The activation of the primary transcription factor NF-kB (nuclear factor kappa-light-chain enhancer of activated B cells) capable of translocating into the nucleus and binding to the promoters of several genes coding for pro-inflammatory mediators; this factor appears significantly more expressed in OLP than in the cutaneous LP, and it has been observed that the greater nuclear expression of NF-kB by epithelial cells corresponds to an increase in cytotoxic cell infiltration (this may explain why OLP is typically more recalcitrant than cutaneous LP) [63].
- Inhibition of the TGF-β (transforming growth factor-beta)/Smad control signal, which can cause keratinocyte hyperproliferation leading to the development of white lesions [86].

CD8+ T lymphocytes cause the death of self-cells present on their membrane with foreign antigens associated with MHC-I molecules, recognized through the TCR receptor and the co-receptor CD8: antigen binding promotes activation and the mechanism of clonal expansion clonal expansion. These are usually peptide antigens derived from the degradation of bacterial, viral or bacterial, viral, or altered proteins due to neoplastic transformation of a cell population [38]. In OLP, the CD8+ T lymphocyte infiltrate is mainly located in the intraepithelial region and in areas of basement membrane degeneration, adjacent to the destruction of basal keratinocytes [12, 55, 87].

Identification of the antigen expressed by the basal keratinocytes can occur either through routine surveillance of T lymphocytes or through an attraction promoted by chemokines produced by the activated keratinocytes themselves [4]. The migration of T lymphocytes into the oral epithelium is further enhanced by molecules of intercellular adhesion molecules (ICAM-1 and VCAM). The attraction and migration of activated T cells in the oral epithelium are further enhanced by intercellular adhesion molecules (ICAM-1 and VCAM), by the upregulation of extracellular basement membrane matrix proteins (collagen types IV and VII, laminin, and integrins) and potentially by the signal transduction pathways of CXCR3 and CCR5 (two chemokine receptors) [88]. The activated cytotoxic lymphocyte, once it makes contact with the target cell, conveys secretion vesicles containing perforin and protease. The former promotes in the target cell membrane the formation of pores through which proteases can penetrate. One of these is called granzyme B and is able to activate a pro-caspase in the target cell, which in turn initiates apoptosis. In addition, the cytotoxic T lymphocyte can induce the caspase cascade through a counterreceptor, called Fas ligand (FasL), that binds to the Fas receptor on the target membrane [38], and also through the release of TNF-α that binds to the TNF-R1 receptor expressed on the keratinocyte membrane [63]; TNF-α is also able to stimulate the activation of nuclear factor kappa (NF-kB) whose overexpression has been demonstrated in OLP as partially responsible for the chronic production of pro-inflammatory cytokines [40].

These three mechanisms (granzyme B, FasL, and TNF- α) by which the cytotoxic T lymphocyte induces programmed cell death constitute a form of extrinsic pathway of apoptosis. We speak of an extrinsic pathway of apoptosis when the death stimuli originate from the external environment and the intrinsic pathway when the stimuli originate from within the cell itself.

The sequence of events culminating in the formation of apoptotic bodies takes place in three stages: induction, execution, and disruption. The intrinsic and extrinsic pathways of apoptosis converge in the activation phase of the executing caspases:

1. Induction phase

   The stimuli that trigger the extrinsic pathway (in addition to the action of proteases and granzyme B in particular) are mainly provided by pro-apoptotic cytokines, i.e., those belonging to the tumor necrosis factor (TNF) family: the best known are TNF-α, TNF-β, and FasL. These cytokines in turn interact with specific receptors expressed on the membrane of the target cell, which are referred to as death receptors (DR): TNF-R1, TNF-R2, and Fas (or CD95). The ligand-receptor interaction enables the activation of procaspase 8 and consequently the enzymatic cascade of caspases (proteolytic enzymes).

   In addition to activating the effector procaspases (e.g., 3, 6, and 7), caspase 8 acts proteolytically on the BID protein, from which it detaches the t-BID fragment that translocates into the outer mitochondrial membrane (assisted by other pro-apoptotic proteins such as BAX and BAK and other caspases), leading to the formation of megapores through which cytochrome C and other moleculesthat participate in the execution phase. In addition, executor caspase 3 acts on the protein cytoplasmic CAD (caspase-activated deoxyribonuclease) protein by releasing it from its inhibitor: the CAD protein translocates into the nucleus where, together with other deoxyribonucleases, it participates in the specific degradation of DNA (see Degradation step).

   The intrinsic pathway, on the other hand, is triggered by various types of cell damage such as:

   (a) The prolonged lack of growth factors, which promotes the release of the BAD protein which translocates to the mitochondrial membrane, where, in association with other pro-apoptotic proteins such as BID, BAK, and BAX, it forms pores from which various mitochondrial constituents are released, including cytochrome C. The process is also facilitated by the simultaneous inactivation of certain anti-apoptotic proteins such as BCL-2 and BCL-XL. Cell survival in fact depends on the balance of a number of pro-apoptotic proteins (e.g., BAX, BAD, BAK, BCL-XS, BIK, BID, NOXA) and anti-apoptotic proteins (BCL-2, BCL-XL, BCL-W), all encoded by genes that are part of the BCL-2 gene family, which act on the mitochondrial membrane by modulating the process of mega-spore formation, both through their concentration, but also according to the type of dimers (homodimers or heterodimers) that they form: for example, homodimers formed by two anti-apoptotic proteins block apoptosis, while homodimers formed by two pro-apoptotic proteins stimulate apoptosis and heterodimers formed by one pro-apoptotic and one anti-apoptotic protein are ineffective.

   (b) Sub-lethal DNA damage caused by errors in DNA replication, oxidative stress, radiation, antineoplastic agents, etc. In the case of DNA damage, the cell instead receives signals that activate the P53 protein (a product of the oncosuppressor gene P53), which causes the cell cycle to stop so that repair mechanisms can take place. If these are not sufficient to restore DNA integrity, the P53 protein itself, which is a transcription factor, translocates into the nucleus where it activates certain pro-apoptotic genes, in particular bax, which encodes for the BAX protein, which, upon reaching the mitochondria, promotes its membrane permeabilization.

2. Execution phase

   All proteins activated in the induction phase have as their main targets the mitochondria and the nucleus. Moreover, in the extrinsic pathway, the ligand-receptor interaction can lead in the context of the plasma membrane to the production of ceramide, which directly damages directly the mitochondrial membrane in a caspase-independent manner. Cytochrome C (also called Apaf-2, apoptosis protease-activating factor) binds to a cytoplasmic protein, called Apaf-1, and this eventually allows the formation of a polymer known as the apoptosome, which recruits effector caspases causing an amplification of the process. The AIF proteins (apoptosis-inducing factor) and Smac/DIABLO also play an important role in controlling apoptosis. The AIF protein promotes the release of cytochrome C from the mitochondria and, by translocating into the nucleus, induces chromatin condensation and activates certain procaspases. The protein Smac/DIABLO is considered a supercontroller of the apoptotic process, as it inactivates IAP (inhibitors of apoptosis proteins) by preventing their inhibitory effect on several caspases.

3. Degradation phase

   It consists of DNA fragmentation, which is the phenomenon culminating in cell apoptosis. This process is operated by certain endonucleases activated by caspases or by calcium ions, whose intracellular concentration gradually increases in the course of the process. In addition, the caspases that perform this process further contribute to nuclear and cytoplasmic breakdown [40].

Finally, with regard to OLP, according to a review of the literature, the main changes, morphological changes, observed in the epidermal basal layer are more suggestive of necrosis, rather than apoptosis [69]. It is therefore conceivable that the liquefactive degeneration observed in OLP and traditionally considered as an expression of the cytotoxic effects of CD8+ T lymphocytes does not unequivocally indicate apoptosis [89].

Thus, in the pathogenesis of oral lichen, T lymphocytes (CD4+ and CD8+) play an essential role. As already explained CD4+ T cells are activated by antigens presented via MHC-II molecules, whereas CD8+ T cells are activated by antigens presented via MHC-I molecules (see Sect. 4.1.2).

MHC-II-associated antigens are processed via an endosomal cellular pathway, whereas antigens associated with MHC-I are processed through a cytosolic cellular pathway. MHC-I-associated antigen presentation alone elicits a rapid cytotoxic T-cell response, a phenomenon observed, for example, in oral herpes infections and in recurrent aphthous stomatitis. In contrast, presentation of the MHC-II-associated antigen alone can promote MHC-II and may favor the activation of Th1 cells, which, in the absence of MHC-I-associated antigen presentation to CD8+ cells, would be cytotoxically inert. Thus, the putative antigen presented by MHC-II molecules to CD4+ T lymphocytes in OLP might differ from that presented by MHC-I molecules to CD8+ T lymphocytes [31]. The second antigen could be a self-antigen, such as an HSP induced on basal keratinocytes through activation of the innate immune response [4, 11]. Alternatively, a single antigen could access both the endosomal and cytosolic cellular pathways of antigen presentation [4]. For example, in patients with HCV-OLP association, the recruitment of HCV-specific CD4+ and/or CD8+ T lymphocytes into OLP-affected tissue has been demonstrated [90].

Another category of T cells is the regulatory (Treg) or suppressor T lymphocytes, which, like all other subpopulations of T lymphocytes, express on their membrane the TCR and CD3 proteins, acquired during the thymic maturation process.

However, what distinguishes Treg lymphocytes is the contextual expression of CD4 and CD25 molecules, and they are therefore also called CD4+ CD25+ lymphocytes, but their specific molecular marker is given by the presence of the transcription factor Foxp3, which is essential for their functioning. The main function of these cells is to allow the maintenance of immunological tolerance to the self, acting at the peripheral level on self-reactive T cells that have escaped the central deletion processes: thus, their role is fundamental in preventing autoimmune diseases. They also perform other repressive functions on the immune system, such as the induction of tolerance on the intestinal mucosa of the bacterial flora: MICI seems to be linked precisely to alterations in this tolerance mechanism. Treg cells are also crucial in pregnancy as they induce maternal tolerance toward the fetus (which is genetically different from the mother) [38]. Indeed, it is not surprising that Treg lymphocytes, which perform an inflammation suppressing function, are rare in both erosive and non-erosive OLP lesions [43]. Several recent studies have been performed on the Foxp3 marker of Treg lymphocytes (see Sect. 4.3.1 "IL-17").

4.1.4 Natural Killer (NK) Lymphocytes

NK cells constitute a lymphocyte population that is morphologically characterized by being larger than other lymphocytes [40]. They do not express the antigens that characterize T lymphocytes (CD3 and TCR) nor do they express surface immunoglobulins such as B lymphocytes (BCR). Rather, they express specific surface markers such as CD16 and CD56 (see Table 4.2). They are called natural killer cells as they do not require activation of antigens associated with MHC-I molecules [38] but are stimulated by the action of certain cytokines such as IL-2 and IL-12. NK lymphocytes kill organism cells lacking antigens of histocompatibility antigens (either because they are modified by neoplastic transformation or because they are infected by viruses), through the production of perforins and certain serine proteases [40]. Thus, they make contact (defined by some authors as a "deadly kiss") with target cells, causing their death following the introduction of molecules with lytic action [38].

Table 4.2 Summary of the distribution of the main markers in the lymphocyte subtypes

Cells	Main proteins expressed on the membrane
B lymphocytes	BCR, MHC-II, CD19, CD21
T lymphocytes	TRC, CD3
1. Cytotoxic T lymphocytes	1. TCR, CD3, CD8
2. T helper lymphocytes	2. TCR, CD3, CD4
3. Regulatory T lymphocytes	3. TCR, CD3, CD4, CD25
Natural killer lymphocytes	CD16, CD56

From Monesi V., Histology, PICCIN, 6th edition, Padua, 2012

The literature data on the role of NK cells in OLP are controversial. CD16+ CD56+ cells, i.e., NK lymphocytes, were identified in OLP lesions, and only a minor fraction (<2%) co-expressed the marker CD94 (another NK cell receptor with an inhibitory function on NK cells), indicating their true nature as natural killers [45] which are also capable of producing TNF-α and IFN-γ [91, 92]. Furthermore, it is possible that IFN-γ+ cells may be Th1 and/or NK lymphocytes [44]. Killer cell immunoglobulin-like receptor (KIR) family genes, coding for a series of inhibitory and activating receptors expressed mainly in NK cells, do not appear to be involved in the pathogenesis of OLP [93]. Instead, it has been observed that NK lymphocytes are able to selectively express the functional receptor ChemR23 (mainly expressed by mononuclear phagocytes and DCs), whose agonist ligand is chemerin which performs a chemotactic function. According to the results of this study, the chemerin/ChemR23 axis could play an important role in the recruitment of NK cells into the blood, and chemerin constitutes a key factor in the co-localization of NK cells and myeloid and plasmacytoid DCs [45]. However, the functions of NK lymphocytes in OLP are not yet defined [44].

4.1.5 Mast Cells (MCs)

Mast cells (MCs) are large (20–30 μm in diameter) and motile, bone marrow-derived cells that have in their cytoplasm numerous granules [38] rich in inflammatory mediators, which expel when they are reached by physical stimuli (e.g., trauma, heat, radiation), chemical stimuli (e.g., toxins and other microbial molecules), and immunological stimuli. This release is called "explosive degranulation" [40]. These cells are mainly located in the loose connective tissue and are scattered along the blood vessels [38] and perform a wide range of functions including inflammatory, immunomodulatory, tissue repair, and remodeling [46]. Within the granules contain heparin with an anticoagulant function and histamine, which causes vasodilation and increases the permeability of capillaries.

MCs, during the biological response, also secrete numerous interleukins (IL-4, IL-5, IL-6), other cytokines (TNF-α, TGF-β), and various chemotactic factors for eosinophilic and neutrophilic granulocytes.

Mast cell activation also leads to a rapid production of leukotrienes from the metabolism of arachidonic acid contained in lipid bodies: leukotrienes (also known as SRS-A, slow-reacting substance of anaphylaxis) induce smooth muscle contraction and bronchoconstriction (typical of asthma crisis). MCs also release other substances including nitric oxide (another vasodilator) and proteolytic enzymes such as tryptase and chymase [38]. Immunological stimuli that activate mast cell degranulation include reactions of immediate hypersensitivity reactions that occur when an individual already sensitized against an antigen comes into contact with it again. These immune reactions include allergic, anaphylactic, and delayed hypersensitivity reactions. Following exposure to certain types of antigens, called allergens, the secretion of plasma cell IgE occurs, which, by binding (at least two IgEs) to the antigen and also to contiguous receptors on the membrane of basophils and of the MCs, make the latter capable of recognizing the antigen by triggering explosive degranulation.

This very fast and effective reaction is usually confined to a local district. This reaction is very fast and effective and is usually confined to a local area. In some situations pathological situations, however, the response may extend to become generalized: in these cases, anaphylactic shock can occur, which can lead to death [38].

The role of MCs in allergic diseases, anaphylaxis, autoimmunity, and reproductive disorders has been well documented in the medical literature. However, their role in the etiopathogenesis of oral diseases is still under discussion [46]. Furthermore, the literature on the role of T-cell populations in OLP is extensive, whereas other immunocompetent cells have attracted less scholarly attention [94]. It has long been known that the number of MCs is elevated in OLP lesions compared to healthy oral mucosa [95]. In particular, the presence of activated degranulated mast cells has been found [96], which promote the migration of various inflammatory cells from the circulatory stream [44] and co-assist T lymphocytes in disrupting the epidermal basement membrane [31]. In OLP lesions the increased density of MCs is mainly observed in the lamina propria, near blood vessels, and nerves [15, 97] but also, in a marked manner, at the sites of basement membrane rupture: this already suggests a direct role of MCs in basement membrane disruption as well as in the migration of CD8+ T lymphocytes into the intraepithelial zone [2]. However, one study found more mast cells in the deeper connective tissue than in the subepithelial zone. According to the authors, this could be explained by the fact that the mastocytes migrated from the blood vessels into the deeper connective tissue move to the subepithelial zone where they exert their biological effect on the blood vessels and increase the recruitment of other inflammatory cells to the site of injury [95].

At least 60% of tissue MCs are degranulated in the context of tissues with PLO, compared to the 20% mast cell degranulation observed in normal control mucosa [15], releasing a number of cytokines such as IL-3, IL-4, IL-5, IL-6, IL-8, IL-10, IL-13, IL-16, and TNF-α, the chemokine RANTES, as well as other molecules such as chymase, tryptase, and histamine [4, 15, 46–48].

Mast cell degranulation in OLP can be triggered by two different mechanisms:

1. The interaction of the antigen via MHC-I or MHC-II molecules with T lymphocytes leads to the activation of the latter, which in turn activates the T lymphocytes. T lymphocytes in turn stimulate degranulation and the release of cytokines mast cells.
2. The presence of chemokines could induce an increased influx of calcium capable of causing direct degranulation of mast cells, which in turn stimulate T lymphocytes in the production of other cytokines and chemokines.

Indeed, there is a growing realization that T lymphocytes and mast cells in the oral mucosa interact bidirectionally in maintaining the chronicity and pathogenesis of OLP [96]. IL-16 is known to stimulate the migration of T lymphocytes through connective tissue [98]. TNF-α regulates the expression of vascular adhesion molecules such as CD62E (E-selectin), CD54 (ICAM-1), and CD106 (VCAM-1) by endothelial cells of the subepithelial vascular plexus: the expression of vascular adhesion molecules is required for the adhesion of lymphocytes to the luminal surfaces of blood vessels and their subsequent extravasation [5, 99]. It is indeed known that, in response to inflammatory stimuli, endothelial cells transiently express an increase of adhesion molecules such as ICAMs (intercellular adhesion molecules), VCAMs (vascular cell adhesion molecules), and E-selectin, which promote leukocyte transmigration [100].TNF-α also stimulates the secretion of RANTES and MMP-9 from T cells [1]. RANTES (also produced by antigenically altered basal epithelial cells [46]) further stimulates degranulation of mast cells, while MMP-9 degrades extracellular matrix proteins and prepares the endothelium to allow inflammatory cells to pass through it [3, 99].

In particular, MMP-9 cleaves type IV collagen fibers resulting in degeneration of the basement membrane [12, 13]. Mast cell density is more pronounced at the sites of basement membrane colliquation, suggesting that mast cells may play a direct role in the basal degenerative process and intraepithelial migration of CD8+ T lymphocytes [13]. Indeed, the release of tryptase and chymase directly damage the epithelial basement membrane but also indirectly as these substances stimulate the production of MMP-9 by T lymphocytes, thus demonstrating the indirect role of mast cells in basement membrane destruction [14, 95, 99]. In contrast, histamine induces vessel permeability resulting in submucosal edema and antigen-induced T lymphocyte proliferation [94]. Histamine has recently become the subject of interest and study by some researchers, and its role in the pathogenesis of OLP is currently being investigated (see Sect. 4.4.4).

Finally, there are some studies that have evaluated mast cell counts (MCC) not only in OLPs but also in OLLs (oral lichenoid lesions). Sharma et al. found, compared to healthy oral mucosa, an increase in MCC in both OLP and OLL but without significant differences between these two conditions [46, 95]. In contrast, a more recent study found that the increase in MCC is greater in OLP than in OLL, to the point that the authors suggested that mast cell count is an essential histopathological element for the differentiation of OLP and OLL [46]. Thus, mast cells act directly and indirectly in the degeneration of the oral epithelium, interacting with T lymphocytes in a bidirectionally activating manner and leading to the establishment of vicious circles that favor the progression and chronification of the disease.

4.2 Pathogenic Hypotheses of the OLP

Although OLP is not considered a typical autoimmune disease, it is believed that basal keratinocytes express one or more antigens involved in the disease. It has long been known that antigens presented by MHC-II are processed through an endosomal cellular pathway, while those presented by MHC-I are processed through a cytosolic cellular pathway [4]. Thus, the antigen presented by cells with MHC-II to CD4+ T lymphocytes may differ from that presented by cells with MHC-I to CD8+ T lymphocytes. The second antigen could be a self-antigen such as a heat shock protein induced on basal keratinocytes through activation of the response innate immune response [4]. Alternatively, a single antigen could be processed through both endosomal and cytosolic cellular pathways of antigen presentation [4], such as some viral proteins [31]. For example, recruitment of HCV-specific CD4+ and/or DC8+ T lymphocytes has been demonstrated in OLP tissue [90]. Regardless of the number of antigens involved, it has been suggested that for the development of the persistent infiltrate of CD8+ T lymphocytes, simultaneal presentation of antigens to CD8+ and CD4+ T lymphocytes, respectively, is required by MHC-I and MHC-II [4] (see Sect. 4.3.1).

4.2.1 Sugerman's Unifying Hypothesis

The first unifying hypothesis for antigen presentation and T-cell activation in OLP was introduced by Sugerman et al. in 2002 [4]. This hypothesis is based on a theoretical interaction between CD4+ and CD8+ T lymphocytes through a cell surface molecule called RCA (request cytotoxic activity) expressed by CD8+ T lymphocytes and an RCA receptor (RCAR) expressed by CD4+ T lymphocytes: this interaction enables the initiation of cytotoxic activity by CD8+ T lymphocytes. According to the authors, this interaction can occur only after MHC receptors (class I for CD8+ cells and class II for CD4+ cells) have engaged with the foreign antigen (Ag) in both cell populations. This hypothesis has not yet been proven.

According to the pathogenetic hypothesis of Sugerman et al., initially the antigen receptor of CD8+ T lymphocytes engages, via MHC-I, a specific antigen foreign (Ag 1) on the target cell of basal keratinocytes [5]. The CD8+ T lymphocyte can then seek confirmation of the CD4+ T cell by expressing the hypothetical cell surface molecule RCA [14]. The CD4+ T lymphocyte expresses the hypothetical RCAR [101] only after engagement of its antigen receptor with a related foreign antigen (Ag2) in the context of MHC-II expressed by the keratinocyte or LC [102].

RCA-RCAR binding in combination with co-stimulatory signals of the APC MHC-II+ cell (e.g., CD40, CD80, and IL-12 binding of CD154, CD28, and IL-12R, respectively, on CD4+ cells) initiates Th1-directed differentiation of the CD4+ T lymphocyte that secretes IL-2 and IFN-γ [5]. Receptors for IL-2 and IFN-γ are expressed by the CD8+ T lymphocyte but only upon following specific antigen receptor engagement (with Ag1) of CD8+ T cells in the MHC-I context and/or RCA-RCAR binding. Th1 cytokines (IL-2 and IFN-γ) promote cytotoxic activation of CD8+ T lymphocytes against basal keratinocytes, resulting in their lysis. The activation of keratinocytes (by CD4+ or CD8+ T lymphocyte resulting from the antigen-MHC receptor trimerization or by exogenous agents such as viruses, products bacteria, mechanical trauma, systemic drugs, or contact sensitivity) regulates the secretion of keratinocyte cytokines and chemokines 6 which promotes extravasation and migration lymphocytes at the site of the developing OLP lesion.

4.2.2 Modificate Hypothesis of Carrozzo

APC cells, which may be stromal DCs or LCs, and basal keratinocytes are "activated" by, for example, viral infection (such as HCV), systemic contact sensitivity drugs (e.g., amalgam), or an unidentified agent [5]. The different subgroups of DCs (LC, myeloid, and plasmacytoid DCs) can also be recruited through the expression of the chemotactic agonist chemerin by endothelial cells lining the blood vessels [31]. APC cells and activated keratinocytes secrete chemokines, such as CXCR3/CCL20/CCR6 [88], which attract lymphocytes into the lesion developing OLP. Plasmacytoid DCs, through the production of IFN-α [37], could amplify the activating effects of such stimuli. APC cells present MHC-II-associated antigen to CD4+ T lymphocytes (2a). Activated basal keratinocytes present MHC-I-associated antigen to CD8+ T lymphocytes (2b). APC cell co-stimulatory signals such as the expression of CD40, CD80, and IL-12 (which bind CD154, CD28, and IL-12R, respectively, on CD4+ cells) initiate differentiation in the Th1 direction of the CD4+ T lymphocyte, which secretes IL-2 and IFN-γ (3a) which bind to their respective receptors on CD8+ T cells (3b). It is possible that Th0 and/or Th17 lymphocytes may play a role in this stage, the latter especially in erosive forms of OLP. Activated antigen-specific CD8+ cytotoxic T lymphocytes, express FasL/granzyme B/TNF-α [101] that trigger apoptosis of basal keratinocytes [5]. Mast cell degranulation could further stimulate T-cell activity by aiding them in basement membrane damage. The author of this pathogenetic hypothesis still left open questions: what is the event initial in the formation of the OLP lesion? Does the OLP antigen vary from site to site or from patient to patient?

4.3 Soluble Factors Involved in the OLP Pathogenesis

Many molecules intervene in the OLP modulating the immuno-inflammatory reaction. Among these, the most studied soluble factors are cytokines, chemokines, and matrix metalloproteases (MMPs).

4.3.1 Cytokine

Cytokines constitute a large group of small peptide molecules synthesized and secreted by various immune and nonimmune cells [103]. They behave as signal-transport molecules by binding to specific receptors expressed on the surface of target cells, initiating signal transduction that, through various factors regulating gene transcription, cause phenotypic and functional alteration of them [104, 105]. Several cytokines have been termed interleukins because they were initially identified in leukocytes and were thought to be able to transduce signals only in such cells. Other cytokines, on the other hand, have been defined based on the first effect highlighted, such as tumor necrosis factor (TNF) and transforming growth factor-β (TGF-β). In addition, some cytokines that exert chemotactic effect on leukocytes are named chemokines [40]. Interferons also belong to the large family of cytokines. Most cytokines have pleiotropic action: this term indicates that they can produce different effects depending on target cell types and environment [106]. Cytokines can also induce reciprocal productions and can act by autocrine (effect on the secreting cell itself), paracrine (effect on neighboring cells reached by contact and via interstitial fluids), and endocrine (effect at a distance mediated by circulatory stream transport) mechanisms [40, 103, 104], Regarding the immunological role, cytokines are potent regulators and play a central role in controlling the extent and duration of innate and acquired immune responses [106]. Aberrant cytokine productions are linked to the onset of immunodeficiency, allergic, autoimmune, and inflammatory diseases [106, 107]. The literature on expression abnormalities of various cytokines in OLP at the level of lesions, saliva, serum, and peripheral blood mononuclear cells (PBMCs) is vast [108] (Table 4.3).

1. *Interleukin 1 (IL-1)*
   (a) *Characteristics*. There are two variants of IL-1, called IL-1α and IL-1β, which are encoded by two distinct genes but bind to the same receptor complex and perform the same biological function. IL-1 is synthesized by different cell populations: IL-1β is secreted mainly by monocyte-macrophage, while IL-1α is expressed by keratinocytes and endothelial cells [176]. IL-1 constitutes an important mediator of the immune-inflammatory response; in fact, it causes rapid activation of T lymphocytes (especially stimulates CD4+ T lymphocytes in IL-2 production and IL-2 receptor expression), neutrophils, monocytes, eosinophils, and macrophages. IL-1 stimulates the production of itself and other cytokines such as TNF-α, IL-6, and IL-8 (all NF-kB-dependent cytokines [109]). Finally, IL-1 stimulates the proliferation of bone marrow cells, such as B lymphocytes, neutrophil granulocytes, macrophages, and platelets [176–178].
   (b) *Role of IL-1 in OLP*. Some studies have found in OLP lesions an abundant presence of IL-1+ cells with monocyte-macrophage surface characteristics [114] and a positive immunostaining for IL-1β in basal and spinous keratinocyte and lymphocyte infiltrates [179]. In ex vivo studies, performed on cell cultures, an increase in IL-1β concentration and the number of IL-1β producing cells in OLP compared with gingiva healthy and inflamed. In addition, in the same studies, after stimulation with IL-1β, keratinocytes and TIMCs (tissue-infiltrating mononuclear cells) produced more TNF-α, IL-6, and GM-CSF than keratinocytes from healthy gingiva [127, 156]. These studies have noted the role of IL-1β in regulating the cytokine network in OLP [108]. Other authors have detected by ELISA tests the levels of the NF-kB-dependent cytokines TNF-α, IL-1, IL-6, and IL-8 in three types of samples: whole unstimulated saliva (WUS), mixture of saliva and oral sus-

Table 4.3 Main cytokines involved in OLP

Cytokines	Cellular sources	Lesions	Saliva	Serum	PBMC	Polymorphism	References
IL-1α	KC, cell.endot.	–	↑	–	–	/	[32, 109–113]
IL-1β	Monoc./macro f.	↑	–	–	–	/	[32, 112–115]
IL-2	Cell. NK, B, T (CD4+e CD8+)	↑	–	≈	/	/	[31, 108, 113, 116–118]
IL-4	(not in early phase): Th1, Th2, MC	≈	↑	≈	–	−590 (C/C), 1098	[62, 70, 113, 119–124]
IL-5	Th2, T-γδ, MC, basof., eosin	≈	–	/	–	–	[38, 70, 125, 126]
IL-6	DC, linf.B, macr., KC, cell.endot., fibrobl., astroc.	↑	↑ (↑↑ in OED)	↑	/ o ↓	−174 (G/C)	[94, 109, 112, 118, 127–132]
IL-8	Monoc., cell.NK, T, neutr., KC, cell. endot., fibrobl	≈	↑ (↑↑ in EOLP e OSCC, none in OED)	↑	–	↓ −251 (AA) e ↑251A/+781C e −251T/+781C in EOLP; ↑rs4073 A>T.	[35, 109–111, 133, 134]
IL-10	Linf.T CD4+, monoc./macr. e molte cell.imm.	≈	↑	≈	↓	↓ −1082G/A, 819C/T e 592C/A	[135–139]
IL-17	Linf.T, T-γδ, NK, DC, macr	↑ (↑↑ in EOLP)	≈	↑ (↑↑ in EOLP)	↑	Allele G197A (rs2275913)	[80, 81, 140–144]
IL-18	Macr., DC, cell.T, B, KC, astroc., cort. surr cells	/	↑	↑	–	≈ −607 (C/A), ↑ −137 G/G in EOLP	[70, 122, 145–147]
IL-22	Linf. Th17, Th22, CD8+, N	↑↑ (↑ CLP)	↑	↑ (/ in CLP)	–	–	[141, 148–152]
IL-23	Macr., KC, DC	↑↑ (↑↑↑ in EOLP e ↑ in CLP)	/ (↑ con Porph. g.)	/	–	–	[80, 82, 130, 151–155]
TNF-α	Macr., linf.T B, NK, DC, MC, neutr., KC, fibrobl., astroc., glial and neopl. cells	↑	↑ (↑↑ in severe forms)	(/with met. ≠ from ELISA)	↓	≈ −308 (G/A)	[62, 67, 68, 70, 108, 109, 111–113, 119, 127, 128, 133, 156–164]
IFN-γ	B lymph, T CD4+, CD8+, NK, APC	↑ (↑↑ in EOLP)	≈	≈	↓	UTR 5644 (T/T), ≈ +874 (T/T)	[62, 70, 81, 108, 113, 117, 118, 121, 122, 164–173]
TGF-β	Subepithelial infiltrate	≈ (↑ in OSCC)	–	≈	–	/	[31, 43, 62, 67, 113, 160, 163, 174, 175]

↑ increase, ↓ decrease, – not specified, / absent, ≈ unclear

OED oral epithelial dysplasia, *CLP* cutaneous LP, *EOLP* erosive OLP, *OSCC* squamous cell carcinoma, *PBMC* peripheral blood mononuclear cells, *MC* mast cells, *KC* keratinocytes, *DC* dendritic cells, *NK* natural killer, *APC* antigen-presenting cells, *TLR* Toll-like receptor, *WUS* whole unstimulated saliva, *Porph. g. Porphyromonas gingivalis*

pension of isotonic saline (saliva-NaCl), and transudate of injured tissue (TT). These values were found to be much higher in patients with OLP than in healthy controls, and therefore the authors propose NK-kB-dependent cytokine levels in oral fluodes as potential diagnostic and prognostic markers for disease monitoring and therapeutic decision-making and monitoring [109, 110]. Indeed, the increase of these cytokines in WUS decreased (to values equal to healthy subjects for IL-1α and IL-8) after treatment with an oral suspension of dexamethasone 0.1% for 6 weeks [128]. Moreover, IL-1α levels are significantly increased in OLP cases with moderate dysplasia without showing differences with oral squamous cell carcinoma (OSCC) [111]. So, IL-1α values may also be useful in assessing the risk of malignant transformation of OLP lesions [108]. In HCV+ patients with OLP, there is a reduction in IL-1 levels in the oral epithelium compared with patients with OLP, and this suggests that HCV infection may influence cytokine levels and thus result in an indirect effect on the development of OLP [180]. Finally, it is known that cytokine genetic polymorphisms are associated with susceptibility to develop certain immune conditions [108]. Genetic polymorphism is defined as the simultaneous presence, with a prevalence of >1%, in the general population of two or more alleles that exhibit any sequence variation. No genetic polymorphisms of the IL-1 cluster have been found to be associated with the susceptibility to develop OLP [112, 113].

2. *Interleukin 2 (IL-2)*
   (a) *Characteristics.* It is a cytokine involved in the response to microbial infection and in the discrimination between self and non-self antigens [116]. IL-2 is produced mainly by T lymphocytes CD4+, but also CD8+, B lymphocytes, and NK cells [181]. Its effects are mediated by IL-2R receptors, which are expressed on the surface of lymphocytes involved in cellular immunity [116]. IL-2 is a true real growth factor for T cells, since it can induce the expansion of both CD4+ and CD8+ cells [181]. In addition, IL-2 plays a key role in modulating the differentiation of CD4+ T cells; in fact it can trigger the differentiation of Th1 and Th2 lymphocytes and inhibit that of Th17 [115, 182]. IL-2 plays a key role in the maintenance of Treg lymphocytes [182], induces the differentiation and expansion of cytotoxic effector T lymphocytes by increasing their cytolytic activity [115], promotes the proliferation of activated B lymphocytes by stimulating the secretion of antibodies, and promotes the proliferation of NK cells, monocytes, and macrophages [115, 181].
   (b) *Role of IL-2 in the OLP.* The expression of IL-2 and its receptor IL-2R has been found consistently in OLP lesions; especially IL-2R (considered a marker of T lymphocyte activation) has been localized on infiltrated T cells [108]. In an in vitro study, it was also observed that, following pre-treatment with IL-2, TIMCs (tissue-infiltrating mononuclear cells) in OLP lesions generated a higher proportion of IL-6 than the PBMCs (peripheral blood mononuclear cells) [127]. So, the signal transduction induced by IL-2/IL-2R is involved in regulating the expansion and activation of infiltrating T lymphocytes in OLP lesions [108]. Several studies have shown that IL-2/IL-2R signaling is upregulated and may be a possible therapeutic target in the treatment of OLP: for example, cyclosporine induces a decrease in the number of activated IL-2R+ cells [183–185]. About the serum levels of IL-2 in OLP, the studies are discordant. Some authors have noted an increase, while others a decrease [117, 119]. In addition, no statistically significant difference was found in the number of peripheral blood T lymphocytes secreting IL-2 [118]. Such discrepant results could be explained by different research means and measurement techniques. It has not been yet demonstrated the existence of a genetic polymorphism of IL-2 related to OLP has not been yet demonstrated [31, 113].
3. *Interleukin 4 (IL-4)*
   (a) *Characteristics.* IL-4 is the representative cytokine of polarization in the Th2

direction as it induces the differentiation of CD4+ T lymphocytes into Th2 lymphocytes [186]. The cells that produce, at an early stage, IL-4 have not yet been identified, but once activated, Th2 lymphocytes further produce IL-4 by self-stimulating in an autocrine manner to maintain their differentiation state [120]. Mast cells and Th1 lymphocytes are also capable of producing IL-4 [120, 187]. This inflammatory mediator has pleiotropic effects on a large group of cell populations [188], can stimulate the production of other Th2 cytokine profile such as IL-5 and IL-13 [187], and inhibit the production of Th1 and Th17 profile inflammatory mediators such as TNF-α, IFN-γ, and IL-17 [187, 189]. Finally, IL-4 also acts on B lymphocytes by promoting their proliferation, differentiation, and the expression of MHC-II, CD23, and IL-4R [108].

(b) *Role of IL-4 in the OLP*. The role of IL-4 has been widely studied in the literature, but it has not yet been fully elucidated given the sometimes-discordant results. TIMCs isolated from OLP tissue samples showed an increase in IL-4-producing cells compared with the TIMCs isolated from normal or inflamed gingiva [127]. The m-RNA and protein levels of IL-4 are much higher in erosive/ulcerated OLP lesions than in healthy mucosa [70, 121]. But other studies report that IL-4 secretion was not detected by unstimulated T lymphocytes and that molecules of IL-4 m-RNA were detected in only one out of seven T-cell lines cultured from OLP lesions [62, 67]. Studies on salivary and serum levels of IL-4 in patients with OLP also report discordant results. One study reports elevated levels of IL-4 (Th2 cytokine) in the WUS of patients with OLP (ulcerative-erosive species), low levels of IFN-γ (Th1 cytokine), and consequently a lower value of the IFN-γ/IL-4 ratio compared with healthy controls; the authors hypothesized a possible role of the imbalance of salivary Th1/Th2 cytokines with predominance of the Th2 profile and that the salivary IL-4 levels could be a fine biomarker reflecting the degree of severity of OLP [165]. But a high study reports no difference in the salivary IL-4 levels of the affected patients compared with healthy controls [121]. The converse is also similar for serum values. In fact, some authors have found a reduction in the serum concentration of IL-4 in patients with OLP [185], while other studies report comparable or higher serum levels of this cytokine in affected patients [119, 190]. However recent studies may have resolved this issue. A very recent meta-analysis investigated the role of serum and salivary IFN-γ/IL-4 ratio and found that this value does not play a major role in the development and severity of OLP [166]. Another similar, and equally recent, meta-analysis investigated the connection between the severity of OLP variants and serum and salivary levels of IL-4, and the data obtained showed that these values are indeed elevated in OLP patients, so the authors concluded that IL-4 may represent a potential salivary biomarker of disease, but clinicians should keep account that these concentrations may also be modified by other factors such as secondary infections [59]. Finally, two studies have evaluated the possible presence of IL-4 gene polymorphisms in OLP. A significant increase in the frequency of IL-4-590 (C/C) genotype in patients with non-erosive OLP compared with the group control consisting of healthy subjects [122]. In addition, a sixfold increase was also found at a higher frequency of IL-4-1098 genotype (G/G) in patients with OLP than in controls [31]. So, the correlation between the genetic polymorphism of IL-4 and the susceptibility OLP is possible, although further study is needed.

4. *Interleukin 5 (IL-5)*
   (a) *Characteristics*. IL-5 is a Th2 cytokine profile (regulated in fact by the transcription factor Th2-related GATA-3) but can also be produced by CD34+ progenitor cells, basophilic and eosinophilic granulocytes, mast cells, and T-γδ lymphocytes [38, 125]. IL-5 constitutes the main regulator of differentiation, marrow maturation, and eosinophil biology, also modulating their tissue migration, survival, proliferation, and function. It is also involved in the terminal differentiation of B lymphocytes into antibody-secreting plasma cells [40, 191].
   (b) *Role of IL-5 in the OLP*. The evidence for a role of IL-5 in the pathogenesis of OLP is relatively limited [108]. Increased m-RNA expression of IL-5 has been observed in OLP lesions compared with healthy oral mucosa [70, 126], while another reports a decrease in the number of IL-5-secreting cells [118]. In addition, other authors have found not statistically significant in serum IL-5 levels between healthy and affected patients [119]. The possible explanations for these inconsistent results include diversity in the sources of IL-5 and the different composition of the subjects involved in these studies [108].
5. *Interleukin 6 (IL-6)*
   (a) *Characteristics*. IL-6 is mainly produced by APC cells (including DCs, B lymphocytes, and macrophages), but it is also expressed by nonimmune cells such as keratinocytes, fibroblasts, endothelial cells, and astrocytes [34, 129]. IL-6 stimulates target cells through the IL-6R receptor, but only a few cells express it bound to the membrane, while most of them expose gp130, a ligand binding-associated receptor signaling protein, on the cell membrane. In fact, cells expressing only gp130 do not respond exclusively to IL-6 but also to a complex composed of IL-6 associated with a soluble form of IL-6R. Thus, the generation of a soluble form of IL-6R can greatly increase the spectrum of IL-6 target cells. IL-6 expresses a wide variety of biological activities in the regulation of immunity, inflammation, hematopoiesis, and oncogenesis [108]. For example, this cytokine promotes the differentiation and production of plasma cell antibodies and regulates the activity of CD4+ T lymphocytes [192]; especially it exerts anti-apoptotic activity on these cells and prolongs their survival in vitro by maintaining the expression of Bcl-2 [34]. In addition, IL-6 can result in an early expression of IL-4, thus making CD4+ T lymphocytes nonresponsive to IFN-γ and polarizing their differentiation in a Th2 direction [34]. In addition, IL-6 is required for the differentiation of Th17 lymphocytes by overcoming immune suppression mediated by lymphocytes Treg [34]. So, with these functions, this inflammatory mediator plays a key role in modulating the immune response from a tolerant state to active inflammatory conditions [176].
   (b) *Role of IL-6 in OLP*. The literature on the role of IL-6 in OLP is extensive and generally reports a role of this cytokine especially in erosive forms. Already for several years, it has been demonstrated in increased levels of IL-6 in samples of exfoliated oral mucosa cells, especially in ulcerative-erosive forms [193]. The same also occurs in various oral fluids [130, 131] such as WUS [109, 111, 128, 194] saliva-NaCl, and TT [109, 110] from patients with OLP lesions. This phenomenon in several of these studies was also observed for other NF-kB-dependent cytokines such as, in addition to IL-6, TNF-α, IL-1, and IL-8 [110, 128, 177]. Especially one of these shows a reduction in salivary levels of these four cytokines after treatment with a 0.1% dexamethasone oral suspension for 6 weeks, reaching values equal to healthy subjects for IL-1α and IL-8 [128]. In the

forms of OLP associated with dysplasia, an alteration in the levels of NF-kB-dependent cytokines was also detected: as for IL-6, an increase in its levels in the WUS of affected patients (OLP + dysplasia) compared with healthy subjects was shown, but these values were significantly lower than in OSCC. Therefore, the salivary concentrations of IL-6 have been suggested as potential tools for monitoring disease activity, therapeutic response, and to reflect in part the potential for malignant transformation of OLP [109, 128]. The elevated IL-6 values in lesional tissues and saliva may be explained by the fact that various cell types within the local microenvironment of OLP could produce significant amounts of IL-6, including monocytes and infiltrating T lymphocytes, macrophages, fibroblasts, and altered keratinocytes [108, 193]. This is supported by the finding of IL-6 m-RNA localized in infiltrating CD4+ and CD8+ T lymphocytes and basal and suprabasal keratinocytes in OLP lesions [195] and by some tissue culture studies in which it was observed that keratinocytes from OLP lesion tissues produced much more IL-6 than the same from normal or inflamed gingival tissues [127, 156]. In addition, TIMCs in OLP tissues produced more IL-6 than TIMCs in inflamed gingival tissues and PBMCs from OLP patients themselves. Also in affected patients, TIMCs produced a higher proportion of TNF-α and GM-CSF than PBMCs under IL-6 stimulation [127, 156]. Taken together, these results suggested that IL-6 constitutes an important inflammatory mediator responsible for the immune disharmony related to infiltrating lymphocytes and altered keratinocytes, resulting in increased production of pro-inflammatory cytokines and increased local inflammatory response in OLP lesions [108]. In addition to the local environment, many studies have reported elevated serum concentrations of IL-6 in patients with OLP [68, 130, 131, 133, 193]. Moreover, these serum concentrations appear significantly higher in erosive forms of OLP than in non-erosive forms [130, 193]. Researchers have also found that in patients with OLP, after treatment with levamisole or some medicinal Chinese herbs, serum levels of IL-6 decrease [131]. So, it is possible to believe that these values may constitute a useful marker in assessing the progress of OLP and the response to therapy [108]. In fact, IL-6 has also been associated with keratinocyte expression of MRP protein (multidrug resistance protein), which is overexpressed in OLP [196]. Patients with OLP erosive (EOLP) treated with oral mycophenolate mofetil showed a significant reduction of serum level of IL-6 and absence of resistance to therapy, while those treated with methotrexate combined with local application of pimecrolimus showed no such reduction, and treatment resistance was observed in some of these patients, especially in lesions with plaque. This further confirms how IL-6 may be a useful biomarker in the choice of the best possible therapy in the treatment of resistant forms of OLP [196]. Some authors suggest that the elevated serum concentration of IL-6 could be attributed mainly to PBMCs and endothelial cells and partly also to locally secreted IL-6 which can diffuse into the blood capillaries or be drained into the lymphatic vessels to be finally poured into the blood circulation [131]. So, IL-6 secreted locally and IL-6 produced systemically by PBMCs and endothelial cells could be the possible reason for the high serum concentration of IL-6 in LP patients [131]. However, unlike its serum levels, the expression of IL-6 in PBMCs of patients with OLP was similar or even reduced compared with controls, and this could be attributable to a suppressed immune function of PBMCs in the OLP patients [68, 118]. Recently, two meta-analyses were performed that analyzed the role of IL-6 in OLP. One of these evaluating publications up to December 2015 from different databases selected eight studies (five on Asian and three on Caucasian populations) and found an increase in serum IL-6 values in OLP patients: this increase was significant in studies involving Asian patients but not in those performed on Caucasian individuals. However, the limited number of studies included in the survey, together with the small size of the total sample analyzed, may have resulted in an insufficient ability to assess a statistically significant effect [131]. Another meta-analysis studied data drawn from searches from 1983 to October 2016 on different databases, including an overall sample that was somewhat larger than the previous meta-analysis and assessed both serum and salivary levels of IL-6. The authors conclude that the results obtained confirm the role of IL-6 in the pathogenesis of OLP and its usefulness as a pathological marker. However, the higher salivary levels of IL-6 than serum levels suggests that salivary measurement of this marker may be more useful than serum measurement for diagnostic and therapeutic purposes [59]. Xavier et al. studied an IL-6 genetic polymorphism by analyzing a sample of 53 Brazilian patients with OLP and 53 healthy controls, and they found a significantly higher frequency in affected patients of the IL-6-174 (G/C) genotype, thus demonstrating the association between OLP and this polymorphism [112].

6. *Interleukin 8 (IL-8)*
   (a) *Characteristics*. IL-8, also known as CXCL8 or neutrophil chemotactic factor [197], is produced by various cells of the immune system such as monocytes, T lymphocytes, NK cells, and neutrophils and by nonimmune cells such as endothelial cells, fibroblasts, and epithelial cells [35]. IL-8 production is not constitutive but is inducible through the activity of pro-inflammatory cytokines such as IL-1β, IL-17, and TNF-α and by the presence oxidative stress and products of microbial origin [35]. In contrast, some factors such as IL-4 and TGF-β some natural agents (such as lycopene and green tea) inhibit IL-8 synthesis [198, 199]. IL-8 promotes the activity of neutrophil granulocytes, their adhesion to endothelia, and transmigration but also degranulation, bursting respiratory, and the release of defensins and MMPs [200]. IL-8, also known precisely as CXCL8, acts as a chemotactic factor for so many immune cells such as macrophages, granulocytes basophils, and T lymphocytes, also increasing the expression of adhesion molecules [35]. Such cytokine also enhances the metabolism of reactive oxygen species (ROS) and supports the mitosis of epithelial cells and angiogenesis, so it may play a role in various disorders such as arthritis rheumatoid and various cancers [201].
   (b) *Role of IL-8 in the OLP*. One study reports the failure to detect IL-8 in cells of the oral mucosa with OLP lesion: the evaluation was performed by immunohistochemical investigation on frozen biopsy sections [202], so an important review indicates that IL-8 might function primarily in the systemic immune response of patients with OLP rather than in local lesions [108]. However, a more recent study of this review instead detects the presence of IL-8 in the oral mucosa affected by atrophic/erosive OLP through an immunohistochemical investigation, performed by a different method from the previously described study [134]. In particular, the study showed decreased immuno-expression of VEGF and IL-8 in the tissues treated with bevacizumab-based intralesional

injections compared with those treated with 0.1% triamcinolone acetonide topical ointment [134]. So, it is possible that IL-8 plays a role also local in the pathogenesis of OLP, but further studies in this direction are needed to prove this with certainty. Instead, there are many studies that have consistently demonstrated elevated IL-8 values in both serum and oral fluids of patients with OLP [42, 109, 110, 128, 133, 202]. For example, a study performed on a sample of ethnic Chinese patients with OLP showed salivary concentrations of NF-kB-dependent cytokines much higher than that of their respective serum values, among which IL-8 was the most prominent. In addition, the authors found that salivary levels of IL-8 change from the reticular to the erosive form, suggesting that the salivary assay of IL-8 could be a promising biomarker of OLP severity [133]. Similarly, Rhodus et al. found an increase in IL-8 levels in different oral fluids from OLP and that salivary levels decreased significantly after treatment with a 0.1% dexamethasone oral suspension for 6 weeks and that they correlated closely with the VAS score (visual analogue scale or visual analogue pain scale), indicating that salivary analysis of IL-8 can be applied for monitoring the therapeutic response of OLP [109, 110, 128]. They also found a significantly lower salivary IL-8 concentration in OLP associated with dysplasia compared with patients with OSCC, indicating that salivary IL-8 values constitute a useful and non-invasive method for monitoring malignant transformation of OLP [109]. Another study shows that serum levels of IL-8 constitute a more sensitive marker than serum levels of IL-6 in the monitoring of OLP activity and therapeutic effects, since the abnormality of the serum concentration of IL-8 (compared with IL-6) has been detected in more patients affected [42]. A recent meta-analysis further substantiated the increased serum and especially salivary levels of IL-8 in OLP patients: the greater elevation of salivary levels than serum levels demonstrates that the measurement of this marker in the saliva is more useful than the serum measurement for diagnostic and therapeutic purposes [203]. An association has also been demonstrated between OLP and genetic polymorphisms of IL-8. A study performed in Chinese population has found a significantly lower frequency of genotype-251 (AA) in the EOLP group compared with controls. Haplotype analysis revealed a reduced frequency of haplotype −251 A/+781 C and a higher frequency of the −251 T/+781 C haplotype in patients with EOLP compared with healthy controls, suggesting that IL-8 gene polymorphisms may be associated with the severity of OLP [204]. A recent study reveals the higher prevalence of "A allele-containing" genotypes of IL-8 rs4073 A>T in patients with OLP compared with healthy subjects and that HCV+ patients with OLP are more likely to develop active/erosive lesions, but no association was found particular polymorphism in HCV+, HCV-, non-erosive OLP (NEOLP), and EOLP subgroups [80].

7. *Interleukin 10 (IL-10)*
   (a) *Characteristics.* IL-10 was initially described as an inhibitory factor of the synthesis cytokine (CSIF), secreted by Th2 lymphocytes, because of its inhibitory effects on the production of IL-2 and IFN-γ in Th1 lymphocytes, but today it is known as a cytokine widely much more expressed [205]. IL-10 is mainly secreted by CD4+ T lymphocytes, monocytes, and macrophages but also by almost all cell populations of the immune system [167, 206]. The production of IL-10 in CD4+ T lymphocytes is accompanied by the expression also of other specific cytokines necessary for

the development of each subpopulation, which are, however, inhibited by the regulatory presence of IL-10, which, by negative feedback mechanism, limits immune responses. In contrast, in monocytes/macrophages, IL-10 is released in response to various endogenous mediators such as LPS (lipopolysaccharide) bacteria and catecholamines. As an anti-inflammatory cytokine, IL-10 exerts different functions in various target cells. In monocytes/macrophages (the main target cells), IL-10 suppresses the release of pro-inflammatory cytokines and functions to present antigen but increases the efficacy of phagocytosis. IL-10 inhibits the proliferation and synthesis of Th1 and Th2 cytokine profile and promotes the development of a regulatory phenotype by CD4+ T cells but in contrast has no direct inhibitory effect on Th17 and CD8+. IL-10 inhibits the secretion of neutrophil-attracting chemokines and also the release of pro-inflammatory mediators by the latter. Instead, this cytokine promotes proliferation, differentiation, and MHC expression of B lymphocytes and also stimulates the activity cytotoxicity of NK lymphocytes [206].

(b) *Role of IL-10 in the OLP.* One study showed that TIMCs from OLP produced more IL-10 than those from inflamed gingiva and PBMPs and that TIMCs pretreated with IL-4 released a higher proportion of IL-10 [127]. The presence of IL-10 in mononuclear cells adjacent to the basement membrane within the inflammatory infiltrate itself in OLP lesions has been picked up [199]. Therefore, IL-10 was previously considered a critical mediator of the cytokine network involved in the local microenvironment in OLP lesions [108]. However, this has been challenged by a study by Khan et al. who report the absence of IL-10 detection in T lymphocytes in OLP lesions [62]. Studies on serum levels of IL-10 are also discordant. One study shows a decrease in serum IL-10 levels in patients with OLP [187], while other authors have reported an increase in these values in serum and saliva [119]. In addition, a significant reduction in IL-10 production of peripheral blood T lymphocytes and monocytes from patients with OLP has also been observed in vitro [118, 135]. The reason for these inconsistencies remains unclear; however, some researchers have hypothesized that the different expression patterns of IL-10 might be due to different regulatory mechanisms in the various individuals, including the inducing effects of other inflammatory mediators and the various predispositions genetics of this disease [135, 167]. A more recent study found a significant increase in serum IL-10 levels compared with controls: there was no correlation between serum IL-10 levels with the age and sex of the participants; moreover, the results indicated a significant difference between the different types of OLP and serum IL-10 values. So, it is possible that the elevation of IL-10 may play an important role in the immunomodulation of the disease, although the exact mechanism is unclear [207]. Three studies have been performed on IL-10 polymorphisms associated with OLP. Although two of these [112, 157] found no differences in allele and genotype frequencies of IL-10 between patients with OLP and healthy subjects, Bai et al. [157] and Al-Mohaya et al. [158] have revealed that the haplotype of IL-10 polymorphisms −1082G/A, −819C/T, and −592C/A, which are associated with lower serum levels of IL-10, has a lower association with OLP, suggesting that the IL-10 gene polymorphisms might have some influence on susceptibility and progression of the disease. The haplotype is the specific combination of nucleotides, one for each of the polymorphic sites that are present on a single chromosome. Thus, the haplotype indicates the constitution genetics of individuals with respect to a member of an allelic gene pair or set of genes that are closely related and tend to be inherited together such as those in the complex major histocompatibility [208].

8. *Interleukin 12 (IL-12)*
   (a) *Characteristics*. IL-12 is a cytokine produced mainly by monocytes/macrophages, by DCs, by B lymphocytes, and, to a lesser extent, by activated T lymphocytes [136]. The production of IL-12 requires specific priming signals (e.g., from bacterial products) and amplification signals from the cytokines produced by DCs or T lymphocytes, whereas IL-10 and TGF-β inhibit the production of IL-12 [209]. The main functions of this cytokine include the induction of IFN-γ production by NK cells and T lymphocytes, increasing the cytotoxicity of the former and the proliferation of the latter [136, 209]. It can also increase the effects of cytotoxic T lymphocytes by inducing the production of cytolytic factors such as perforin and granzymes [209]. Of fundamental importance is the role of IL-12, produced by macrophages and DCs in response to microbial pathogens, as a key cytokine in the differentiation of virgin T lymphocytes into Th1 lymphocytes, indicating its central role in the mechanism in which innate immune cells drive the adaptive immune response by polarizing virgin CD4+ T lymphocytes toward the Th1 phenotype [209]. Therefore, IL-12 is required for resistance to bacterial and intracellular parasites and for the establishment of organ-specific autoimmunity [136].
   (b) *Role of IL-12 in the OLP*. Studies on IL-12 in OLP are few. A higher amount of IL-12 in peripheral blood monocytes of patients with OLP compared with healthy controls, has been observed [135]. In addition, salivary epithelial cells of affected subjects secrete a higher proportion of IL-12 [135]. The increased expression of IL-12 was found to be always contextual to a strong expression of TLRs [135, 139]. In contrast, other authors have reported a lower levels of IL-12, secreted in the peripheral blood of patients with OLP [118]. Lu et al. [108] believe that these results suggest that the main producers of IL-12 in OLP are probably monocytes and epithelial cells and that the production of this cytokine depends, at least partially, on the expression of TLRs in different cells: consequently, IL-12 would act as a promoter, but not as an actual effector in the Th1 immune response both in the local environment and in the peripheral blood. However, it has long been known that the expression of CD40 and CD80 and the production of IL-12 by APC cells can promote an activation of CD4+ T lymphocytes into Th1 lymphocytes [210]. Supporting this hypothesis is the fact that LCs and keratinocytes are capable of producing IL-12 [137, 211]. Although IL-12 activity in OLP has not been directly measured, the Th1 cytokine profile in OLP suggests the co-stimulation of IL-12 on CD4+ T cells with subsequent production of IFN-γ and IL-2, a key event in the pathogenesis of OLP 9, [4]. In this context, the reduction of IL-12 activity could be of clinical benefit in OLP [4]. A recent study showed increased serum levels of IL-12 and IL-27, and this expression increase did not seem to correlate with the clinical features of OLP [138]. Therefore, as mentioned before, it is likely that the expression of IL-12 (as well as IL-27) is synergized [209] and that this cytokine may actually promote the development of the inflammatory process in OLP. Finally, a study performed on a sample of ethnic Chinese individuals assessed the presence of possible IL-12A gene polymorphisms and found a significant difference in the distributions of the rs568408 genotype

between the affected patients and controls. In addition, a highly significant in the distributions of that genotype and in the frequencies of the A allele in the OLP group compared with the control group. Therefore, this study indicates that the rs568408 variation in the IL-12A gene might influence disease susceptibility and be related to the severity of OLP [212].

9. *Interleukin 17 (IL-17)*
   (a) *Characteristics*. IL-17 (also known as IL-17A) is part of the Th17 cytokines and is secreted mainly by T lymphocytes but also by DCs, macrophages, NK cells, and T-γδ lymphocytes [213]. IL-17 represents the cytokine that defined the new subclass of T helper cells named Th17 and distinguished from Th1 and Th2 [214]. IL-17 constitutes a crucial mediator in the functioning of the immune system [108]. Although mainly produced by T lymphocytes in acquired immunity, IL-17 also plays a key role in innate immunity by triggering the production of numerous chemokines, resulting in the recruitment of neutrophils and macrophages to eliminate pathogens. Therefore, IL-17 is considered an important "molecular bridge" between innate and acquired immunity [214]. The pleiotropic effects of this cytokine on different tissue and immune target cells have also been demonstrated [108]. IL-17 stimulates the production of various inflammatory mediators such as IL-1β, IL-6, IL-8, TNF-α, MCP-1 (monocyte chemoattractant protein-1 or CCL2), GM-CSF, and MMP in monocytes, endothelial cells, keratinocytes, and fibroblasts. So, IL-17, together with its downstream molecules, is involved in the formation and maintenance of the local inflammatory microenvironment [213]. IL-17 is very important in the clearance of bacterial and fungal pathogens and leads to severe inflammation with marked tissue destruction [75].
   (b) *Role of IL-17 in the OLP*. Studies on IL-17 and Th17 cytokines are all recent and in early stages. In a DNA microarray study, the IL-17 gene was identified over sevenfold upregulated in OLP lesions compared with healthy oral mucosa [140]. Th17 cells were detected in OLP lesions, especially in atrophic-erosive forms [81]. Increased m-RNA levels of IL-17 have been shown in biopsies of EOLP lesions [70]. The authors of the latter study (who detected Th17 and Th0 cytokines in erosive forms and Th2 in reticular forms) hypothesized that in EOLP, Th17 cytokines (which play a role in inflammation) and Th0-type cytokines (which include the production of IFN-γ capable of activating CD8+ T lymphocytes) may be responsible for the most obvious oral mucosal damage, while the reduced number of Th0 cells and increased Th2 cells (which are not pathogenic) may explain the less obvious epithelial damage associated with reticular OLP [70]. The role of Th2 cytokines in OLP is still debated, but a recent meta-analysis [166] showed that serum levels of IL-4 (cardinal Th2 cytokine) are indeed positively associated with OLP. The plasticity of Th17 lymphocytes toward Th1 cells or not is related to prolonged exposure to IL-12 (toward Th1) or IL-23 (toward Th17) activity [215, 216]. So virgin CD4+CD161+ T lymphocytes, precursors of Th17 lymphocytes [217], can differentiate into Th17, Th17/Th1, and finally Th1 cells in response to environmental IL-12. However, the respective role of Th17, Th17/Th1, and Th1 cells in the pathogenesis of chronic inflammatory disorders is still debated [70]. Several recent studies are helping to better understand the role of Th17 cells and their cytokines in OLP. For example, one study showed a significantly higher proportion of Th1 and Th17 cells and serum levels of IL-17 than controls, especially in atrophic-

erosive rather than reticular forms [81]. A strong increase in epithelial immunostaining for IL-17 and IL-23 was also observed in OLP lesions and significantly more IL-23+ lymphocytes (detection with cytoplasmic immunostaining) in erosive forms [82]. The IL-23/IL-17 axis has recently been discovered as a signaling pathway implicated in several chronic inflammatory diseases and immune disorders, and the immunoexpression of these cytokines is elevated in OLP lesions [153]. Furthermore, in vitro studies have shown that exogenous IL-23 increases the percentage of Th17 cells and IL-17 production and that exogenous IL-17 can significantly increase in oral keratinocytes the m-RNA expression of defensin-2 and defensin-3, CCL-20, IL-8, and TNF-, but not defensin-1, CXCL-9, CXCL-10, CXCL-11, CCL-5, and IL-6 [153]. IL-17 immunoexpression levels correlate positively with those of Foxp3 (a specific marker of Treg lymphocytes; see Sect. 4.1.3 "Treg lymphocytes") [218]. The latter marker is also more expressed in OLP than in cutaneous LP, pointing to it as a possible association with the different clinical behavior of these two disease variants [218]. Another study also found greater immuno-expression of Foxp3+ cells, especially in the subepithelial infiltrate, whereas IL-17+ cells localize mainly more deeply in stromal tissues [219]. Overexpression has been observed (and positive inter-correlation) of Foxp3 and the long noncoding RNA DQ786243 in peripheral blood CD4+ T lymphocytes of OLP patients. The overexpression of DQ786243 in CD4+ T lymphocytes resulted in the upregulation of Foxp3 and Foxp3+ Treg cells [220]. Furthermore, DQ786243-induced Foxp3+ Treg cell induction greatly increased its suppressive function on other CD4+ T cells such as Th1 and Th17 by decreasing the levels of IFN-γ and IL-17. In addition, overexpression of DQ786243 also greatly increased the expression of miR-146A through upregulation of Foxp3, thus inhibiting NF-kB factor activity [220]. Recently, renin (induced by the NF-kB pathway), through promoting STAT4 phosphorylation, was also found to be able to induce IL-17 production in keratinocytes of OLP patients (opening avenues for new potential therapeutic targets) [221]. The salivary concentration of IL-17 is significantly increased in patients with EOLP lesions, but not in cases of reticular OLP [80]. In contrast, another study reports that the salivary concentration of IL-17 is not significantly increased in patients with OLP and that there are no differences with erosive forms [141]. The same study reports an increase in salivary values of IL-22, but with no differences between reticular and atrophic-erosive subtypes; the authors noted the lack of correlation between the levels of IL-17 and IL-22 [141]. Several studies, on the other hand, report increased serum levels of IL-17 in OLP patients [142, 222, 223]: some of these detect differences between levels in NEOLP and EOLP cases [222], while others do not [142]. Another study reports an increase in serum values of IL-17 in the forms of EOLP but not NEOLP compared with control subjects [143]. The serum and tissue levels mean IL-17 and the mean IL-17R levels in the OLP were significantly higher than in the controls, and a statistically significant positive (direct) correlation was observed between serum IL-17 serum and both tissue levels of IL-17 and IL-17R [143]. Furthermore, in one study, the levels of IL-17 m-RNA in peripheral blood, which were higher in OLP and even higher in EOLP, were positively correlated with mi-RNA-155 levels [222]. In contrast, no correlation was found between serum levels of IL-17 and vitamin D (the latter not significantly increased in patients with OLP according to a recent study). The single nucleotide polymorphism (SNP) of the IL-17A has been associated with increased susceptibility of several systemic diseases such as carcinoma gastric [224], Crohn's disease and ulcerative recto colitis [225], juvenile systemic lupus erythematosus [226], and pulmonary tuberculosis [227], but little is still known about its role in oral diseases. A single paper evaluates this polymorphism in OLP [142]. The SNP of the IL-17A gene allele G197A (rs2275913) has been associated with increased susceptibility to the development of OLP and increased serum levels of IL-17 [142].

10. *Interleukin 18 (IL-18)*
    (a) *Characteristics*. IL-18 was originally identified as "IFN-γ induction factor" (IGIF) for its potent induction function on IFN-γ production by T cells and NK cells [228]. IL-18 is released mainly by immature macrophages and DCs during acute immune responses but also by various immune and nonimmune cells, including T and B lymphocytes, keratinocytes, adrenal cortex cells, and astrocytes [145]. IL-18 is a cytokine characterized by a pleiotropic function in inflammation and autoimmunity, which can promote the differentiation and activation of different subgroups of Th lymphocytes depending on its surrounding cytokine. In synergy with IL-12, IL-18 shows a potent ability to induce the IFN-γ production by T and NK lymphocytes and to polarize the development of Th1 lymphocytes. However, in the absence of IL-12, IL-18 instead promotes differentiation in the Th2 direction by inducing NK and T cells to produce Th2-type cytokines such as IL-4, IL-5, IL-10, and IL-13 [229]. Therefore, IL-18 constitutes a balancing factor between the Th1 and Th2 immune responses and plays a fundamental role in the modulation of immune status. IL-18 is also capable of mediating the acquired immune responses, also being involved in the recruitment of DCs to the inflammatory site and in the maturation process of myeloid DCs [229]. In addition, IL-18 can activate multiple cell populations that are themselves sources of additional IL-18 in an autocrine manner, indicating its important role in sustaining many chronic inflammatory diseases [228]. High serum levels of IL-18 have been found to be associated with disease severity and poor clinical outcomes of many inflammatory and autoimmune disorders [145].
    (b) *Role of IL-18 in the OLP*. Although the mechanisms of IL-18 activity in many other inflammatory and autoimmune disorders have been widely explored, to date, there are only a few studies concerning IL-18 in OLP [108], which may have similar effects on cytotoxicity and IFN-γ production to those of IL-12 [44]. The sources of IL-18 have not yet been defined in OLP [44]. No difference was found between OLP lesion and normal oral mucosa in the m-RNA expression of IL-18, but significant increases of IL-18 protein have been shown in both serum and saliva of affected patients [70, 146]. In addition, serum and salivary levels of IL-18 were found to be positively correlated with disease severity, indicating the importance of its values in predicting the prognosis of the disease [146]. Regarding polymorphisms, the data have shown a significant difference in IL-18 −607 genotype distributions between affected patients and controls [230]. In addition, the polymorphisms identified in the promoter region of the IL-18 gene (i.e., −137 G/G) appear to be statistically associated with the more severe erosive subtype of OLP and exert a positive effect on IL-18 protein production in the serum of affected patients, suggesting that the overproduction of IL-18 in the

patient's body might have a genetic basis which could be involved in the pathogenesis of OLP [230]. Another more recent one performed on a sample of Indian patients shows a significant increase in the mean serum levels of IL-18 in patients with OLP [147] and assesses the presence of some polymorphisms. More specifically, the genotypic and allelic frequencies of IL-18 at position −137 (G/C) have shown that the GG genotype and G allele were significantly higher in patients with OLP, while the GC genotype and C allele were high in the control group. The polymorphism of IL-18 at the −607 (C/A) position, on the other hand, showed no significant differences [147]. These results cast somewhat question those of the previous study, but the authors specify that the study lacks a clear statistical correlation, that the observed differences could be caused by problems in sampling, and that the results may not be fully representative of Indian patients with OLP [147]. Further studies are therefore needed on the role of these polymorphisms in the development of OLP but also on the sources of IL-18 production and its specific role in the pathogenesis of the disease.

11. *Interleukin 22 (IL-22)*
    (a) *Characteristics.* IL-22 is a cytokine belonging to the IL-10 superfamily that transduces signal into target cells through IL-22R1 and IL-10R2 receptors, and it is produced by Th17, Th22, NK lymphocytes, innate lymphoid cells, and various types of CD4+ and CD8+ T lymphocytes [231]. In fact, IL-22 is the characteristic cytokine of a new subgroup of CD4+ helper T lymphocytes that has been given the name Th22 [232]. Subsets are defined according to their cytokine production and their functions: most notably, these are a class of lymphocytes Th initially identified as infiltrating the epidermis of subjects with skin inflammatory disorders and producing IL-22 and TNF-α, but not IFN-γ, IL-4, or IL-17 [232]. In fact, among T helper lymphocytes, in addition to Th1, Th2, Th17, Treg (see Sect. 4.1.3), and Th22, there are also Th3, TR1, Th9, and T follicular helper (Tfh) cells, which, except for the latter category, are considered more than variants within the main categories [233]. Several studies have shown that IL-23, IL-18, and IL-6 increase the release of IL-22 [234, 235]. The regulation of IL-22 expression is mediated by several transcription factors such as RORγt (retinoid acid-related orphan receptor γt) and STAT3 (signal transducer and activator of transcription 3), and more recently it has been discovered that this is done also by the work of micro-RNAs (mi-RNAs) [236]. The known activity of IL-22, explicated through binding to its receptors, consists mainly of tissue repair and defense of the host [236]. During wound healing (including in the oral cavity), various cytokines are useful in the removal of damaged tissue and microbes [237]. Keratinocytes are the main target cells of IL-22 which could modulate, via STAT3, the expression gene in wounds involving keratinocytes by promoting the expression of collagen type I and MMP-1, which may contribute to reepithelialization and healing without any scarring. So, it is possible that IL-22 promotes keratinocyte proliferation but not fibroblasts [237]. In the intestine, the main function of IL-22 is to stimulate epithelial proliferation to support and maintain the gastrointestinal epithelial barrier [235]. In addition, Th22 lymphocytes promote barrier defense against bacterial pathogens, and thus IL-22, through stimulation of antimicrobial peptide production, plays a key role in protecting against bacterial infection at barrier sites [238, 239]. In addition, IL-22 might be involved in defense against viruses [240,

241] and *Candida albicans* [242]. However, evidence has demonstrated both protective and pathogenic properties of IL22 in autoimmune diseases, infections, and malignancy [231]. Previous studies have demonstrated the involvement of IL-22 in the development and pathogenesis of several autoimmune diseases such as systemic lupus erythematosus, rheumatoid arthritis, multiple sclerosis, Sjögren's syndrome, and psoriasis [243]. IL-22 also has a protective role in liver disease and graft-versus-host disease (GvHD) [244], an anti-apoptotic role in rheumatoid arthritis [245] and an anti-inflammatory role in asthma [246]. In addition, IL-22 induces psoriasis-like lesions in mice [247]. The activity of IL-22 is closely related to IL-23, since IL-22 is a downstream cytokine effector of IL-23 [159]. Recent studies have revealed that IL-23 is required to produce IL-22 and IL23 is also considered a key cytokine in the pathogenesis of inflammatory and autoimmune diseases [247, 248].

(b) *Role of IL-22 in the OLP*. The role of IL-22 in OLP is at an early stage of study. Increased immuno-expression of IL-22 and IL-23 was found in tissue samples from OLP patients compared with samples from healthy patients, and these expressions were higher in OLP samples than in skin LP samples [249]. The expression of IL-22 was correlated with that of IL-23 [148]. The higher values of OLP than those of cutaneous LP probably resulted from the presence of Th22 cells as an important component of oral mucosal host defense against the oral microbiota and tissue antigens [249]. Another study reports in OLP patients a correlation between high IL-22 expression and altered expression levels of some mi-RNAs (especially decreased miR-562 and increased miR-203) compared with controls, suggesting that IL-22 and its target mi-RNAs may contribute to the pathogenesis of OLP [249]. Regarding the investigation in saliva, the salivary concentration of IL-22 was significantly higher in the control group than in affected patients, but no significant difference was observed between the reticular and atrophic-erosive forms. These results suggest that the protective effect of IL-22 may be reduced in patients with OLP [141]. One study also showed elevated serum IL-22 levels in patients with OLP but not in patients with cutaneous LP [148]. Moreover, these values undergo important changes in the acute relapse and chronic phases of OLP [149]. So, IL-22 could be a diagnostic marker of OLP, and IL-22 antagonists could be potential therapeutic options [148].

12. *Interleukin 23 (IL-23)*

(a) *Characteristics*. IL-23 is secreted by various cell populations such as macrophages, keratinocytes, and activated DCs [154]. IL-23 plays a key role in the induction and maintenance of Th17 lymphocytes [250, 251], but it may not be involved in the differentiation initial differentiation of such cells [160]. In addition, IL-23 also induces the production of IL-17 by Th17 lymphocytes [75]. The IL-23/IL-17 axis is widely involved in chronic inflammatory processes in various pathological states [213]. Indeed, its involvement in the pathogenesis of several diseases has been observed in chronic inflammatory [252] and immune disorders such as rheumatoid arthritis [253], psoriasis [254], allergic contact dermatitis [255], chronic inflammatory bowel diseases [256, 257], MICI or IBD (including Crohn's disease [258] and ulcerative rectocolitis), and periodontal disease [259, 260]. It has been also observed that IL-23-deficient mice fail to resist infection by intestinal pathogens or pulmonary bacteria [261]. Furthermore, as mentioned earlier (see

"IL-22"), IL-23 is required to produce IL-22, which constitutes a downstream cytokine effector of IL-23 [159].

(b) *Role of IL-23 in the OLP*. The role of this cytokine in lichen is still under study. A strong increase in epithelial immunostaining for IL-17 and IL-23 has been observed in OLP lesions and significantly more IL-23+ lymphocytes (detection by cytoplasmic immunostaining) in erosive forms [82]. Another study also reports high immuno-expression of IL-23 and IL-17 in OLP [153]. The expressions of IL-23 and IL-17 were found to be positively correlated with lesion progression. IL-23 increases the percentage of Th17 cells and IL-17 production in CD4+ T cells from OLP patients [153]. Other authors report increased immuno-expression of IL-22 and IL-23 in OLP patients compared with samples from healthy patients, and these expressions were higher in OLP samples than in skin LP samples [249]. The expression of IL-22 was found to be correlated with that of IL-23 [249]. No significant increase in IL-23 concentrations was observed in the saliva of patients with reticular and erosive OLP compared with healthy controls [80], but another study showed that the bacterium *Porphyromonas gingivalis* can influence the salivary levels of IL-17 and IL-23 of patients with OLP [155]. Nor do serum levels of IL-23 increase in affected patients compared with controls [161]. However, further studies are needed to better understand the functioning and alterations of this cytokine in OLP.

13. *Tumor Necrosis Factor-alpha (TNF-α)*

(a) *Characteristics*. Tumor necrosis factor-alpha (TNF-α) is produced primarily by activated macrophages and T lymphocytes but also by a wide range of cell populations including immune cells (B lymphocytes, DCs, NK cells, and neutrophils), nonimmune cells (keratinocytes, fibroblasts, astrocytes, and glial cells), and various tumor cells [262]. TNF-α is undetectable in healthy subjects but is rapidly released following trauma, infection, or exposure to pathogenic stimuli and becomes one of the most abundant early mediators in the inflamed tissue [263]. It constitutes a key regulator of innate immunity and almost always augments that type of response. Indeed, it plays an important role in the maturation of DCs and can activate the migration and phagocytosis of macrophages, which in turn are both major producers of TNF-α [262, 263]. Such a positive feedback loop may be important in the maintenance of innate immune responses [108]. TNF-α also assumes an important role in acquired immunity. The effects of TNF-α on T lymphocytes depend on the timing of exposure [264]. Short-term stimulation of TNF-α causes proliferation and activation of T cells. In contrast, long-term exposure induces reversible loss of the surface TCR complex, leading to hypo-responsiveness of T cells, without affecting their IL-2-mediated proliferation [264]. TNF-α is an amplifier of the Th1 response by stimulating the production of IL-12 and IL-18, which are potent inducers of IFN-γ [265]. In addition, TNF-α promotes the growth and activities of B lymphocytes and induces the production of IL-1 and IL-6. Conversely, B lymphocytes can produce TNF-α within an autocrine cycle [264]. In addition, TNF-α appears to be a potent modulator of cell apoptosis through binding to TNFR1 expressed in various cell types, a TNFR receptor-associated death domain (DD). This function occurs not only during normal development but also under pathological conditions characterized by increased TNF-α production [265].

(b) *Role of TNF-α in OLP*. TNF-α is the cytokine most studied by researchers in OLP. TNF-α is overproduced in OLP lesions compared with healthy mucosa

[162, 266–268]. The elevated expression of TNF-α in OLP lesions is inhibited after topical application of 0.1% of fluocinolone acetonide in orabase, suggesting that overexpression of this cytokine is linked to the immunopathogenesis of OLP [162]. Several cells, such as keratinocytes, mast cells, and CD4+T lymphocytes, have been identified as hyperactive sources in the production of TNF-α in OLP lesions [87, 127, 156, 162, 252, 268, 269]. Compared with the keratinocytes of healthy and chronically inflamed gingiva, those of OLP lesions produce much more TNF-α [127, 156]. Similarly, the CD4+ T lymphocytes infiltrates produce much more TNF-α in OLP lesions than their counterparts from healthy oral mucosa [70, 127, 156]. In OLP, degranulated mast cells are also characterized by overproduction of this cytokine [13]. All this confirms the role of TNF-α in the local inflammatory environment [108]. Indeed, in OLP lesions, TNFR expression is observed from mononuclear cells and from epithelial keratinocytes [87, 266]. It has long been known that in OLP, the stimulation of TNF-α on cell populations induces the production of various inflammatory mediators such as RANTES, MMP-9, and further TNF-α itself [13, 87]. Some authors have proposed the hypothesis that TNF-α, present also in basal epithelial cell apoptosis and LC activation mechanisms, are typically present as hallmarks of OLP lesions, but further studies are needed to confirm these mechanisms [6, 168]. Many authors have consistently observed increased levels of salivary TNF-α in patients with OLP [111, 128, 133, 163, 270, 271], and it appears that the increase in these values correlates with disease severity [270], so salivary TNF-α analysis may be a useful diagnostic tool and a potential prognostic marker in OLP. In addition, elevated salivary levels of TNF-α decreased to normal values after glucocorticoid treatment such as prednisone and dexamethasone, suggesting that the salivary TNF-α level may be useful in monitoring the activity of the disease and the effectiveness of therapy [128, 256]. Most studies have consistently also observed elevated serum levels of TNF-α in patients with OLP by using mean method ELISA [68, 267, 272–275]. However, it does not appear that serum levels correlate with the degree of oral mucosal involvement [276]. According to a survey by Pekiner et al. [159], using a measurement method other than ELISA, there were no statistically significant differences in serum TNF-α levels between patients with OLP and controls. This indicates that the different method of detection may influence the results [108]. It has been observed that elevated serum levels of TNF-α can decrease to a normal level after treatment with levamisole in patients with EOLP [275], suggesting that the serum level of this cytokine, like its salivary counterpart, may have value in assessing therapeutic efficiency [108]. The elevation of serum levels of TNF-α, a decreased expression of it was observed in patients with OLP in PBMCs which exhibited an inhibitory state, suggesting an impaired lymphocyte function in patients [277]. Finally, a recent meta-analysis that studied the results of different studies on serum and salivary levels of TNF-α concludes that salivary levels of this cytokine are more useful than serum levels for diagnostic and therapeutic purposes [278]. Regarding studies on the genetic polymorphisms of the TNF-α gene, a biallelic SNP at the −308 locus has been reported at the promoter, which is associated with elevated levels of TNF-α and therefore increased susceptibility to a wide variety of human diseases [164]. So many studies have evaluated the association between the −308 (G/A) polymorphism in the TNF-α gene and susceptibility to OLP, but the results are mixed [108]. Although most authors have found higher frequencies of the A allele (G/A or A/A genotype) of the TNF-α −308 polymorphism in patients with OLP, other authors, on the other hand, have found no differences in allele and genotype frequencies of TNF-α between patients with OLP and healthy controls [112, 113, 169, 279–281]. A meta-analysis on this topic showed no association between this polymorphism and lichen risk in the combined analyses [281]. In addition, in subgroup analysis by subtypes for CLP (cutaneous lichen planus) and OLP, ethnicity, and HCV infection, the authors found no significant risk connections from the CLP or OLP groups for the AA+GA vs. GG comparison but found significantly increased risks of OLP among the population with mixed ethnicity and among patients without HCV infection. However, the authors stated that the negative results could have been biased due to the lack of some information on HCV status and clinical variety in some previous studies and suggested that further studies are needed to validate these associations [281]. A recent meta-analysis [282] on the subject found a subgroup analysis by ethnicity, a significantly positive association of TNF-α −308 (G/A) polymorphism in patients with OLP of mixed ethnicity, but not in Asians and Caucasians (for AA+GA vs. GG comparison). These results indicate that carriers of A alleles (AA + AG) have a significantly higher risk of OLP in the mixed ethnic population, but not in Asians and Caucasians. Regarding subgroup analysis based on HCV infection status, a significantly increased risk of OLP was found among patients with mixed HCV infection status (study population with or without HCV infection or HCV information not mentioned), but not in patients without HCV infection and patients with HCV infection. HCV infection also induces increased TNF-α production and thus may be a confounding factor in studies of association between OLP risk and cytokine gene polymorphisms, indicating the need for future studies to investigate the HCV status of patients with OLP [282]. The results of this recent meta-analysis suggest that the substitution of G into A of the TNF-α −308 (G/A) polymorphism is a risk factor for the development of OLP. Its effect is mainly detected among mixed populations with mixed HCV status. This polymorphism may be a useful genomic marker for OLP [282]. Although TNF-α antagonists (anti-TNF-α) have been approved therapies in some immune-mediated inflammatory diseases for many years, their off-label use in inflammatory diseases of the oral mucosa is only beginning [170]. Several case reports have shown beneficial effects of anti-TNF-α use in patients with OLP refractory to glucocorticoids and immunosuppressants [283, 284]. For example, a case of a successful treatment with etanercept in a patient with severe EOLP, with infliximab in another case with severe orogenital OLP, and with adalimumab in two other cases with severe orogenital OLP has been reported: this shows the real feasibility of the clinical use of anti-TNF-α in the treatment of OLP [171, 283]. However, these drugs may have important side effects such as headache, inducing a lichenoid reaction, lupus-like syndrome (SLE, systemic lupus erythematosus), promoting viral infections, and the risk of carcinogenesis. These potentially adverse events may be a barrier to future application of anti-TNF-α and should always be noted in clinical use [171].

14. *Interferon gamma (IFN-γ)*
    (a) *Characteristics*. Interferon-γ (IFN-γ) is the only type II interferon (whereas IFN-α and IFN-β are type I IFNs) and is

the specific cytokine of Th1 profile. Initially, it was thought that IFN-γ was produced exclusively by CD4+ T lymphocytes and CD8+ and NK cells, but later tests have shown that B lymphocytes and APC cells can also produce it. IFN-γ is produced by these cells only when activated by other cytokines, particularly IL-2, IL-12, and IL-18. At contrary, its production is inhibited by the action of IL-4, IL-10, TGF-β, glucocorticoids, and cyclosporine A [285]. IFN-γ is one of the most critical mediators of immunity and inflammation, e.g., in promoting innate immune responses through the activation of macrophages [286]. IFN-γ also regulates various proinflammatory mediators by disrupting various anti-inflammatory feedback loops. Other important mechanisms of innate immune response mediated by IFN-γ are provided by its direct inhibition of downstream expression and signaling pathways of anti-inflammatory molecules [286]. As the main effector cytokine of Th1 profile, IFN-γ autoamplifies Th1 responses by activating NK cells and macrophages and promoting specific cytotoxic immunity through the interaction between T lymphocytes and APCs [287]. In addition, IFN-γ inhibits the differentiations and functions of Th2 and Th17 lymphocytes [288, 289] and through these mechanisms promotes the maintenance of the Th1 phenotype. In addition, IFN-γ exerts functions to limit tissue damage at the site of inflammation and to inhibit the proliferation of various cell types [286]. The literature has revealed both the promoting and suppressing roles of IFN-γ in various inflammatory and autoimmune diseases [286, 290].

(b) *Role of IFN-γ in OLP*. As mentioned above, in OLP inflammation, there is believed to be a predominant Th1 profile [4, 87, 121], and IFN-γ is one of the most studied cytokines in this pathology. In early studies, positive staining of both m-RNA and IFN-γ proteins was observed in mononuclear cells throughout the subepithelial infiltrate in OLP lesions [87, 291]. Recently, in OLP lesions, IFN-γ expression has also been localized to CD4+ T lymphocytes [81]. Some studies have also shown high levels of IFN-γ expression in EOLP lesions, but not in reticular lesions, compared with healthy oral mucosa [70, 140]. It has also been hypothesized that IFN-γ overexpression may be involved in the activation of CD8+ T lymphocytes and may maintain MHC expression on oral keratinocytes in advanced stages of OLP development [4]. In addition, the number of IFN-γ-positive mononuclear cells in OLP lesions is decreased after 1 month of treatment with 0.1% fluocinolone acetonide, indicating an association between IFN-γ expression and the clinical manifestation of OLP lesions [292]. The data on salivary IFN-γ levels in OLP patients are inconsistent. Liu et al. [165] observed a significantly lower level of salivary IFN-γ in patients with OLP. In contrast, Tao et al. reported that these values were significantly higher in patients with ulcerative-erosive OLP compared with patients with reticular form and the control group [140]. In addition, Ghallab et al. [271] found an elevated salivary IFN-γ level in patients with EOLP, which could be significantly reduced after treatment with prednisone. The reason for these differences in results is still unclear. Furthermore, although there is an increase in IFN-γ levels in the local lesion of OLP, its production is found to be suppressed in PBMCs of patients with OLP [108]. In fact, numerous studies have consistently found reduced IFN-γ production in PBMCs of OLP patients compared with those of healthy donors or compared with those subjected to other stimuli such as IL-2, or purified protein derivatives [118, 123, 190, 277]. These data indicated that peripheral cellular immunosuppression may be a hallmark of OLP [108]. Data on serum IFN-γ levels are also inconsistent. Hu et al. [117] reported an increase in the serum level of IFN-γ in patients with OLP, but other researchers have found no statistical differences in serum IFN-γ levels between patients with OLP and controls [119, 172]. The discrepancy in these results may be because of some other sources of IFN-γ production in peripheral blood (except for PBMCs), but further studies are still needed [108]. One study reports a profile of high expression of salivary and serum levels of IL-10 and poor expression of IFN-γ levels and consequently a decrease in the IFN-γ/IL-10 ratio in both fluids of patients with OLP, compared with healthy controls [167]. A recent meta-analysis found that the serum IFN-γ/IL-4 ratio and salivary may not play a major role in the development and severity of OLP [59]. Another recent meta-analysis by the same study group (including 11 papers from the literature) finally found that there were no statistically significant differences in serum and salivary levels of IFN-γ between the OLP group and the control group and between the EOLP and NEOLP groups at the salivary levels; therefore, this cytokine, according to the authors, might not be considered important in the pathogenesis or severity of OLP [166]. About genetic studies, several works have evaluated the influence of IFN-γ genetic polymorphism on OLP susceptibility. Polymorphisms within regulatory sequences or introns can have a significant effect on the transcription as they usually result in an alteration of the promoter region, changing accordingly the structure of the transcription binding site or the structure of enhancers and silencers within introns [293]. To date, two possible polymorphisms have been found in the first intron of the IFN-γ gene promoter, genotype UTR 5644 (T/T) [113, 169], and genotype +874 (T/T) [122, 173, 294], but not all results agree in the latter polymorphism. Carrozzo et al. [113] report a significant increase in the number of homozygotes (T/T) of the IFN-γ UTR 5644 genotype in patients with OLP compared with healthy controls. The same study group also reports an increase (close to statistical significance) in the number of heterozygotes (A/T) in OLP-HCV+ patients compared with those with OLP but HCV-380. Two studies report the involvement of genotype +874 (T/T) (rs2430561), that is, an increased risk of developing OLP compared with subjects with the A allele (AA or AT genotype) [122, 294], but a more recent study [173] does not detect a statistically significant between patients with OLP and healthy subjects, although the T allele is prevalent in affected individuals.

15. *Transforming growth factor-beta (TGF-β)*
    (a) *Characteristics*. There are three highly homologous isoforms of TGF-β in humans, TGF-β1, TGF-β2, and TGF-β3, which share a receptor complex and signaling pathways but are expressed differently in different tissues [174]. Initially, all TGF-β ligands are synthesized as inactive precursors. After dimerization, TGF-β precursors are cleaved by proteases and interact with LAPs (latency-associated peptides) to form SLCs (small latent complexes). These are subsequently transported into the extracellular matrix and further bind to LTBPs (latent TGF-β-binding proteins) forming LLCs (large latent complexes). Release of active, signal-inducing TGF-β occurs through proteolysis of LAPs and LTBPs [295, 296]. The most potent functions of TGF-β consist of growth inhibition and induction of apoptosis in many cell types, including epithelial, endothelial, fibroblastic,

hematopoietic, and immune cells [295, 296]. TGF-β also has a marked effect on extracellular matrix composition, angiogenesis, and induction of epithelial-mesenchymal transition, so it is probably responsible for many physiological and pathological features in the mesenchyme [174, 295].TGF-β exerts suppressive function on the immune system and has wide effects on most immune cells [108]. Regarding acquired immunity, TGF-β can repress the proliferation of T lymphocytes and induce apoptosis of B cells, to suppress immune responses. In addition, TGF-β can suppress the differentiation of Th1 and Th2 lymphocytes and instead promote the development of Treg, which are crucial for the maintenance of immune tolerance. Regarding immunity innate, TGF-β can repress IFN-γ production by NK cells and polarize the macrophage pro-inflammatory type (M1) toward the anti-inflammatory type (M2) phenotype [295].

(b) *Role of TGF-β in OLP*. Although m-RNA expression of TGF-β1 was identified in all OLP biopsies studied, TGF-β1 immunostaining was variable in the subepithelial infiltrate of OLP lesions [62, 87, 297]. In vitro, TGF-β1 secretion was not detected in any T-cell lineage from OLP [62]. In the erythematous lesions of OLP, overexpression of Smad7 (an inhibitor of TGF-β signaling) was also detected, along with reduced expressions of phosphorylated Smad2/3 (pSmad2/3) and Smad4, which are activators of TGF-β signaling. This suggests that the immunosuppressive function of TGF-β is inhibited in the lymphocytic infiltration of OLP lesions, which may contribute to chronic inflammation [174]. The inhibition of TGF-β in OLP T lymphocytes may be partly attributed to the excessive productions of IFN-γ, which block the phosphorylation of Smad3 [174]. Therefore, the balance between the function of TGF-β and IFN-γ may be crucial in the immunological activities of lesions by OLP and could represent a therapeutic target [298]. Several studies have found that the TGF-β1 expressions were significantly elevated in cases of OLP lesions gone through neoplastic transformation [43, 299]. In fact, it is known that TGF-β probably inhibits growth in the early stages but promotes it in the later stages of carcinogenesis and acts as an inducer of the epithelial-mesenchymal transition, a significant step in malignant transformation [296]. Therefore, TGF-β may play an important role in OLP carcinogenesis, but the underlying mechanisms remain unclear [108]. Studies on serum TGF-β levels in patients with OLP report conflicting results. Zhou et al. [272] observed a slight increase in serum TGF-β1 levels in OLP patients, while Taghavi Zenouz et al. [300] reported a significant reduction in serum TGF-β levels in affected patients. Furthermore, in a study on genetic polymorphisms in OLP, no significant differences were observed in the frequencies of allelic or genotypic TGF-β between subjects with OLP and healthy controls [113].

16. *Other cytokines*
    (a) Other cytokines have also been studied in OLP.
    (b) *IL-15*. One study shows in patients with OLP an increase in serum levels of IL-15 and the percentage of Treg lymphocytes (CD4+, CD25+, Foxp3+) compared with healthy controls but without differences among the clinical subtypes of the disease. In addition, the authors observed a positive correlation between the percentage of Treg lymphocytes and IL-15 levels; thus the high serum expression of Treg cells and IL-15 may be responsible for the pathogenesis of OLP [175].
    (c) *IL-16*. Significantly increased serum levels of RANTES and IL-16 have been observed in OLP patients compared with

healthy subjects, and a positive correlation has been reported between the levels of RANTES, IL-16, and clinical severity; thus the levels of RANTES and IL-16 may be useful biomarkers for the severity of OLP [55].

(d) *IL-21*. Recently, the role of follicular T helper (Tfh) cells in several autoimmune diseases has been highlighted for their pivotal regulation on humoral immunity. One study evaluated the expression of circulating Tfh-like cells and its correlations with IL-21 and B cells in OLP. This study showed a significant increase in circulating Tfh-like cells and B cells, as well as a reduction in serum IL-21 expression in OLP. An increase of circulating Tfh-like cells may be involved in the pathogenesis of OLP through abnormal modulation on B-cell proliferation and IL-21 production and may be associated with different clinical forms of OLP [301].

(e) *IL-25*. The m-RNA levels of IL-25 and IL-4 were elevated and significantly correlated with each other in specific subtypes of OLP lesions compared with controls, and the number of IL-25+ cells was locally increased in local OLP lesions. It is possible that increased levels of IL-4, IL-8, and CCL20 in the oral keratinocytes are induced by IL-25 but not IL-17. IL-25 may mediate the Th2 response in the reticular subtype of OLP and be related to disease severity [302].

(f) *IL-27*. One study reports in patients with OLP an increase and positive correlation of serum levels of IL-12 and IL-27, while no correlation of these values with clinical features of OLP was found. So, it is possible that the high expressions of IL-12 and IL-27 are synergized and promote the development of the inflammatory process in OLP [138].

(g) *IL-33 and IL-35*. IL-33 appears to be the Th2 profile counterpart of IL-18 (instead of considering a Th1 cytokine of the IL-1 family) [228] and functions as an alarmin released after cell necrosis to alert the immune system of tissue damage or stress [303]. IL-35, a member of the IL-12 cytokine family, is produced by Treg lymphocytes and suppresses the immune response. A recent study showed positive immunostaining of IL-33 and IL-35 in OLP, and significantly more IL-33+ cells were observed in the deeper connective tissue region than at the epithelial-connective tissue interface [303]. In addition, all IL-35+ cells showed ovoid/plasmacytoid morphology. Gene expression experiments showed significantly higher expression of EBI3 (a dimeric IL-35 chain) in OLP compared with non-specific inflammatory controls. IL-33 gene expression was not, on the other hand, different between the groups. However, within OLP tissues, the expression of IL-33 was significantly higher than EBI3. These data demonstrate the expression of IL-33 and IL-35 in OLP [303]. Another recent study reports increased expression of IFN-γ and IL-33 in the OLP lesions compared with non-specific inflammatory lesions (NSILs), and these lesions differed in oral microbiota composition as well [304].

(h) *TNF-β*. In the TNF-β (+252A/G) polymorphism (rs909253) within the first intron of the TNF-β gene, the presence of G (guanine) at this position defines the mutated allele known as TNF-β1 (allele-1), which is a less frequent allele and associated with higher production of TNF-α and TNF-β [305]. One study showed that the frequency of the GA genotype of TNF-β (+252 A/G) was significantly higher in OLP patients than in controls, while the AA genotype was completely absent in affected patients. This polymorphism could therefore be significantly associated with the risk of susceptibility to OLP; however, further studies using a larger sample size are needed to confirm this association [158].

The roles of the main cytokines involved in OLP have been summarized in Table 4.3.

4.3.2 Chemokine

Chemokines constitute a group of cytokines that exert a recall action toward cells other than those that produced them: they thus play an important role in the phenomenon known as "chemotaxis," which in physiology allows, for example, the landing of lymphocytes in secondary lymphoid organs, while in pathology it allows the fixation of leukocytes on the endothelial wall, their subsequent extravasation, and their influx in each direction. Some chemokines exert other effects on target cells besides the chemotactic one. Chemokines are distinguished into four families, depending on the position of the cysteine pairs (two pairs joined by bridges disulfide for each molecule):

- *First* family: each of the two cysteine pairs is separated by only one amino acid, and they are called CXC chemokines and are active on neutrophils, andT and B lymphocytes.
- *Second* family: the two cysteines of each pair are contiguous with each other, and they are therefore called CC chemokines and are active on PBMCs (monocytes, NK cells, and lymphocytes).
- *Third* family: there is only one cysteine pair in the molecule, and it includes only the lymphotactin, referred to as chemokine C, which is active only on T lymphocytes and NK cells.
- *Fourth* family: it is characterized by a single cysteine pair in which the two cysteines are separated by three amino acids, including only fractalkine, termed CX3C, also active on lymphocytes T cells and NK cells.

In the nomenclature, an L is added after the second C, possibly followed by a progressive numbering [40].

Recent evidence has shown the role of chemokines in various autoimmune diseases such as rheumatoid arthritis and multiple sclerosis [306]. RANTES (Regulated on Activation, Normal T cells Expressed and Secreted) or CCL5 is a member of the CC chemokine family produced by various cells, including activated T lymphocytes, which plays a critical role in the recruitment of various inflammatory cells and especially lymphocytes and mast cells in OLP [307]. Its main receptor is CCR5 [3], but other surface receptors for RANTES have also been identified in OLP, such as CCR1, CCR3, CCR4, CCR9, and CCR10 [4, 13]. These chemokines are associated with increased mast cell density in OLP and LP skin lesions [3]. RANTES is secreted by activated T lymphocytes, keratinocytes, and numerous other cells [14]. Its effect causes recruitment and degranulation of mast cells that in turn release TNF-α and chymase which further upregulate RANTES secretion by T cells, thus establishing a vicious cycle responsible for the chronic course of the disease [13].

Unlike myeloid DCs and mast cells, NK cells and plasmacytoid DCs are not normal residents of the oral mucosa. Depending on the condition, myeloid DCs differentially express Th1-recruiting chemokines such as CXCL9, CXCL10, and CXCL1 or Th2-recruiting chemokines [308]. In OLP lesions and peripheral blood, CXCL9, CXCL10, and other different chemokines associated with inflammation were indeed identical [117]. It was also found that in OLP, CD8+ T lymphocytes express CXCR3 and CCR5 receptors and produce their own CXCL10, probably leading to self-reclosure [309]. In the vast majority of OLP cases analyzed in one study, NK cells, unlike T lymphocytes, expressed ChemR23, a chemotactic (chemotactic-acting) chemerin receptor produced by mucosal vessel endothelial cells [45]. In OLP lesions, overall, chemokines and chemokine receptors are consistent with a Th1 immune response [44].

4.3.3 Matrix Metalloprotease (MMP)

MMPs constitute a family of zinc-dependent proteases of at least 20 members involved in cell migration, angiogenesis, and proteolytic activation of growth factors, events necessary for normal tissue repair, as well as in wound healing and invasion tumor [310]. Their action consists in the degradation of extracellular matrix proteins by allowing cells to pass through them: a process that allows, for example, leukocytes to invade tissues in inflammatory processes but also occurs in carcinomas with marked metastatic spread [3]. Their function is regulated in part by tissue inhibitors of metalloproteinases (TIMPs), of which the best known are TIMP-1, TIMP-2, and TIMP-3. The MMP/TIMP imbalance is associated with tissue destruction, as seen in some diseases such as cancer, arthritis, and cardiovascular diseases [311, 312]. MMPs from T lymphocytes promote the movement of these cells into extravascular tissues and their migration across the basement [4]. The possible role of MMPs and TIMPs in the genesis and maintenance of OLP has been studied. High concentrations of MMP-9 and TIMP-1. MMP-9, together with its activators released by T lymphocytes, cleaves fibers' type IV collagen resulting in degeneration of the basement membrane, thus facilitating the intraepithelial degradation of T cells [7, 13]. Sutinen et al. [313] observed low expression of MMP-1, limited to fibroblasts of the subepithelial region, while MMP-2 was not detected in the ten samples studied. Zhou et al. found that MMP-2 and MMP-3 were mainly expressed in the epithelial region, while MMP-9 was identified in the infiltrate subepithelial inflammatory layer. In another study, has been observed an increased expression of MMP-2 and MMP-7 in the epithelium and connective tissues of OLP lesions compared with healthy oral mucosa [314]. Furthermore, in the affected patient group, the MMP-2/TIMP-1 and MMP-7/TIMP-1 ratios were greater than in the control group. These results confirm that an increase in the expression of MMPs and imbalance between MMPs and TIMPs plays a role in the pathogenesis of OLP. In addition, there were significant differences found in the expression levels of MMPs in different variant clinical OLPs; in particular, it was seen that MMP-1, MMP-2, MMP-3, and MMP-4 appear to be more associated with the development of erosive lesions [299, 315].

4.3.4 Role of OLP Immunopathogenesis in Response to Therapy

The immunopathogenesis of OLP can influence the response to treatment, which basically consists of immunosuppression. The most widely used class of drugs are topical corticosteroids or systems whose efficacy is related to inhibition of DC and T-cell activity, Th1 cytokine secretion [316, 317], and stimulation of the Th2 cytokine IL-10, which also acts by interfering with Th1 cytokine activity [318]. However, provided the diagnosis of OLP is accurate and no other complicating conditions are present, some patients with OLP may be resistant to steroids [44]. This phenomenon can also occur in other non-infectious inflammatory conditions such as in OICs, rheumatoid arthritis, asthma, etc. [316, 319]. Steroid resistance has a genetic basis, related, in part, by the wide variation in the sensitivity of lymphocytes to these drugs even in healthy subjects [319–321]. Because functional genetic polymorphisms influence the production of inflammatory mediators responsible for disease severity, the presence of additional polymorphisms may alter the response to corticosteroid treatment and thus affect treatment options [44]. For example, it is known that a specific polymorphism in the regulatory sequence of the TNF-α gene can induce steroid resistance in several systemic inflammatory disorders. In these cases, the therapeutic choice should aim at the use of other molecules that act by a different mechanism of action, such as calcineurin inhibitors, which are often useful because they directly target T lymphocyte activation and proliferation [44]. In more complex cases, it is possible to consider treatment with biologic drugs (e.g., anti-TNF-α), which can target individual cytokines or their receptors [170], but the possibilities of using these drugs are still being evaluated. This confirms what physician Armand Trousseau said several years ago, "There are no diseases. There are only sick people."

4.4 Other Factors Involved in the Pathogenesis of OLP

Recent studies are increasingly highlighting the complexity of the immunopathogenesis of OLP and how it involves a wide variety of immunological modulators.

4.4.1 Micro-RNA (mi-RNA or miR)

Micro-RNAs (mi-RNAs or miRs) represent a class of small endogenous single-stranded non-coding RNA molecules which are 17–24 nt (nucleotides) long [322, 323]. They are molecules widely present in the body and involved in the regulation of many biological functions [324].

MiRs can repress protein expression at the post-transcriptional level through imperfect coupling of nitrogenous bases with the 3′UTR (untranslated region, 3′ end) region of the target m-RNA, leading to the reduction of its translation and/or its degradation [325]. Currently, about 1000 human miRs have been identified and are believed to regulate the expression of as many as 30% of human genes [322]. MiRs are implicated in the modulation of many biological functions such as regulation of cell growth and cycle, differentiation, apoptosis, and immunity [322, 326].

Studies have shown that altered expression of miRs is closely associated with inflammatory and autoimmune diseases [327, 328]. For example, the expression of miR-155 is found to be significantly increased in patients with rheumatoid arthritis, and its levels have been closely associated with disease activity [329]. It has also been shown that miR-29 can modulate innate and acquired responses to intracellular bacterial infection by acting on IFN-γ [323]. In addition, miR-155 can inhibit IFN-γ signaling in CD4+ T lymphocytes [330].

Recently, several authors are investigating the function of these molecules in OLP. A microarray analysis of mi-RNAs performed on patients with OLP and healthy subjects showed substantial changes (with a more than twofold difference) in the expression of about 70 mi-RNAs [331]. A follow-up study found significant alterations in the expression of nine mi-RNAs (miR-21, 26b, 121, 137, 146a, 155, 203, 375, and 4484) in patients with OLP [332]. It was observed that the expression of miR-155 in PBMCs and plasma of patients with OLP was higher than in healthy controls; furthermore, the plasma concentrations of miR-155 and miR-146a were significantly higher in patients with EOLP than in those with NEOLP, while there was no difference in the expression of the two molecules in PBMCs between these two groups [332]. Increased expression of miR-155 and miR-146a, analyzed by real-time polymerase chain reaction (RT-PCR), was also observed in OLP lesions [333]. All these data suggest the involvement of mi-RNA/m-RNA interaction in the pathogenesis of OLP. A recent study shows increased serum m-RNA levels of IL-17 and miR-155 in OLP patients compared with healthy controls, and these values were higher in patients with EOLP than in NEOLP, so these indices could be used as potential biomarkers to predict the degree of injury [222]. Since miRs are known to regulate inflammation-related cytokine expression, recently some researchers have reviewed in the literature the role of miRs involved in the regulation of several primary cytokines in OLP (IL-10, IL-17, IL-22, IFN-γ, and TNF-α) [334]. Another study also evaluated the influence of certain mi-RNAs on the production of TLRs (Toll-like receptors) and eNOS (endothelial nitric oxide synthase) [322]. Indeed, it has been shown that the activation of DCs by TLR3 and TLR4 can lead to the production of various cytokines that eventually trigger different Th1 and Th2 reactions, respectively [323]. eNOS and their catalytic product, NO (nitric oxide), have been shown to be able to suppress inflammatory reactions by maintaining a balance between the Th1 and Th2 profiles [335]. Instead TLR2 would be able to promote inflammatory reactions by inducing a Th1/Th2 imbalance [336, 337], and it is known that this imbalance may participate in the pathogenesis of OLP [110]. This study therefore detected in PBMCs of OLP patients an altered expression profile of miR-155 and miR-19a which, in turn, directly affected the production of eNOS and TLR2, respectively [335]. The simultaneous alteration of miR-155/eNOS and miR-19a/TLR2 is thus able to synergistically induce Th1/Th2 imbalance and is responsible for an elevated risk of OLP [335].

All these new aspects that are emerging may allow for new alternatives to cytokine therapies (which while effective increase the risk of infection and cancer); in fact, mi-RNAs can disrupt several immune-inflammatory pathological pathways by directly or indirectly targeting cytokines [334]. Several mi-RNA-related therapies are currently under investigation. The functions of the main mi-RNAs involved in OLP are summarized in Table 4.4.

4.4.2 Vitamin D (VIT.D)

Vitamin D is a fat-soluble vitamin. From a biochemical point of view, it is possible to distinguish between vitamin D2 or ergocalciferol (from plant sources) and vitamin D3 or cholecalciferol [338]. Vitamin D3 (vitamin D or vit.D) can be obtained from the diet (i.e., from animal sources such as deep-sea fatty fish, egg yolks, or liver) or from supplements [338]. In addition, vit.D is synthesized ex novo in the skin by the action of UVB rays from sunlight, which promote the formation of 7-dehydrocholesterol from lanolin [339]. The effectiveness of this mechanism depends on multiple factors such as sunlight exposure time, air pollution, clothing, and skin pigmentation. It is estimated that about one billion people have vitamin D deficiency or insufficiency worldwide [339]. Vit.D from the skin (7-dehydrocholesterol) and from the diet is metabolized in the liver into 25-hydroxyvitamin D (or 25-hydroxycholecalciferol or calcidiol) [25(OH)

Table 4.4 Main mi-RNAs involved in OLP

mi-RNA	Target	Main functions	Role in the OLP	Alterations
miR-146a	(TNF-α), (IL-17)	↓ transcription of TNF-α in T lymph. lymph; ↑proinflamm. genes via NF-kB; ↑inflamm. persistence in psoriasis, role in periodontitis	–	↑ (EOLP serum)
miR-155	(IFN-γ), (IL-17), (TNF-α), eNOS	Role in unstable angina; autoimm. inflammation; vasc. inflammation; ↓ NF-kB in lymph. T lymph; prolif. regulation; modulation of Treg and Th17	↑ m-RNA of IL-17 (↑↑ in EOLP), ↑eNOS	↑ (PBMC and serum), ↑↑ (serum in EOLP
miR-21	TNF-α, (TNF-α), (IL-10), (IL-17)	Anti-apopt. effect; ↓ vascular damage by ox-LDL; ↓ via NF-kB-TNFα; ↓antimicr. rep. by TLR2/1; balancem. activ. imm./toller. imm.	–	↑(lesion)
miR-19a	TLR2	–	↑ TLR2	↑ (PBMC)
miR-203	TNF-α, (TNF-α)	Anti-inflamm. effect; cytokine signaling and imm. resp. in neopl.	–	↑(lesion)
miR-121	–	–	–	↓ (lesion)
miR-26b	–	–	–	↓ (lesion)
miR-375	(TNF-α)	Diff. adipoc. promotion, ↑ TNF-α-induced apoptosis in lingual OSCC.	–	↓ (lesion)
miR-4484	–	–	–	↑(lesion)
miR-137	–	–	–	↑(lesion)

Taken and modified from Ma et al. [334]

In the "Target" column, the cytokine/factor in brackets indicates an indirect effect, outside the brackets a direct effect by the miR. For further details, please refer to the cited study. ↑ stimulation/increase, ↓ inhibition/decrease, – not specified

D] [340], which in turn is metabolized in the kidneys by the enzyme 25-hydroxyvitamin D-1α-hydroxylase (CYP27B1) into its active form, 1,25-hydroxyvitaminD (or 1,25-dihydroxycholecalciferol or calcitriol) [1,25-$(OH)_2$D] [328, 339], which exerts a wide range of biological activities by entering the target cell and binding to the vitamin D receptor (VDR) [341]. Renal production of 1,25-dihydroxyvitamin D is tightly regulated by plasma levels of parathormone and serum levels of calcium and phosphorus [339]. VDR is a member of the nuclear hormone receptor superfamily, including receptors for steroid, thyroid, and retinoic acid hormones. VDR functions as a heterodimer bound generally with the retinoid X receptor (RXR) for regulation of the target genes of vitamin D. These heterodimer complexes interact with specific DNA sequences, the vitamin D-responsive elements (VDREs), generally within the promoter of target genes, resulting in activation or repression of gene transcription [21]. Vitamin D acts mainly on the duodenum (increasing calcium absorption) and on bone tissues, modulating the activity of osteoblasts and osteoclasts to mobilize calcium [338]. It has been shown that the signaling induced by the vit.D/VDR interaction regulates numerous pathological activities, including the immune reaction, inflammatory response, and cell apoptosis [152]. The presence of VDR in various immune cells, such as APCs and B and T lymphocytes, [342], has shown that vitamin D is able to modulate innate and acquired immune responses [343]. Its action is to inhibit the differentiation and maturation of DCs, consequently leading to the inhibition of T lymphocyte-dependent activation [344].

It has been confirmed that vit.D/VDR interaction-induced signaling possesses regulatory functions in inflammatory diseases [340] and that vit.D has potential therapeutic benefit in autoimmune diseases, psoriasis, and neoplasms [345]. Vit.D deficiency is closely related to an increased risk of several autoimmune diseases such as systemic lupus erythematosus, rheumatoid arthritis, multiple sclerosis, MICIs, type I diabetes mellitus, Hashimoto's thyroiditis, Graves' disease, and autoimmune gastritis and also OLP [346, 347]. Vitamin D deficiency also has an influence in the pathogenesis of autoimmune mucocutaneous vesiculo-bullous diseases [348, 349]. For example, a low serum concentration of the vitamin has been observed in patients with pemphigus vulgaris [350]. Vit.D also influences periodontal health status [351, 352]; in fact a lowering of its serum levels is associated with an increase in gingival inflammation [353]. An inverse relationship between loss of periodontal attachment and serum levels of vit.D has also been observed, regardless of the presence of aggravating factors such as smoking or diabetes [354]. Vit.D may increase the production of antimicrobial peptides in gingival epithelial cells that are invaded by bacteria and may regulate the production of pro-inflammatory cytokines by gingival oral keratinocytes and infected periodontal ligament cells [355, 356]. A recent study [357] evaluated the role of vit.D on the development of adherens junctions (E-cadherin-dependent) of oral keratinocytes which form the first line of defense as a barrier epithelial against the attack of microorganisms [358]. The authors have shown the inhibitory action of TNF-α on the development of adherens junctions in gingival keratinocytes [357], and the dissociation of these junctions by TNF-α has been accompanied by an upregulation of MMP-9 production [357]: the dissociation of E-cadherins increases the permeability of intercellular junctions in gingival keratinocytes [355]. For example, elevated TNF-α production has been found in gingival epithelial cells infected with oral bacteria such as *Porphyromonas gingivalis* [355], and it is possible that TNF-α-secreting gingival keratinocytes may affect themselves in an autocrine manner [357]. Researchers in this recent study observed that vit.D reduces TNF-α-induced MMP-9 and NF-kB production in gingival keratinocytes, resulting in an overall protective and maintenance effect of adherens junctions [357]. Since factors such as TNF-α, NF-kB, and MMP-9 are also involved in OLP inflammation, this could substantiate the role of vit.D in this pathology. A recent study found a reduction of VDR levels in the oral mucosa affected by OLP by almost 50%, and this is associated with an induction of immune reactivity [347]. Given that VDR in intestinal cells helps maintain the integrity of the intestinal mucosal barrier through inhibition of cell apoptosis and regulation of the adherens junction of the intestinal epithelium [340, 359], some authors hypothesized that VDR located in the oral epithelium could preserve its homeostasis [23]. They demonstrated that lipopolysaccharide (LPS) significantly reduced keratinocyte VDR expression and that this reduction was dependent on the TNF-α/miR-346 pathway [22]. Indeed, VDR levels in the mucosa of OLP patients decreased substantially while there was a robust induction of TNF-α and miR-346, compared with healthy tissues [22]. In contrast, vit.D/VDR-induced signaling inhibited in keratinocytes the PUMA factor (p53-upregulated modulator of apoptosis, a proapoptotic protein of the Bcl-2 family [360, 361]) induced by LPS through blocking the activation of NF-kB factor, resulting in decreased apoptosis of these cells. This mechanism is summarized in Fig. 4.2. PUMA activity was indeed very intense in OLP-affected epithelium, with an inverse correlation with the expression of VDR [22].

These data indicate that LPS is responsible for the inhibition of VDR expression in the oral keratinocytes, which is associated with the development of OLP [22].

Regarding serum levels of vit.D in patients with OLP, data are conflicting, but there is still little research on this aspect. Du et al. [347] found

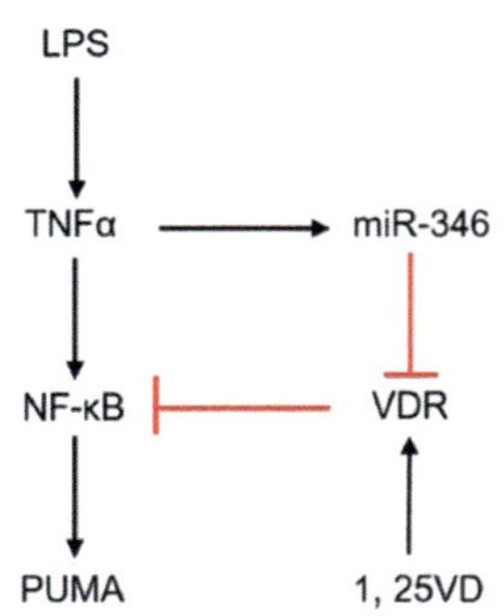

Fig. 4.2 Schematic illustration of the role of vit.D/VDR signaling in inhibiting LPS-induced PUMA activation. In OLP tissues, overexpression of TNF-α/miR-346 inhibits VDR expression, resulting in NF-kB → PUMA → keratinocyte apoptosis activation

a consistent reduction in serum calcidiol levels in patients with OLP. Ahmed et al. [362] found vit.D deficiency in 60% of patients with OLP and 22.5% of healthy patients, but the latter presented more deficient values than the affected; the authors found therefore that the deficiency of serum vit.D level was not only related to the development of OLP, but it was also related to the symptoms and clinical forms of OLP. In any case, given that vit.D/VDR signaling has a protective role from OLP by suppressing the immune reaction and apoptosis of epithelial cells [22, 347], the mechanism remains unclear [23]. One study showed that vit.D can suppress LPS-induced keratinocyte production of IFN-γ and IL-1β through HIF-1α (hypoxia-inducible factor-1α) and that HIF-1α, IFN-γ, and IL-1β are highly induced in the epithelia of OLP patients [221]. Another research showed the role of miR-802 in apoptosis of oral keratinocytes, as well as the protective mechanism of vit.D/VDR signaling in OLP, attenuating keratinocyte apoptosis and repressing the expression of miR-802 [23]. Some researchers have detected a decrease in the expression of miR-27a and miR-27b (miR-27a/b) in oral tissues and serum and saliva samples of patients with OLP, while vit.D/VDR signaling (binding sites for VDR were found in the miR-27a/b gene promoters) induces the expression of these mi-RNAs in OLP [363]. The same has also been shown to occur for miR-26a/b [25]. Analyses performed by the researchers have shown that miR-26a/b blocks keratinocyte apoptosis by acting on protein kinase C-δ (PKC-δ) that promotes cellular apoptotic processes. In addition, miR-26a/b can suppress the secretion of Th1 cytokines by acting on CD38: in fact, in OLP patients decreases in miR-26a/b (due to suppression of vit.D/VDR) and very high levels of PKC-δ and CD38 are detected. These new findings may pave the way for new therapeutic approaches in the clinical management of OLP [25].

Regarding genetic studies, growing evidence suggests that SNPs in genes associated with vit.D could influence its properties, such as its anti-carcinogenic effects [24]. A study performed in a Chinese population sample showed that the risk of OLP increases in subjects with TT genotype (rs2239185) and CC genotype (rs7975232). These polymorphisms also showed significant cumulative effects on the risk of OLP. Haplotype analysis showed that haplotype CC (rs2239185-rs7975232) was associated with an increased risk of OLP, compared with haplotype AC. So VDR gene polymorphisms may be associated with OLP [364]. A single study evaluated vit.D supplementation in the treatment of patients with OLP. The authors observed statistically significant improvement of subjective and objective symptoms in patients who were supplemented with vit.D with or without psychological counselling in addition to topical application of steroids for a short period. So the marked improvement and long-term remission of symptoms in patients with vit.D deficiency after restoration of its normal levels further corroborate its role in the pathogenesis of OLP like other autoimmune diseases [342].

4.4.3 Beta-Defensin

In order to provide effective defense, the oral cavity is equipped with various defense mechanisms against invading microbial pathogens: non-specific barriers, innate immunity, and immunity adaptive [365]:

- Non-specific barriers in the oral cavity are represented by the stratified squamous epithelium which acts as a physical barrier and by saliva which acts as a chemical (neutral pH) and mechanical barrier (action of salivary flow on mucosal and tooth surfaces) [365].
- Innate immunity is provided by innate immune cells and salivary secretion of adverse molecules that limit microbial growth such as lysozyme (cleavage of cell wall bacteria), lactoferrin, salivary amylase, cystatins, proline-rich proteins, mucins, peroxidases, and some molecules known as oral antimicrobial peptides (AMPs) [366].
- Adaptive immunity in the oral cavity is determined by lymphocytes and the production of IgA secretory which are constitutively excreted in saliva and perform the exclusion immune exclusion of antigens [365, 367].

Antimicrobial peptides (AMPs) constitute a wide range of host defense molecules that exert their action early to combat microbial invasion. They are small cationic peptides, produced by the oral epithelium and salivary glands, which play an important defense role in oral innate immunity [368]. AMPs, in addition to antimicrobial action, act as effective biological molecules in immune activation, inflammation, and wound healing [369–371]. So, these molecules perform and protect against pathogens either through direct antimicrobial action or by stimulating the immune response:

- Some AMPs directly damage the membrane or cellular components of pathogens.
- Many AMPs are also capable of inducing the innate immune response by stimulating the activity of monocytes/macrophages, polymorphonuclear leukocytes, and keratinocytes, inducing the production of chemokines and cytokines, and promoting the recruitment activation and differentiation of immune cells. These molecules also induce wound healing and polarization of adaptive immunity.

So, the overall effect of AMPs is to promote immune efficacy against infection and to have an immunobulking effect without exacerbating the pro-inflammatory response [372]. AMPs are classified into different classes based on amino acid composition, molecular size, and conformational structures [368]:

1. *Defensins*. They are classified into three forms (α, β, and θ) according to their chemical structure [373–375]. The junctional epithelium is protected by the action of α-defensins (hAD) and LL-37 (cathelicidin), while β-defensins 1 and 2 (hBD-1 and hBD-2), also localized in healthy noninflamed tissues, protect stratified and differentiated epithelia [27, 28]. Especially hBD-1 and hBD-2 have been localized in the suprabasal layer of normal gingiva, while hBD-3 is expressed in undifferentiated

epithelial cells within the basal layer [29]. It is believed that hBD-1 is continuously expressed (constitutive) and prevents normal flora from becoming opportunistic. In contrast, hBD-2 and hBD-3 are inducible in response to LPS, IL-1β, TNF-α, and IFN-γ and are most effective against almost all pathogens [27].

2. *Histatins*. We distinguish three principal members (His-1, His-3, and His-5) that exert predominantly antifungal action [376, 377]. In addition to inhibiting the growth of *Candida*, they perform other functions such as regulating oral hemostasis and binding metal ions in the saliva [378, 379].
3. *Cathelicidins*. The only molecule in this class is LL-37 [365] which exerts similar activity to that of defensins against gram-positive and gram-negative bacteria and *Candida albicans* [380].
4. *Adrenomedullin*. It is a potent long-acting peptide vasodilator [381]. It is produced to a greater extent in periodontally compromised areas than in healthy areas [382].
5. *Statherin*. It hinders the growth of anaerobic bacteria isolated from the oral cavity and also limits the crystallization of calcium phosphate, thus having a protective role against the formation of plaque [383–385].
6. *C-C motif chemokine 28 (CCL-28)*. It acts as both a broad-spectrum antimicrobial agent and a chemokine [386].
7. *Azurocidin*. It is a protein consisting of 251 amino acids that possesses strong antibacterial properties against gram-negative bacteria because of its strong affinity for LPS [386, 387].
8. *Neuropeptides*. Their antimicrobial role is extremely limited because their concentrations, ranging from 2 to 45 pg/ml, are several orders of magnitude lower than the minimum inhibitors needed to be effective against bacteria and *Candida albicans* [388].

Several researchers have found altered expression of hBD-2 in OLP. A recent study showed, compared with healthy epithelium, increased expression of hBD-2 in OLP lesions and OTSCC (oral tongue squamous cell carcinoma), but the expression of this peptide was attenuated in cancer cells compared with OLP lesions, suggesting an association between hBD-2 expression and the initiation and progression of OTSCC [389].

These results agree with previous studies showing decreased levels of hBD-2 m-RNA in samples obtained from OSCC patients [390, 391]. Strong positive immunostaining of hBD-2 was observed in OLP lesions, while healthy controls showed a weak signal. The m-RNA expression levels of hBD-2 were also found to be significantly higher in affected patients than in healthy controls. It is therefore possible that the low levels of hBD-2 expression on healthy oral mucosa play a role in maintaining the health of the oral mucosa as part of innate immunity, while overproduction of this peptide may participate in the immune inflammation of OLP. In fact, the expression of hBDs appears to be correlated with epithelial integrity in OLP, and the loss of epithelial cells due to erosion has caused a concomitant decrease in hBDs and an increase in i biofilm in vitro [392]. Regarding hBD levels in oral fluids, one study showed increased salivary levels of hBD-1 in patients with OLP, Behcet's disease, and recurrent aphthous stomatitis compared with healthy subjects, and furthermore, in subjects with these diseases, these values decreased after therapy [393]. In contrast, hBD-2 levels in oral fluids showed a dichotomous with higher values in patients with red OLP (atrophic-erosive forms) compared with those with white OLP (hyperplastic reticular forms), suggesting that hBD-2 may represent an index for assessing active inflammation and is probably related to the presence of the typical CD8+-banded T lymphocyte infiltrate in the OLP [394]. Two SNPs of the DEFB1 gene have been identified (5′UTR) in patients with OLP [395]. The same study found increased salivary levels of hBD-1 in patients with OLP; in particular SNP −52 G> A (rs1799946) was correlated with the salivary concentration of hBD-1 in both healthy subjects and patients with OLP, and the SNP −44C> G (rs1800972) was correlated with the salivary concentration of hBD-1 in patients with OLP [395]. So hBD-1 production was different between OLP and healthy subjects and the polymorphisms of the

DEFB1 gene, −52G> A, and −44C> G were correlated with salivary concentrations of hBD-1 [395].

Recent research has also found in OLP a correlation between hBD-2 expression and histaminergic transmission. First, it seems that LPS and histamine (HA) mainly influenced the expression of hBD-2, which was strongly induced in OLP] [389]. hBD-2 has also been implicated in the pathogenesis and progression of OSCC [396, 397]; however, unexpectedly, the hBD-2 protein was attenuated in OTSCC tissues with a marked downregulation of its transcription in tumor cells [389], and this, as mentioned before, is in agreement with the results of previous studies showing decreased m-RNA levels of hBD-2 in samples obtained from OSCC patients [390, 391]. Researchers have shown in oral keratinocytes that hBD-2 is induced, and partially regulated, by mediators derived from LPS and MC. Specifically, MCs influence hBD-2-mediated OLP pathogenesis through two pathways: (1) as the main "non-epithelial" source, they directly release hBD-2 once activated, and (2) MCs also release HA, which can induce the release of hBD-2 from the oral epithelium [398] via the action of TNF-α and IFN-γ [389]. The hBD-2 produced can subsequently stimulate MCs to release even more histamine, which leads to further production of hBD-2 in a vicious pro-inflammatory [389, 399, 400]. In fact, HA has a synergistic effect on hBD-2 production via TNF-α and IFN-γ, probably through overregulation of the region of the hBD-2 promoter which contains two binding sites for NF-kB and one for STAT-1 [389, 401].

Interestingly, activation of the histamine receptor H4R in oral keratinocytes regulates the m-RNA level of hBD-2, and pharmacological targeting of H4R can modulate the expressions of hBD-2 mediated by TNF-α and LPS [389]. In particular, the use of an agonist of H4R (HST10) appears to inhibit HA/TNF-α- and HA/LPS-mediated signaling pathways, while the reverse agonist (ST-1007) potentiated their effect [389]. In this regard, H4R shows a suppressive effect on both STAT-1- and TNF-α-mediated effects [402], and thus it is logical to assume that such an effect mediated by HST10 may also be mediated by interfering with one or both pathways [389].

These results suggest the involvement of hBD-2 in the pathogenesis of OLP and may therefore be exploited for therapeutic interventions in this pathology [403].

4.4.4 Histamine

Histamine (HA) or beta-imidazole ethylamine is an endogenous pleiotropic amine with a potent and short-lived action [403] that can mediate various pathophysiological mechanisms, including the proliferation of various normal and malignant cells [404–407]. HA is synthesized only by the enzyme histidine decarboxylase (HDC), which converts the amino acid L-histidine to HA [408]. HDC is widely expressed in different types of cells and tissues such as the central nervous system (CNS), the neurons, gastric mucosal tissue, MCs, basophils, and similar enterochromaffin cells [409, 410]. A wide range of cell populations can produce and release HA. Basically, it is possible to distinguish them into two categories: "professional" and "nonprofessional" histamine-producing cells [411]. Professional cells (MCs, basophils, and similar enterochromaffin cells) use the low-molecular-weight (53 kDa), post-translationally cleaved HDC enzyme to produce HA in large quantities, which is stored within cytoplasmic granules and rapidly released by exocytosis in response to stimuli (e.g., allergens). In contrast, nonprofessional cells use the high-molecular-weight (74 kDa), full-length, to produce basal amounts of HA, with a lower rate of 100–1000 times of MCs. Moreover, in these cells, HA is not stored in granules but is transported through histamine channels (such as OCTs or organic cation transporters) according to concentration gradient [411, 412]. HA degradation is operated by two enzymes: histamine N-methyl transferase (HNMT) and diamine oxidase (DAO) [413]. The former is a cytosolic and therefore degrades HA only intracellularly, while the latter removes HA from the extracellular spaces [414].

HA exerts its physiological and pathological effects by binding to four distinct receptors coupled to G proteins (H1R, H2R, H3R, and H4R) [48]:

- The H1R receptor is associated with a Gq/11 protein with GTPase activity that stimulates the activity of a phospholipase C which in turn induces Ca++-dependent processes and cellular excitation. In addition, activation of this receptor can induce the formation of cGMP and arachidonic acid, the latter through the action of phospholipase A2 [415]. H1R was the first histaminergic receptor subtype identified and is exploited in the treatment of allergic reactions [412].
- Activation of H2R promotes the activity of a Gs protein that causes increased levels of cAMP and PKA (protein kinase A) [415]. This receptor subtype stimulates the secretion of stomach acid and is therefore used to pharmacologically block its excessive production [412].
- H3R is accoupled to a Gi/Go protein that decreases cAMP-dependent PKA activity [412]. This receptor shows high constitutive activity, and its activation inhibits the discharge of histaminergic neurons and exerts negative control over synthesis and release in the CNS (central nervous system CNS) also of other transmitters such as catecholamines, GABA, and peptides [415]. H3R has shown very promising clinical effects and has been involved in studies targeting CNS disorders.
- H4R represents the last characterized receptor subtype of the HA family [416]. Like H3R, H4R is also associated with a Gi protein [415].

H1R and H2R show low affinity for HA and therefore require higher concentrations of that receptor for activation, compared with H3R and H4R, which are high-affinity receptors, so even low concentrations of HA are sufficient for their activation [389].

H4R can exist in two conformations: a resting R (GDP-bound) state indicating the absence of a ligand and an active R* (GTP-bound) state characterized by ligand-receptor binding [389]. In fact, some G-protein-coupled receptors can spontaneously reach the R* conformation and thus promote signal transduction even in the absence of ligand: this phenomenon is known as constitutive, intrinsic, or basal activity [389]. H4R shows high constitutive activity compared with H1R and H2R, indicating sustained and extensive histamine interactions under physiological and inflammatory conditions [411]. The intrinsic activity of H4R (given by the ratio of R*/R) equals about 50% of its total activity, making it sensitive at very low (nanomolar) concentrations of HA [417]. In fact, compared with H1R and H2R, H4R, exhibiting a pronounced constitutive activity, is related to several physiological interactions and inflammatory conditions [411].

Unprofessional cells produce HA concentrations that are too low to stimulate H1R and H2R but high enough to stimulate H4R activity [389]. So, while low-affinity H1R and H2R are activated during acute and transient responses such as allergic reactions and helminthic infestations, on the other hand, the high-affinity H4R receptor regulates the mechanisms responsible for homeostasis and immunity, and thus the latter is also expressed in non-occupational cells such as DCs, T lymphocytes, and monocytes/macrophages [411, 418, 419].

Receptor ligands can act as agonists, neutral antagonists, or reverse agonists. Agonists, by binding to the receptor, promote the active R* conformation by inducing the signal transduction. Binding of a neutral antagonist to a constitutively active receptor does not promote either state (R or R*), but simply competes with the agonist for receptor binding, preventing its effects. In contrast, inverse agonists promote the inactive R conformation, thereby inhibiting the intrinsic activity of the receptor [411].

These recent discoveries about histaminergic transmission have brought new interests in the study of HA and its novel receptor H4R, paving the way for new feasible therapeutic targets in inflammatory disorders and in neoplastic disease [420, 421].

Regarding tumors, imbalanced levels of HA and HDC have been observed in different neoplastic tissues [404, 407, 422, 423]. Indeed, HA regulates several biological processes associated with the growth of the tumor (with different responses depending on its local concentration and receptor subtype), including cell proliferation, migration, differentiation, and apoptosis [424]. In addition, HA produced by MCs promotes the expression of VEGF (vascular endothelial growth factor) and angiogenesis, thereby regulating growth, neoplastic invasion, and distant metastasis formation [425]. In fact, MCs can synthesize and release pro-angiogenic mediators (e.g., VEGF and IL-8) and proteases (e.g., MMP-9, chymase, and tryptase) that can degrade the extracellular matrix and enhance neoplastic invasion [49].

H1R and H2R receptors have been much studied in various neoplastic tissues [407, 426], while little is known about the role of H4R in oral tongue squamous cell carcinoma (OTSCC) [48], and in fact H4R is a very important receptor in oral tongue squamous cell carcinoma [48], is about 10,000 times more sensitive to the effects of HA than to H1R and H2R, and has been reported to be a crucial factor in cancers [48, 410, 411, 427]. In fact, because of its immunomodulatory effects and on the growth and progression of many neoplasms, H4R appears to be one of the most promising HA receptor subtypes that could be used as a molecular therapeutic target in cancer management [428]. And, MCs, which are active in the tumor microenvironment, being professional cells (in HA production), constitute potent regulators of H4R [48, 429]. In addition, this cell population also releases pro-inflammatory cytokines such as IL-17A, which is implicated in the progression of OTSCC [430]. Finally, the factors environmental may influence histamine metabolism; in fact, it has been shown that the oral microbiota, via LPS, can influence HDC levels and stimulate HA release by keratinocytes [20]. Some researchers have found a significant decrease of H4R immunostaining in oral epithelial dysplasia (OED) and OTSCC samples (especially in those with more advanced histopathological grades) and a significant increase in the number of MCs [20]. In addition, gene expression data have indicated that inflammatory and environmental elements relevant to HA (such as IL-17A and LPS) may participate in the regulation of oncogenes (including EGF/EGFR) [20]. These results thus suggest an association between H4R and oral carcinogenesis [20].

Histamine metabolism has also been studied in OLP. Because of the increased number of mast cells in OLP [41], it was believed that HA release could stimulate low-affinity receptors H1R and H2R and damage basal keratinocytes [48]. However, H1R and H2R antagonists (antihistamines) have not proven useful in the treatment of OLP [431], and speculation about the potential of histamine in the pathogenesis of OLP was abandoned [48]. The discovery of H4R receptors (high affinity and high intrinsic activity) [432], expressed in keratinocytes [433], together with the recognition of these as nonprofessional HA-producing cells [434] has revived interest in the potential role of HA in healthy oral mucosa and OLP [41]. Given the high intrinsic activity of H4R, this led to the hypothesis that low amounts of HA continuously released and produced by nonprofessional and interacting cells on H4Rs might participate in the maintenance of oral keratinocyte health [41].

Perturbation of histamine concentrations due to mast cell degranulation in OLP results in activation of low-affinity receptors (H1Rs and H2Rs) and supersaturation of H4Rs that downregulate their expression [48]. The researchers showed that H4R immunoreactivity was weak in OLP and negatively correlated with concomitant mast cell hyperplasia and degranulation [41].

In particular, the most affected areas in the OLP, namely, the basal and suprabasal layers, were H4R negative, while H4R+ cells were found in the more superficial epithelium, starting from the middle of the spinous layer, with weak and irregular staining of the granulosa cell layer. In contrast, immunostaining of healthy epithelium was different, which showed H4R immunoreactivity in all layers except the basal layer and a thin layer of adjacent suprabasal cells. Furthermore, by mast cell tryptase staining, in the healthy epithelium, few MCs were detected in the subepithelial connective tissue, whereas, in OLP, the number of MCs increased in this region, pericellular matrix staining also being present, probably due to tryptase degranulation by MCs [48].

Furthermore, it has been shown that nanomolar levels of H4R agonists (HST-10) led to rapid internalization of these receptors in a dose-dependent manner and that high concentrations of HA and IFN-γ lead to a decrease in H4R gene transcripts, so cytokines may also lead to a decrease in H4R production [48]. It is therefore possible that H4R may be involved in the maintenance of healthy oral mucosa [48]. It has also been shown that oral keratinocytes possess a true functional HA metabolization and transport apparatus [48]. Specifically, m-RNA levels of HDC and OCT-3 transporter increase, and HNMT immunoreactivity decreases in oral keratinocytes of OLP patients compared with healthy controls [20].

In contrast, neither OCT-1/OCT-2 nor DAO was detected in tissue sections nor in oral keratinocytes [20]. This shows that oral keratinocytes release HA through OCT-3 channels in concentrations too low to activate low-affinity H1R and H2R receptors but high enough to stimulate high-affinity H4R in an autocrine and paracrine manner [20]. In addition, it was observed that LPS induced a dose-dependent release of HA in keratinocytes, while a high concentration of HA inhibited the expression of epithelial adhesion proteins (integrin-α6 and integrin-β4). This confirms that substantially deranged HA metabolism and transport in OLP could compromise epithelial integrity and, in part, contribute to disease pathogenesis [20]. Recently, it has also been shown that the expression of claudins 1 and 4 and E-cadherin is decreased in OLP, leading to a disturbance of adherens junctions, cell-cell connections, and epithelial permeability [435]. As mentioned before, vit.D exerts a protective on such junctions, while TNF-α alters their development [436] (see Sect. 4.4.2).

The effect of HA and the H4R receptor on hBD-2 production has already been discussed (see Sect. 4.4.3).

Altered expression of TLRs is also observed in OLP lesions.

Bacterial cell wall components are mainly detected by membrane TLRs, while nucleic acids are detected by intracellular TLRs [437]. Specifically, in OLP, the immunoreactivity of all TLRs (TLR1 to TLR10) except TLR5, which instead appears to be significantly reduced, increases [389]. These results suggest a fundamental role of the response mediated by TLRs to invading pathogens in the initiation and perpetuation of OLP lesions [389].

Indeed, the high concentration of HA in patients with OLP, by inducing hypo-expression of the epithelial adhesion proteins, could promote subsequent bacterial invasion, and thus the TLRs that intercept bacterial components (such as LPS) could increase further immune response and HA production [389], establishing a vicious cycle. In addition, the interference of HA/H4R signaling given by MCs and the presence of LPS could be partially involved in the pathogenesis of OTSCC, and this is further supported by the altered expression of H4R and by its ability to regulate cell apoptosis and modulate antibacterial response in keratinocytes [389].

Indeed, recently, several researches have been carried out on the suppression of the apoptotic process of oral keratinocytes [23, 430] which is the key process in the pathogenesis of OLP and may also modulate its potential for transformation into OSCC [23, 438]. In fact, apoptosis, by causing the loss of keratinocytes, compromises the protective epithelial barrier and, if not adequately eliminated, perpetuates the precancerous inflammatory reaction, even leading to cancerization [23, 438, 439]. H4R activation has been shown to modulate the oral cell proliferation in a dose-dependent manner; in fact, the H4R agonist HST-10 exhibits a dual effect depending on its concentration: low nanomolar concentrations of HST-10 inhibit apoptosis in a dose-dependent manner [389]. In fact, HST-10 has a protective against TNF-α-mediated cell death [389], and it has been observed that the attenuation of H4R-induced cell apoptosis occurs through suppression of the BCL-2 protein [389].

Finally, Salem et al. [403] provided a possible scenario of the role of the HA/hBD-2 axis in the perpetuation of chronic inflammation in OLP (Fig. 4.3).

Fig. 4.3 Intensity of TLR immunoreactivity in different epithelial layers of OLP samples (taken from Salem et al. [403])

	Basal/suprabasal layers		Intermediate layers		Superficial layers	
	Control	*OLP*	*Control*	*OLP*	*Control*	*OLP*
TLR1	+++	+++	+	++	-	++
TLR2	+++	+++	+	+++	-	+++
TLR3	+++	+++	+	+++	+	++
TLR4	+++	+++	+	+++	-	+++
TLR5	+++	+	++	-	+	+
TLR6	+++	++	+	++	-	+++
TLR7	+++	+++	+	+++	-	+++
TLR8	+++	+++	-	++	-	++
TLR9	+++	+++	+	+++	-	+++
TLR10	+	+	-	+	-	-

Further studies on H4R signal transduction will be used to evaluate its role as a potential molecular target in the therapy of OLP and OTSCC.

4.4.5 Other Factors

The vast literature on OLP has also identified other factors that might intervene in the OLP pathogenesis and are still being studied and investigated in depth.

Among these factors is, for example, the multifunctional pro-inflammatory protein YLK-40 (also known as chitinase-3-like protein 1). It is one of 18 known glycosidases [436], produced by various inflammatory (neutrophils, macrophages) and non-inflammatory cells (fibroblasts, cells endothelial and smooth muscle, chondrocytes) [440], and, although its biological role is still unclear, some studies report that YKL-40 is related to innate and adaptive type 2 immunity and that it plays a role in inflammation, angiogenesis, tissue remodeling, and proliferation cells [441–445]. This protein has been evaluated in several diseases such as dermatitis atopic, psoriasis, and Behcet's disease [446–448]. Some researchers have evaluated the role of YKL-40 in LP as well and found a significant increase in serum levels of YKL-40 in affected patients compared with healthy controls, and these levels were significantly higher in OLP patients than in those with cutaneous LP; these results, although only a beginning, support the role of YKL-40 in the pathogenesis of lichen planus and could contribute to the treatment of this condition [449].

Several studies have also been performed that have attempted to identify potential salivary markers in OLP, and, among these, cortisol and nitric oxide (NO) stand out. A recent systematic review of the literature (which included 15 articles related to the analysis of these two mediators) showed that 55.5% of selected studies on cortisol and 100% of studies on NO showed increased salivary levels of these markers in patients with OLP compared with healthy controls [450]. While the results remain controversial for salivary cortisol levels, instead the salivary NO measurement may be a potential and significant diagnostic, therapeutic, and prognostic marker for monitoring OLP activity and therapeutic response [450].

The VEGF (vascular endothelial growth factor) family contains large amounts of growth factors [36], and VEGF is believed to be the main regulator of endothelial cell proliferation and differentiation involved in OLP pathogenesis and progression [451, 452]. Each type of VEGF binds to a VEGFR receptor and has its own specific effects. VEGFR-3 is related to lymph angiogenesis, and the role is through binding of certain types of VEGF, particularly VEGFC and VEGFD, which increase the network of lymphatic vessels [36]. A group of researchers demonstrated the presence of increased immuno-expression of VEGFR-3 and blood vessels in OLP tissues compared with healthy tissues, with no differences between the various clinical subtypes of lichen [36]. So, it is likely that suppression of new blood vessel formation would delay disease progression [134]. Prevention of angiogenesis could minimize immune cell extravasation and inhibit the release of pro-inflammatory cytokines. A group of researchers showed the decrease of VEGF and IL-8 immuno-expression in tissues treated with intralesional injections of bevacizumab (anti-angiogenic) [134].

Some researchers have also shown a correlation between dysbiosis and OLP. In general, patients with OLP show lower salivary levels of mycetes and higher levels of bacteria [453]. The presence of *Campylobacter rectus*, *Fusobacterium nucleatum*, and *Neisseria mucosa* has been shown to be associated with OLP [304]. Fungal species *Candida* and *Aspergillus* are significantly more abundant in reticular forms, while *Alternaria* and *Sclerotiniaceae* in erosive forms, compared with healthy controls [453]. In addition, several fungal species (such as *Bovista*, *Erysiphe*, *Psathyrella*, etc.) have shown significant correlations with IL-17 levels [453]. Thus, researchers have shown that fungal dysbiosis can associate with the exacerbation of OLP and alter the salivary bacteriome or result in a direct effect on the host immune response [453]. Further studies will improve the understanding of these findings.

Periostin is a soluble extracellular matrix protein that plays various roles in embryonic development, in wounds, and in tooth and bone formation [454], and its overexpression has been detected in several types of cancer such as breast, lung, ovarian, prostate carcinoma, gastric, colon, and pancreatic. In fact, it is involved in several biological processes such as cell survival, proliferation, adhesion, angiogenesis, epitheliomesenchymal transition, neoplastic invasion, and metastasis [455]. A group of researchers has detected a significant increase in tissue immuno-expression and serum levels of periostin in most majority of patients in the OLP group, and it was observed that this elevated expression was associated with increased serum levels of IL-6, TNF-α, TSLP (thymic stromal lymphopoietin), an increase in tissue mast cell density, and a decrease in the IFN-γ/IL-4 ratio [456]. Modulation of periostin could therefore represent a new therapeutic target [456].

4.5 Pathogenesis Related to the Malignant Transformation OF OLP, Prognosis, and Follow-Up

4.5.1 Epidemiology of Neoplastic Risk in OLP

In 1978, the World Health Organization (WHO) classified OLP as a precancerous condition [457]. However, the possibility of malignant transformation of OLP lesions is the subject of debate among various scholars. In fact, there are studies that have shown no malignant potential of OLP [458–461], while others report highly variable rates of OSCC risk (0.07–12.5%) in OLP lesions [462–474]. These wide fluctuations are due to several factors, including insufficient documentation of all relevant information (e.g., data on previous exposure to carcinogens such as tobacco, arsenicals, irradiation, thorium) [44, 102] and lack of appropriate control populations and long-term follow-up programs 38 but especially inconsistent application of diagnostic criteria and the lack of histological confirmation of clinical diagnosis [44, 102, 475]. Indeed, Krutchkoff et al. [476] and van Der Meij et al. [464] had warned that nearly two-thirds of the cases published until then on the OLP malignant transformation were not sufficiently documented to be considered reliable. But in fact, as early as 1978, WHO had developed standardized diagnostic clinical and histopathological criteria for OLP [477] and then had been modified in 2003 by van der Meij and van der Waal to differentiate OLP from other lichenoid lesions, such as lichenoid dysplasia, which has a significantly higher risk of malignant transformation than OLP [478, 479] (see Sect. 5.5.16). To overcome the problem of the risk of cancerization of OLP, several systematic reviews have recently been published on the subject. The studies reviewed by Fitzpatrick et al. (which included, until 2014, those reporting histologic confirmation of diagnosis) [468] report an overall risk of malignant transformation of OLP of 1.09%. A 2017 meta-analysis [475], on the other hand, reports an overall risk of 1.1% by analyzing 57 studies, with a total of 19,676 patients, while considering the only 14 recent studies that used the WHO diagnostic criteria, the overall risk of cancerization stands at 0.9%. The authors also found a higher risk of malignant transformation in patients with OLL (419 individuals) but also in smokers (odds ratio, OR = 2), alcoholics (OR = 3.52), and HCV+ patients (OR = 5), compared with patients without these risk factors [475]. However, some unresolved questions remained, such as which clinical subtype of OLP is associated with higher neoplastic risk, the role played by therapy, and what frequency of follow-up recall should be adopted, so other authors performed further insights. For example, Giuliani et al. reported an overall risk of cancerization of 1.40% (1.37% for OLP and 2.43% for OLL), which increases in the female gender, in clinical red forms (probably because these lesions may predispose the mucosa to the carcinogen-induced damage to a greater extent than healthy oral mucosa [102]), and when the tongue is the site of the lesion [480]. Another recent systematic review also reported values similar percentages and identified as risk factors: tongue location (OR = 1.82), atrophic-erosive lesions (OR = 4.09), tobacco (OR = 1.98), alcohol (OR = 2.28), and HCV (RR = 4.46) [481], substantially confirming the results of the other reviews cited above. It must be kept in mind that in these reviews, an important factor influencing in the overall percentage risk resulting (in addition to the prevalence of certain risk factors, such as HCV and carcinogens, in the individual study's sample of patients) is the follow-up times of the individual studies taken considered since, as this increases, so does the probability of finding new cases OSCC and recurrences. It has also been observed that the risk of neoplastic transformation is highly elevated between the sixth and seventh decades of life [150], in *Candida albicans* infections (as they produce nitrosamines, a carcinogen) [102] and HPV [16], in cases of changes in diet (such as reduced consumption of fresh fruits and vegetables imposed by symptoms) [482, 483], and also the immunosuppressive drugs could influence severity and promote cancerization [459, 463]. For HPV in the past, a true correlation with OLP (see Sect. 3.1.1). However, a recent meta-analysis may overturn this conception [484]. Indeed, an increased prevalence of HPV in patients with OLP compared with healthy controls was demonstrated (OR, 6.83), and this association varied significantly by geographic populations (OR, 2.43–132.04); in addition, the data showed a greater association with EOLP forms (OR, 9.34) than NEOLP forms (OR, 4.32); and finally, among the genotypes of OLP, HPV-16 showed an extremely strong association with OLP (OR, 11.27), and HPV-18 showed a relatively strong one (OR, 6.54) [484]. So, the researchers concluded that the results suggest that HPV might play an important causal role in OLP and its malignant transformation [484]. Another recent study also advances that p16 protein expression (see Sect. 4.5.4) could be useful in predicting HPV-16/HPV-18 infection in OLP and that HPV-16/HPV-18 (E6) infection could contribute to malignant transformation of OLP [485]. Some researchers also believe that it is possible that malignant transformation rates may be underestimated due to restrictive diagnostic criteria (e.g., in several studies, considering the WHO diagnostic criteria, including those modified by van der Meij in 2003, the presence of epithelial dysplasia was considered an exclusion criterion for the diagnosis of OLP [479], inadequate follow-up periods (less than 12 months), and low quality of the studies) [481]. In this regard, it is now commonly accepted that lichenoid dysplasia (see Sect. 5.5.16) and OLP represent as two different entities [459, 486, 487]. However, it is also likely that "lichenoid dysplasia" may constitute an early stage in the pathway of malignant transformation from "true" OLP to OSCC, that is, a form of OLP lesion capable of becoming dysplastic, and this is suggested by a series of clinical observations by Mignogna et al. [488–490] who performed a large retrospective study of a sample of 45 patients with OLP confirmed histologically without dysplasia at the time of initial diagnosis: 20 patients subsequently went through a single transformation event, and 25 had multiple transformation events including multifocal dysplasia and/or malignancy. These results suggest that not only does OLP itself constitute a risk factor for malignant transformation but that there may also be field cancerization in

OLP [489]. The term "cancerization of field" was first used in 1953 by Slaughter et al. in their studies on oral carcinoma [491]. The authors did not provide a clear definition, but by performing several histological examinations, a description of the characteristics of the term cancerization of field are as follows: (a) oral carcinoma develops in multifocal areas of preneoplastic alteration; (b) the abnormal tissue surrounds the tumor; (c) oral carcinoma often consists of multiple independent lesions that may sometimes merge; and (d) the persistence of abnormal tissue after surgery may explain the appearance of additional primary tumors and local recurrences [492]. It has been shown that in the early stages, a stem cell acquires genetic alterations and forms a "patch," a clonal unit of altered daughter cells with the same DNA modification. These patches can be recognized based on mutations in the oncosuppressor gene TP53. The next critical step in epithelial carcinogenesis is the conversion of the patch into a "field of expansion." This step requires the presence of additional genetic alterations and is facilitated by the growth advantage of these cells over normal cells, so such a proliferating field will go on to gradually replace the normal mucosa. It has been shown that in the mucous membranes of the testacollo (also including the esophagus), such fields assume dimensions of more than 7 cm in diameter.

The important clinical consequence is that such fields often persist after surgery of the primary tumor and can lead to new carcinomas, marked by clinicians as a "second" primary tumor or "local recurrence," depending on the exact site and time interval. Therefore, the diagnosis and treatment of epithelial carcinomas should focus not only on the tumor but also on the field in which it developed [492], and as mentioned above, this concept could be also relevant in OLP lesions that become complicated. With regard to OLP as a lesion capable of becoming dysplastic, however, it must also be taken into account that it is not uncommon to find microscopic "lichenoid" features in oral dysplasia and OSCC [468, 476] and that therefore misdiagnoses of OLP may occur, especially when limited clinical information is provided or when atypical cellular changes of a precancerous nature of mild degree and/or accompanied by a lichenoid infiltrate occur [493]. Currently, there are still no widely accepted diagnostic criteria for OLP [493]. Some pathologists use WHO criteria, which have not addressed a way to distinguish or exclude epithelial dysplasia from the diagnosis of OLP [494]. Application of the WHO criteria has revealed, among other things, great interobserver and intraobserver variability [495]. Others therefore use the modified diagnostic criteria proposed by van der Meij and van der Waal [478], in which as well the presence of epithelial dysplasia excludes a diagnosis of OLP. The absence of broad consensus in the selection of diagnostic criteria has been identified as the main obstacle to ensuring the validity of studies investigating the potential for the malignant transformation of OLP [481]. Therefore, considerable efforts should be made to establish strict clinical and histological criteria for diagnosing OLP and perform observational studies that are methodologically more robust [480]. This issue will be better addressed in Sect. 5.3.

4.5.2 Characteristics of Carcinoma Arising from the OLP Lesion

Oral squamous cell carcinoma (OSCC) is the most common form (90%) of oral carcinoma, with increasing prevalence on a global scale [496]. Clinically, carcinomas arising from OLP mainly present as exophytic keratotic lesions [497], although they sometimes show endophytic growth [498]. In addition, carcinomas evolving from OLP lesions tend to multifocality (according to the concept of field cancerization, as a tendential character of oropharyngeal neoplasms [499]); in fact Mignogna et al. [500] found that 29% of patients with carcinoma in the context of OLP had two or three independent neoplastic lesions (19% with a secondary tumor, 10% with two metachronous tumors, i.e., of later appearance). Finally, from a histopathological point of view, most neoplastic lesions are represented by well-differentiated squamous carcinoma [501].

4.5.3 Pathogenetic Mechanisms of the Transformation Neoplastic OLP

Regarding the pathogenetic mechanisms leading to neoplastic transformation of OLP, it is known that chronic inflammation of long duration is associated with an increased risk of cancerization [502, 503]. Indeed, chronic inflammation can stimulate mucosal healing and repair processes, promote cell survival and proliferation, and thus predispose to mutagenesis, which can be induced by exogenous (e.g., chemical carcinogens such as smoke and tobacco, HPV, *Candida*) or endogenous (e.g., ROS or reactive oxygen species) triggers [16, 44]. So in OLP, it is possible that certain genetic predispositions combined with chronic activation of inflammation-related anti-apoptotic factors promote the process of carcinogenesis: under these conditions, the triggers of mutagenesis (endogenous and/or exogenous) are less likely to kill epithelial cells, thus being able to lead to a malignant transformation [44].

Regarding molecular mechanisms, several chemical mediators are released during chronic inflammation, which in the long term can affect gene expression related to the control of proliferation and apoptosis, thus promoting carcinogenesis [17, 502, 504]. Among the major pro-inflammatory cytokines involved in this process are those derived from tumor-associated macrophages (TAMs) and Th17 cytokines, such as TNF, IL-1β, IL-6, IL-12, and IL-23. These can activate several transcription factors such as AP-1 (activator protein), NF-kB (nuclear factor kB), and STAT-3 (signal transducer and activator of transcription 3), which in turn promote the expression of many other pro-inflammatory and pro-angiogenic mediators and immunoregulatory activities, thus playing an important role in neoplastic OLP transformation [17, 502, 504]. In addition, some pleiotropic cytokines may have different effects depending on their concentration [168] and the stage of tumor development [311]. For example, TGF-β inhibits tumor growth in early stages of carcinogenesis, but in more advanced stages, it can instead stimulate it by inducing angiogenesis and MMP-9 expression [505]. Some studies have also shown the role of chemokines and their receptors in oral carcinogenesis [506]; e.g., RANTES can induce the expression of important cellular enzymes such as PI3K (phosphatidylinositol 3-kinase) and Akt/PKB (protein kinase B), which induce signals of cell survival and proliferation, promoting neoplastic transformation [507, 508]. In addition, an imbalance between MMP and TIMP may be associated with malignant transformation of OLP, MMP-2, and MMP-9 being possible markers of the potential for malignant transformation of OLP [299, 314]. Chronic inflammatory processes also induce activation of COXs (cyclooxygenases), which are enzymes that convert arachidonic acid into prostaglandins, and it has been shown that the inducible COX-2 isoform, when overexpressed, can associate with important mechanisms of carcinogenesis [509] such as angiogenesis [510] and apoptosis [511]. In fact, overexpression of COX-2 has been identified in OLP, so it has been suggested that this enzyme may increase the risk of malignant transformation [512]. Several studies have also shown altered oxidoreductive balance in OLP lesions. For example, low salivary levels of uric acid and an increase in serum gamma-glutamyl transferase (GGT) enzyme and total antioxidant capacity of saliva were found in OLP patients compared with the control group [513]. Ergun et al. [514] showed that the serum level of total antioxidant activity (TAA) defense in OLP patients was significantly lower than that in healthy subjects and that salivary levels of the lipid peroxidation product malondialdehyde (MDA) were significantly higher in the OLP group than in the controls. Some researchers have also detected expression in epithelial and inflammatory cells at the site of carcinogenesis of nitric and oxidative DNA injury products [515]. All these factors contribute to genetic DNA damage and inflammation-associated carcinogenesis [16]. In addition, CD4+ T lymphocyte cytokines, such as IFN-γ, TNF-α, and IL-12, and CD8+ T lymphocyte cytotoxic activity play an important role in the inhibition and death of malignant cells, so neoplastic transformation of OLP lesions may correlate with an imbalance in the activity of different cell types and the expression of different inflammatory mediators, inhibitors, and promoters of carcinogenesis [16].

4.5.4 Genetic Alterations Related to the Malignant Transformation of OLP

Regarding genetic studies on neoplastic transformation of OLP, one of the first molecular genetic investigations of OLP examined the frequency of LOH (loss of heterozygosity) in nine loci of oncosuppressor genes located on chromosomes 3p, 9p, and 17 p, which occurs frequently in most oral cancers, and it was observed that the OLP lesions were characterized by minimal genetic deviation, whereas the various dysplastic and malignant OSCC had steadily increasing frequencies of LOH on multiple chromosomes [516]. Kim et al. [517] found a statistically significant difference in the degree of genetic instability between OLP and lichenoid dysplasia, with an increase in partial imbalance on chromosome [3]. This might suggest that monosomy of chromosome 9 might play a critical role in the malignant transformation of OLP [518]. Other studies have also evaluated the role of allelic imbalance in OLP and lichenoid dysplastic lesions [519, 520]. Other genetic alterations in epithelial cells that promote malignant degeneration include increased content of DNA [521] and cytogenetic abnormalities given by the presence of aneuploidy [522] (a chromosomal aberration chromosome due to the alteration in the number of chromosomes in excess or defects compared to the normal diploid set-up). By immunohistochemistry investigations, p53 oncosuppressor gene expression was upper expressed in OLP and in malignant and metastatic OSCC, along with gradually increasing levels of expression of the proliferating cell nuclear antigen (PCNA) within these lesions, has also been detected [523]. The increase in the number of p53+ biopsies is significantly correlated with the degree of dysplasia and loss of differentiation in the OLP [524]. Most OLP lesions are characterized by the expression of p53+ nuclei confined to the basal layer of the epithelium [519], and one study showed that 9/27 cases of OLP lesions contained mutations at p53 when screened for mutations in exons 5 an 8. In addition, the percentage of p53+ epithelial cells at first diagnosis was significantly higher in cases of OLP+OSCC patients or those who developed OSCC several months or years after the diagnosis of OLP, compared with OLP patients with no dysplastic changes or neoplastic transformation during the follow-up period [525]. This indicates that immunohistochemical evaluation of p53 expression could be practical for selecting OLP cases at high risk of neoplastic transformation [525]. Some studies have also revealed a loss of c-erbB2 protein expression or HER2/neu (proto-oncogene EGFR, epidermal growth factor receptor family member) in the serial biopsies of progressive OLP and OSCC lesions, suggesting that the loss of cerbB2 function could indicate potential neoplastic transformation and be involved in carcinogenesis [526, 527]. In addition, keratinocytes in OLP lesions show a strong activity of the telomerase, which could be another indicator of the potential for transformation neoplastic. Recently, a group of researchers performed a retrospective study in which OLP and LP skin tissue samples were used, and in each sample, a positivity index (PI) for the expression of p16, BUB3, Ki-67, and SOX4 667. Ki-67 is a nuclear protein associated with cell proliferation and recognized as a risk factor in neoplastic transformation of precancerous lesions [528, 529]. p16 is a cell cycle progression inhibitor involved in the inactivation of cyclin-dependent kinase (CDK)-4 and CDK6 and studied as a diagnostic and predictive marker in several tumor types, in particular, that of the cervix, although its value as a predictor of malignancy progression remains controversial and depends on the anatomical site, for example, in cervical or breast carcinoma [530]. BUB3 (budding uninhibited by benzimidazole 3) is a cell cycle checkpoint gene that inhibits mitosis [531]; its expression has been associated with luminal breast carcinoma of low grade, as opposed to high-grade breast cancer [532], and its mutations have been associated with colon-rectal carcinoma [33]. SOX4 (sex-determining region Y-related high mobility group box 4), a marker of proliferation, is considered an unfavorable prognostic factor in patients with carcinoma breast [533] and is widely expressed in small-cell lung carcinoma and in esophageal squamous cell carcinoma [533, 534]. Researchers in this recent retrospective study found a PI for p16 of 20.65% for OLP and 86.59% for cutaneous LP, while the PI for Ki-67 stood at 11.6% for OLP and 8.24% for cutaneous LP. According to the authors, the levels of expression of p16 and Ki-67 suggest that specific OLP lesions may have potential intermediate malignancy and should be closely followed up. No statistically significant different levels of BUB3 expression were observed between groups (including also oral dysplasia and oral fibrous hyperplasia). SOX4 levels were elevated in cutaneous OLP, indicating a different proliferation pattern of the epithelium than in oral mucosal cells, so SOX4 expression may also be associated with the different clinical courses of cutaneous OLP and LP [535]. Other molecular mechanisms possibly involved in carcinogenesis may be related to other cell cycle regulatory proteins and genes (besides p53 and p16) such as p21, Bcl-2, BAX, MdM2 (p53 inhibitor), and SUMO1 (small ubiquitin-related modifier 1) and to chromosomal regions known as AgNORs (argyrophilic nucleolus organizer regions) [493].

4.5.5 Prognosis and Follow-Up of OLP

The typical clinical course of OLP is chronicity and persistence of the injury with periods of exacerbation and quiescence 18: only a low percentage of patients achieve complete and definitive recovery (2.5%–17%) [534]. Patients with OLP have an increased risk of OSCC, but this risk can be reduced with appropriate therapy and follow-up. In this context, the prognosis for most patients with OLP is excellent [41]. The general advice under these circumstances is to schedule an oral examination preferably twice a year [536]. The follow-up interval can range from 2 months to once a year [534]. Patients with a reticular form of OLP could also be evaluated one time per year, whereas the presence of dysplasia requires recalls more frequent, e.g., every 2–3 months [489, 490]. If, during follow-up visits, there are evidence of erosive changes in the lesions, additional biopsies are required, and follow-up intervals will have to be shortened [534]. About the prognosis of patients presenting with neoplasia, Mignogna et al. [489] reported a survival rate of 100% at 3 years and 97% at 5 years, and these authors recommend rigorous follow-up with inspection of head and neck lymph nodes every 2 months during the 5–9 months after the diagnosis of oral carcinoma, when the risk of metastasis or a second primary tumor is highest. Other authors propose regular follow-up for these patients with cancerous lichen [475] for long periods or even for life [481]. However, malignant evolution cannot be easily discovered in the entire population of patients with OLP, and this may be reflected in a rapid progression from intraepithelial neoplasia to invasive carcinoma [102]. In addition, screening for oral carcinoma in patients with OLP has a significant on final costs and effectiveness, considering that a system of recall of all OLP patients requires economic resources and that the malignant potential of OLP is probably very low [465]. To elucidate the true malignant potential of this pathology, follow-up studies will be needed over the long term with strict, unified, and universally accepted diagnostic criteria.

References

1. Lavanya N, et al. Oral lichen planus: an update on pathogenesis and treatment. J Oral Maxillof Pathol. 2011;15(2):127.
2. Zhou XJ, et al. Intra-epithelial CD8+ T cells and basement membrane disruption in oral lichen planus. J Oral Pathol Med. 2002;31(1):23–7.
3. Spadari F, et al. Lichen planus orale: revisione della letteratura, Doctor Os • aprile 2017 • XXVIII 04.
4. Sugerman P, et al. The pathogenesis of oral lichen planus. Crit Rev Oral Biol Med. 2002;13(4):350–65.
5. Gupta S, Jawanda MK. Oral lichen planus: an update on etiology, pathogenesis, clinical presentation, diagnosis and management. Indian J Dermatol. 2015;60(3):222.
6. Sugerman P, Satterwhite K, Bigby M. Autocytotoxic T-cell clones in lichen planus. Br J Dermatol. 2000;142(3):449–56.

7. Roopashree M, et al. Pathogenesis of oral lichen planus–a review. J Oral Pathol Med. 2010;39(10):729–34.
8. Lukač J, et al. Serum autoantibodies to desmogleins 1 and 3 in patients with oral lichen planus. Croat Med J. 2006;47(1):53–8.
9. Biočina-Lukenda D, et al. Serum immunoglobulins IgG, IgA and IgM in patients with oral lichen ruber. Coll Antropol. 2008;32(1):161–3.
10. Srinivasan M, Kodumudi KN, Zunt SL. Soluble CD14 and toll-like receptor-2 are potential salivary biomarkers for oral lichen planus and burning mouth syndrome. Clin Immunol. 2008;126(1):31–7.
11. Lodi G, et al. Current controversies in oral lichen planus: report of an international consensus meeting. Part 1. Viral infections and etiopathogenesis. Oral Surg Oral Med Oral Pathol Oral Radiol Endod. 2005;100(1):40–51.
12. Zhou XJ, et al. Matrix metalloproteinases and their inhibitors in oral lichen planus. J Cutan Pathol. 2001;28(2):72–82.
13. Zhao Z, et al. Mast cell degranulation and the role of T cell RANTES in oral lichen planus. Oral Dis. 2001;7(4):246–51.
14. Mutafchieva MZ, et al. Oral lichen planus–known and unknown: a review. Folia Med. 2018;60(4):528–35.
15. Jose M, Raghu A, Rao N. Evaluation of mast cells in oral lichen planus and oral lichenoid reaction. Indian J Dent Res. 2001;12(3):175–9.
16. Payeras MR, et al. Oral lichen planus: focus on etiopathogenesis. Arch Oral Biol. 2013;58(9):1057–69.
17. Merry R, et al. Oral health and pathology: a macrophage account. Br J Oral Maxillofac Surg. 2012;50(1):2–7.
18. Squier CA, Kremer MJ. Biology of oral mucosa and esophagus. JNCI Monogr. 2001;2001(29):7–15.
19. Ficarra G. Manuale di patologia e medicina orale. Milano: McGraw-Hill; 2007.
20. Salem A, et al. Histamine metabolism and transport are deranged in human keratinocytes in oral lichen planus. Br J Dermatol. 2017;176(5):1213–23.
21. Bikle D. Nonclassic actions of vitamin D. J Clin Endocrinol Metab. 2009;94(1):26–34.
22. Zhao B, et al. LPS-induced vitamin D receptor decrease in oral keratinocytes is associated with oral lichen planus. Sci Rep. 2018;8(1):1–9.
23. Zhao B, et al. Vitamin D/VDR signaling suppresses microRNA-802-induced apoptosis of keratinocytes in oral lichen planus. FASEB J. 2019;33(1):1042–50.
24. Deeb KK, Trump DL, Johnson CS. Vitamin D signalling pathways in cancer: potential for anticancer therapeutics. Nat Rev Cancer. 2007;7(9):684–700.
25. Du J, et al. MicroRNA-26a/b have protective roles in oral lichen planus. Cell Death Dis. 2020;11(1):1–13.
26. Ge X, et al. Vitamin D/VDR signaling inhibits LPS-induced IFNγ and IL-1β in Oral epithelia by regulating hypoxia-inducible factor-1α signaling pathway. Cell Commun Signal. 2019;17(1):1–10.
27. Krisanaprakornkit S, et al. Expression of the peptide antibiotic human β-defensin 1 in cultured gingival epithelial cells and gingival tissue. Infect Immun. 1998;66(9):4222–8.
28. Dale BA, et al. Localized antimicrobial peptide expression in human gingiva. J Periodontal Res. 2001;36(5):285–94.
29. Pisano E, et al. Peptides of human gingival crevicular fluid determined by HPLC-ESI-MS. Eur J Oral Sci. 2005;113(6):462–8.
30. Yamauchi M, et al. Myeloid dendritic cells stimulated by thymic stromal lymphopoietin promote Th2 immune responses and the pathogenesis of oral lichen planus. PLoS One. 2017;12(3):e0173017.
31. Carrozzo M. Understanding the pathobiology of oral lichen planus. Curr Oral Health Rep. 2014;1(3):173–9.
32. Dinarello CA. IL-1: discoveries, controversies and future directions. Eur J Immunol. 2010;40(3):599–606.
33. de Voer RM, et al. Germline mutations in the spindle assembly checkpoint genes BUB1 and BUB3 are risk factors for colorectal cancer. Gastroenterology. 2013;145(3):544–7.
34. Dienz O, Rincon M. The effects of IL-6 on CD4 T cell responses. Clin Immunol. 2009;130(1):27–33.
35. Mukaida N. Pathophysiological roles of interleukin-8/CXCL8 in pulmonary diseases. Am J Physiol Lung Cell Mol Physiol. 2003;284(4):L566–77.
36. Saravi ZZ, et al. VEGFR-3 expression in oral lichen planus. Asian Pac J Cancer Prev. 2017;18(2):381.
37. Hervas-Stubbs S, et al. Direct effects of type I interferons on cells of the immune system. Clin Cancer Res. 2011;17(9):2619–27.
38. Monesi V, Adamo S. Istologia. Padova: Piccin; 1975.
39. Mantovani A, et al. The chemokine system in diverse forms of macrophage activation and polarization. Trends Immunol. 2004;25(12):677–86.
40. Pontieri GM, et al. Patologia generale e fisiopatologia generale. Padova: Piccin; 2015.
41. Sugerman PB, Sabage N. Oral lichen planus: causes, diagnosis and management. Aust Dent J. 2002;47(4):290–7.
42. Mozaffari HR, et al. A systematic review and meta-analysis study of salivary and serum interleukin-8 levels in oral lichen planus. Postepy Dermatol Alergol. 2018;35(6):599–604.
43. Vered M, et al. Inflammatory cells of immunosuppressive phenotypes in oral lichen planus have a proinflammatory pattern of expression and are associated with clinical parameters. Clin Oral Investig. 2013;17(5):1365–73.
44. Kurago ZB. Etiology and pathogenesis of oral lichen planus: an overview. Oral Surg Oral Med Oral Pathol Oral Radiol. 2016;122(1):72–80.
45. Parolini S, et al. The role of chemerin in the colocalization of NK and dendritic cell subsets into inflamed tissues. Blood. 2007;109(9):3625–32.
46. Ramalingam S, et al. Role of mast cells in oral lichen planus and oral lichenoid reactions. Autoimmune Dis. 2018;2018:7936564.

47. Galli SJ, Gordon JR, Wershil BK. Cytokine production by mast cells and basophils. Curr Opin Immunol. 1991;3(6):865–73.
48. Salem A, et al. Histamine H4 receptor in oral lichen planus. Oral Dis. 2015;21(3):378–85.
49. Ribatti D, Tamma R, Crivellato E. The dual role of mast cells in tumor fate. Cancer Lett. 2018;433:252–8.
50. De Panfilis G, Manara GC, Allegra F. Remarks on early versus late lichen planus. Arch Dermatol Res. 1981;270(2):163–6.
51. Scully C, El-Kom M. Lichen planus: review and update on pathogenesis. J Oral Pathol Med. 1985;14(6):431–58.
52. Hume W, Potten C. Proliferative units in stratified squamous epithelium. Clin Exp Dermatol. 1983;8(1):95–106.
53. Lichtman AH, Abbas AK, Pillai S. Immunologia cellulare e molecolare. Italia: Elsevier; 2015.
54. Santoro A, et al. Recruitment of dendritic cells in oral lichen planus. J Pathol. 2005;205(4):426–34.
55. Dorrego MV, et al. Oral lichen planus: immunohistology of mucosal lesions. J Oral Pathol Med. 2002;31(7):410–4.
56. Barrett A, Cruchley A, Williams D. Oral mucosal Langerhans' cells. Crit Rev Oral Biol Med. 1996;7(1):36–58.
57. Cruvinel WDM, et al. Immune system: part I. Fundamentals of innate immunity with emphasis on molecular and cellular mechanisms of inflammatory response. Rev Bras Reumatol. 2010;50:434–47.
58. Porter S, et al. Immunologic aspects of dermal and oral lichen planus: a review. Oral Surg Oral Med Oral Pathol Oral Radiol Endod. 1997;83(3):358–66.
59. Mozaffari HR, et al. Serum and salivary IgA, IgG, and IgM levels in oral lichen planus: a systematic review and meta-analysis of case-control studies. Medicina. 2018;54(6):99.
60. Engel P, et al. CD nomenclature 2015: human leukocyte differentiation antigen workshops as a driving force in immunology. J Immunol. 2015;195(10):4555–63.
61. Sugerman PB, et al. Oral lichen planus. Clin Dermatol. 2000;18(5):533–9.
62. Khan A, et al. Th1 cytokines in oral lichen planus. J Oral Pathol Med. 2003;32(2):77–83.
63. Santoro A, et al. NF-κB expression in oral and cutaneous lichen planus. J Pathol. 2003;201(3):466–72.
64. Lage D, et al. Perforin and granzyme B expression in oral and cutaneous lichen planus–a comparative study. J Cutan Pathol. 2011;38(12):973–8.
65. Lu R, et al. Expression of T-bet and GATA-3 in peripheral blood mononuclear cells of patients with oral lichen planus. Arch Oral Biol. 2011;56(5):499–505.
66. Walton L, et al. Intra-epithelial subpopulations of T lymphocytes and Langerhans cells in oral lichen planus. J Oral Pathol Med. 1998;27(3):116–23.
67. Simark-Mattsson C, et al. Distribution of interleukin-2,-4,-10, tumour necrosis factor-α and transforming growth factor-β mRNAs in oral lichen planus. Arch Oral Biol. 1999;44(6):499–507.
68. Karagouni E, Dotsika E, Sklavounou A. Alteration in peripheral blood mononuclear cell function and serum cytokines in oral lichen planus. J Oral Pathol Med. 1994;23(1):28–35.
69. Sontheimer RD. Lichenoid tissue reaction/interface dermatitis: clinical and histological perspectives. J Investig Dermatol. 2009;129(5):1088–99.
70. Piccinni MP, et al. Potential pathogenetic role of Th17, Th0, and Th2 cells in erosive and reticular oral lichen planus. Oral Dis. 2014;20(2):212–8.
71. Alizadeh D, Katsanis E, Larmonier N. The multifaceted role of Th17 lymphocytes and their associated cytokines in cancer. Clin Dev Immunol. 2013;2013:957878.
72. Ivanov II, et al. The orphan nuclear receptor RORγt directs the differentiation program of proinflammatory IL-17+ T helper cells. Cell. 2006;126(6):1121–33.
73. Guglani L, Khader SA. Th17 cytokines in mucosal immunity and inflammation. Curr Opin HIV AIDS. 2010;5(2):120.
74. Tang C, et al. Interleukin-23: as a drug target for autoimmune inflammatory diseases. Immunology. 2012;135(2):112–24.
75. Korn T, et al. IL-17 and Th17 Cells. Annu Rev Immunol. 2009;27:485–517.
76. Muranski P, Restifo NP. Essentials of Th17 cell commitment and plasticity. Blood. 2013;121(13):2402–14.
77. Wilke CM, et al. Deciphering the role of Th17 cells in human disease. Trends Immunol. 2011;32(12):603–11.
78. Tabarkiewicz J, et al. The role of IL-17 and Th17 lymphocytes in autoimmune diseases. Arch Immunol Ther Exp. 2015;63(6):435–49.
79. Cheung PF, Wong CK, Lam CW. Molecular mechanisms of cytokine and chemokine release from eosinophils activated by IL-17A, IL-17F, and IL-23: implication for Th17 lymphocytes-mediated allergic inflammation. J Immunol. 2008;180(8):5625–35.
80. Wang K, et al. Analysis of oral microbial community and Th17-associated cytokines in saliva of patients with oral lichen planus. Microbiol Immunol. 2015;59(3):105–13.
81. Xie S, et al. Implications of Th1 and Th17 cells in pathogenesis of oral lichen planus. J Huazhong Univ Sci Technol Med Sci. 2012;32(3):451–7.
82. Monteiro BV, et al. Immunoexpression of Th17-related cytokines in oral lichen planus. Appl Immunohistochem Mol Morphol. 2015;23(6):409–15.
83. JUNGELL P, et al. Immunoelectron microscopic study of distribution of T cell subsets in oral lichen planus. Eur J Oral Sci. 1989;97(4):361–7.
84. Walsh L, et al. Immunopathogenesis of oral lichen planus. J Oral Pathol Med. 1990;19(9):389–96.

85. Andrea Cavani CA, Girolomoni G. Interferon-γ-stimulated human keratinocytes express the genes necessary for the production of peptide-loaded MHC class II molecules. J Investig Dermatol. 1998;110(2):138–42.
86. Karatsaidis A, et al. Inhibition of the transforming growth factor-β/Smad signaling pathway in the epithelium of oral lichen. J Investig Dermatol. 2003;121(6):1–8.
87. Khan N, et al. Immunopathology of skin lesions. Indian J Dermatol Venereol Leprol. 2001;67(5):234–7.
88. Ichimura M, et al. Expression profile of chemokines and chemokine receptors in epithelial cell layers of oral lichen planus. J Oral Pathol Med. 2006;35(3):167–74.
89. Bascones-Ilundain C, et al. Significance of liquefaction degeneration in oral lichen planus: a study of its relationship with apoptosis and cell cycle arrest markers. Clin Exp Dermatol. 2007;32(5):556–63.
90. Pilli M, et al. Oral lichen planus pathogenesis: a role for the HCV-specific cellular immune response. Hepatology. 2002;36(6):1446–52.
91. Björkström NK, et al. Expression patterns of NKG2A, KIR, and CD57 define a process of CD56dim NK-cell differentiation uncoupled from NK-cell education. Blood. 2010;116(19):3853–64.
92. Moretta L. Dissecting CD56dim human NK cells. Blood. 2010;116(19):3689–91.
93. Carrozzo M, et al. HLA-C/KIR genotypes in oral lichen planus patients infected or non-infected with hepatitis C virus. Oral Dis. 2011;17(3):309–13.
94. Kamal R, et al. Mast cells and oral pathologies: a review. J Nat Sci Biol Med. 2015;6(1):35.
95. Sharma R, et al. Role of mast cells in pathogenesis of oral lichen planus. J Oral Maxillof Pathol. 2011;15(3):267.
96. Jontell M, Hansson HA, Nygren H. Mast cells in oral lichen planus. J Oral Pathol Med. 1986;15(5):273–5.
97. Zhao Z, et al. Immunohistochemical localization of mast cells and mast cell-nerve interactions in oral lichen planus. Oral Dis. 1997;3(2):71–6.
98. Wray D, et al. The role of allergy in oral mucosal diseases. QJM. 2000;93(8):507–11.
99. Zhao Z, et al. Mast cell/T cell interactions in oral lichen planus. J Oral Pathol Med. 2002;31(4):189–95.
100. Masotti L. Endothelial pathophysiology, glycosaminoglycans and glycocalyx. Clin Manag Issues. 2010;4(4S):5–16.
101. Bermejo-Fenoll A, López-Jornet P. Familial oral lichen planus: presentation of six families. Oral Surg Oral Med Oral Pathol Oral Radiol Endod. 2006;102(2):e12–5.
102. Crincoli V, et al. Oral lichen planus: update on etiopathogenesis, diagnosis and treatment. Immunopharmacol Immunotoxicol. 2011;33(1):11–20.
103. Sanchez-Muñoz F, Dominguez-Lopez A, Yamamoto-Furusho JK. Role of cytokines in inflammatory bowel disease. World J Gastroenterol: WJG. 2008;14(27):4280.
104. Preshaw PM, Taylor JJ. How has research into cytokine interactions and their role in driving immune responses impacted our understanding of periodontitis? J Clin Periodontol. 2011;38:60–84.
105. O'Shea JJ, Murray PJ. Cytokine signaling modules in inflammatory responses. Immunity. 2008;28(4):477–87.
106. Roescher N, Tak PP, Illei GG. Cytokines in Sjögren's syndrome. Oral Dis. 2009;15(8):519–26.
107. Moudgil KD, Choubey D. Cytokines in autoimmunity: role in induction, regulation, and treatment. J Interf Cytokine Res. 2011;31(10):695–703.
108. Lu R, et al. Inflammation-related cytokines in oral lichen planus: an overview. J Oral Pathol Med. 2015;44(1):1–14.
109. Rhodus NL, et al. A comparison of the pro-inflammatory, NF-κB-dependent cytokines: TNF-alpha, IL-1-alpha, IL-6, and IL-8 in different oral fluids from oral lichen planus patients. Clin Immunol. 2005;114(3):278–83.
110. Rhodus NL, Cheng B, Ondrey F. Th1/Th2 cytokine ratio in tissue transudates from patients with oral lichen planus. Mediat Inflamm. 2007;2007:19854.
111. Rhodus NL, et al. The feasibility of monitoring NF-κB associated cytokines: TNF-α, IL-1α, IL-6, and IL-8 in whole saliva for the malignant transformation of oral lichen planus. Mol Carcinog. 2005;44(2):77–82.
112. Xavier GM, et al. Investigation of functional gene polymorphisms interleukin-1beta, interleukin-6, interleukin-10 and tumor necrosis factor in individuals with oral lichen planus. J Oral Pathol Med. 2007;36(8):476–81.
113. Carrozzo M, et al. Tumor necrosis factor-alpha and interferon-gamma polymorphisms contribute to susceptibility to oral lichen planus. J Invest Dermatol. 2004;122(1):87–94.
114. Takeuchi Y, et al. Immunohistochemical analysis of cells in mucosal lesions of oral lichen planus. J Oral Pathol Med. 1988;17(8):367–73.
115. Liao W, Lin J-X, Leonard WJ. IL-2 family cytokines: new insights into the complex roles of IL-2 as a broad regulator of T helper cell differentiation. Curr Opin Immunol. 2011;23(5):598–604.
116. Malek TR, Castro I. Interleukin-2 receptor signaling: at the interface between tolerance and immunity. Immunity. 2010;33(2):153–65.
117. Hu J-Y, et al. Increasing CCL5/CCR5 on CD4+ T cells in peripheral blood of oral lichen planus. Cytokine. 2013;62(1):141–5.
118. Kalogerakou F, et al. Detection of T cells secreting type 1 and type 2 cytokines in the peripheral blood of patients with oral lichen planus. Hippokratia. 2008;12(4):230–5.
119. Pekiner FN, et al. Cytokine profiles in serum of patients with oral lichen planus. Cytokine. 2012;60(3):701–6.

120. Amin K. The role of mast cells in allergic inflammation. Respir Med. 2012;106(1):9–14.
121. Tao XA, et al. Simultaneous detection of IFN-gamma and IL-4 in lesional tissues and whole unstimulated saliva from patients with oral lichen planus. J Oral Pathol Med. 2008;37(2):83–7.
122. Bai J, et al. Association of polymorphisms in the human IFN-gamma and IL-4 gene with oral lichen planus: a study in an ethnic Chinese cohort. J Interf Cytokine Res. 2008;28(6):351–8.
123. Yamamoto T, et al. Cellular immunosuppression in oral lichen planus. J Oral Pathol Med. 1990;19(10):464–70.
124. Zhu J, Paul WE. Heterogeneity and plasticity of T helper cells. Cell Res. 2010;20(1):4–12.
125. Takatsu K. Interleukin-5 and IL-5 receptor in health and diseases. Proc Jpn Acad Ser B Phys Biol Sci. 2011;87(8):463–85.
126. Gotoh A, et al. Skew in T cell receptor usage with polyclonal expansion in lesions of oral lichen planus without hepatitis C virus infection. Clin Exp Immunol. 2008;154(2):192–201.
127. Yamamoto T, Osaki T. Characteristic cytokines generated by keratinocytes and mononuclear infiltrates in oral lichen planus. J Investig Dermatol. 1995;104(5):784–8.
128. Rhodus N, et al. Proinflammatory cytokine levels in saliva before and after treatment of (erosive) oral lichen planus with dexamethasone. Oral Dis. 2006;12(2):112–6.
129. Kamimura D, Ishihara K, Hirano T. IL-6 signal transduction and its physiological roles: the signal orchestration model. Rev Physiol Biochem Pharmacol. 2003;149:1–38.
130. Abdel-Haq A, et al. Interleukin-6 and neopterin levels in the serum and saliva of patients with Lichen planus and oral Lichen planus. J Oral Pathol Med. 2014;43(10):734–9.
131. Yin M, et al. Identifying the association between interleukin-6 and lichen planus: a meta-analysis. Biomed Rep. 2017;6(5):571–5.
132. Sun A, et al. Serum interleukin-6 level is a useful marker in evaluating therapeutic effects of levamisole and Chinese medicinal herbs on patients with oral lichen planus. J Oral Pathol Med. 2002;31(4):196–203.
133. Zhang Y, et al. NF-kappaB-dependent cytokines in saliva and serum from patients with oral lichen planus: a study in an ethnic Chinese population. Cytokine. 2008;41(2):144–9.
134. Sun A, et al. Serum interleukin-8 level is a more sensitive marker than serum interleukin-6 level in monitoring the disease activity of oral lichen planus. Br J Dermatol. 2005;152(6):1187–92.
135. Ohno S, et al. Enhanced expression of Toll-like receptor 2 in lesional tissues and peripheral blood monocytes of patients with oral lichen planus. J Dermatol. 2011;38(4):335–44.
136. Gee K, et al. The IL-12 family of cytokines in infection, inflammation and autoimmune disorders. Inflamm Allergy Drug Targets. 2009;8(1):40–52.
137. Müller G, et al. Identification and induction of human keratinocyte-derived IL-12. J Clin Invest. 1994;94(5):1799–805.
138. Huang Y, Zhou S, Cai Y. Expression of interleukin-12 and interleukin-27 proteins and immune status in serum of patients with oral lichen planus. Hua Xi Kou Qiang Yi Xue Za Zhi. 2016;34(2):140–4.
139. Janardhanam SB, et al. Differential expression of TLR-2 and TLR-4 in the epithelial cells in oral lichen planus. Arch Oral Biol. 2012;57(5):495–502.
140. Tao XA, et al. Differential gene expression profiles of whole lesions from patients with oral lichen planus. J Oral Pathol Med. 2009;38(5):427–33.
141. Shirazian S, et al. Comparison of interleukin 17 and 22 in saliva of oral lichen planus patients with healthy people. Biosci Biotechnol Res Commun. 2017;10:587–91.
142. Gueiros LA, et al. IL17A polymorphism and elevated IL17A serum levels are associated with oral lichen planus. Oral Dis. 2018;24(3):377–83.
143. Chen Q, Cai Y, Feng Q. Expression of IFN-γ, IL-4 and IL-1 7 proteins in peripheral blood of patients with oral lichen planu. J Pract Stomatol. 2014:698–700.
144. Wang R, et al. Re-evaluation of transcription factor function in tomato fruit development and ripening with CRISPR/Cas9-mutagenesis. Sci Rep. 2019;9(1):1–10.
145. Boraschi D, Dinarello CA. IL-18 in autoimmunity. Eur Cytokine Netw. 2006;17(4):224–52.
146. Zhang Y, et al. Salivary and serum interleukin-18 in patients with oral lichen planus: a study in an ethnic Chinese population. Inflammation. 2012;35(2):399–404.
147. Negi D, et al. Assessment of Interleukin-18 gene polymorphism and serum levels in oral lichen planus in an Indian population. J Oral Pathol Med. 2019;48(3):244–50.
148. Mardani M, et al. Serum levels of IL-22 in patients with oral lichen planus and cutaneous lichen planus. J Dent. 2020;21(4):330.
149. Kurchenko A, et al. Assessment of select serum cytokines TNF-A and IL-22 in oral lichen planus patients. Ann Allergy Asthma Immunol. 2018;121(5):S50.
150. Lanfranchi-Tizeira HE, Aguas SC, Sano SM. Malignant transformation of atypical oral lichen planus: a review of 32 cases. Med Oral. 2003;8(1):2–9.
151. Abbate G, et al. Neoplastic transformation of oral lichen: case report and review of the literature. Acta Otorhinolaryngol Ital. 2006;26(1):47.
152. Chen Y, et al. 1, 25-Dihydroxyvitamin D promotes negative feedback regulation of TLR signaling via targeting MicroRNA-155–SOCS1 in macrophages. J Immunol. 2013;190(7):3687–95.
153. Lu R, et al. Overexpression and selectively regulatory roles of IL-23/IL-17 axis in the

lesions of oral lichen planus. Mediat Inflamm. 2014;2014:701094.
154. Tan ZY, et al. Interleukin-23: immunological roles and clinical implications. Int J Biochem Cell Biol. 2009;41(4):733–5.
155. Wang K, et al. Preliminary analysis of salivary microbiome and their potential roles in oral lichen planus. Sci Rep. 2016;6(1):1–10.
156. Yamamoto T, et al. Cytokine production by keratinocytes and mononuclear infiltrates in oral lichen planus. J Oral Pathol Med. 1994;23(7):309–15.
157. Bai J, et al. Association of polymorphisms in the tumor necrosis factor-alpha and interleukin-10 genes with oral lichen planus: a study in a chinese cohort with Han ethnicity. J Interf Cytokine Res. 2009;29(7):381–8.
158. Al-Mohaya MA, et al. TNF-α, TNF-β and IL-10 gene polymorphism and association with oral lichen planus risk in Saudi patients. J Appl Oral Sci. 2015;23(3):295–301.
159. Ciccia F, et al. Potential involvement of IL-22 and IL-22-producing cells in the inflamed salivary glands of patients with Sjögren's syndrome. Ann Rheum Dis. 2012;71(2):295–301.
160. Ghilardi N, Ouyang W. Targeting the development and effector functions of TH17 cells. In: Seminars in immunology. London: Elsevier; 2007.
161. Wang H, et al. Interaction between oral lichen planus and chronic periodontitis with Th17-associated cytokines in serum. Inflammation. 2013;36(3):696–704.
162. Thongprasom K, et al. Expression of TNF-α in oral lichen planus treated with fluocinolone acetonide 0.1%. J Oral Pathol Med. 2006;35(3):161–6.
163. Nandhini J, et al. Estimation of the level of salivary proinflammatory cytokine in oral lichen planus–A case–control study in cuddalore-based population. J Indian Acad Oral Med Radiol. 2019;31(2):128.
164. Qidwai T, Khan F. Tumour necrosis factor gene polymorphism and disease prevalence. Scand J Immunol. 2011;74(6):522–47.
165. Liu W, et al. IFN-gamma and IL-4 in saliva of patients with oral lichen planus: a study in an ethnic Chinese population. Inflammation. 2009;32(3):176–81.
166. Mozaffari HR, et al. Serum and salivary interleukin-4 levels in patients with oral lichen planus: a systematic review and meta-analysis. Oral Surg Oral Med Oral Pathol Oral Radiol. 2019;128(2):123–31.
167. Dan H, et al. Elevated IL-10 concentrations in serum and saliva from patients with oral lichen planus. Quintessence Int. 2011;42(2):157–63.
168. Sugermann P, et al. Is there a role for tumor necrosis factor-alpha (TNF-α) in oral lichen planus? J Oral Pathol Med. 1996;25(5):219–24.
169. Kimkong I, et al. Tumour necrosis factor-alpha gene polymorphisms and susceptibility to oral lichen planus. Oral Dis. 2011;17(2):206–9.
170. O'Neill ID. Off-label use of biologicals in the management of inflammatory oral mucosal disease. J Oral Pathol Med. 2008;37(10):575–81.
171. O'Neill I, Scully C. Biologics in oral medicine: ulcerative disorders. Oral Dis. 2013;19(1):37–45.
172. Bradley J. TNF-mediated inflammatory disease. J Pathol. 2008;214(2):149–60.
173. Azab NA, et al. Interferon gamma and interleukin 8 gene polymorphisms in patients with hepatitis C virus related oral lichen planus. Arch Oral Biol. 2018;96:189–94.
174. Prime S, et al. TGF-β signal transduction in orofacial health and non-malignant disease (part I). Crit Rev Oral Biol Med. 2004;15(6):324–36.
175. Cui-jie W, et al. Correlation of Treg and IL-15 expression in the peripheral blood of patients with oral lichen planus. Shanghai J Stomatol. 2016;25(4):438.
176. Dinarello CA, Simon A, Van Der Meer JW. Treating inflammation by blocking interleukin-1 in a broad spectrum of diseases. Nat Rev Drug Discov. 2012;11(8):633–52.
177. Gabay C, Lamacchia C, Palmer G. IL-1 pathways in inflammation and human diseases. Nat Rev Rheumatol. 2010;6(4):232–41.
178. Sims JE, Smith DE. The IL-1 family: regulators of immunity. Nat Rev Immunol. 2010;10(2):89–102.
179. Ge Y, et al. The molecular mechanisms of the effect of Dexamethasone and Cyclosporin A on TLR4/NF-κB signaling pathway activation in oral lichen planus. Gene. 2012;508(2):157–64.
180. Femiano F, Scully C. Functions of the cytokines in relation oral lichen planus-hepatitis C. Med Oral Patol Oral Cir Bucal. 2005;10(Suppl 1):E40–4.
181. Malek TR. The biology of interleukin-2. Annu Rev Immunol. 2008;26:453–79.
182. Banchereau J, Pascual V, O'garra A. From IL-2 to IL-37: the expanding spectrum of anti-inflammatory cytokines. Nat Immunol. 2012;13(10):925–31.
183. Mozzanica N, et al. Immunohistologic evaluation of the effect of cyclosporine treatment on the lichen planus immune infiltrate. J Am Acad Dermatol. 1991;24(4):550–4.
184. Du GH, et al. The high expression level of programmed death-1 ligand 2 in oral lichen planus and the possible costimulatory effect on human T cells. J Oral Pathol Med. 2011;40(7):525–32.
185. Zhou G, et al. Increased B7-H1 expression on peripheral blood T cells in oral lichen planus correlated with disease severity. J Clin Immunol. 2012;32(4):794–801.
186. Paul WE, Zhu J. How are T(H)2-type immune responses initiated and amplified? Nat Rev Immunol. 2010;10(4):225–35.
187. Zhu LY, et al. Essential role of IL-4 and IL-4Rα interaction in adaptive immunity of zebrafish: insight into the origin of Th2-like regulatory mechanism in ancient vertebrates. J Immunol. 2012;188(11):5571–84.
188. Johnson DJ, et al. Shp1 regulates T cell homeostasis by limiting IL-4 signals. J Exp Med. 2013;210(7):1419–31.
189. Cooney LA, et al. Sensitivity and resistance to regulation by IL-4 during Th17 maturation. J Immunol. 2011;187(9):4440–50.
190. Ding M, et al. Interactions between Golli-MBP and Th1/Th2 cytokines in patients with oral lichen planus. Oral Dis. 2014;20(2):205–11.

191. Kouro T, Takatsu K. IL-5- and eosinophil-mediated inflammation: from discovery to therapy. Int Immunol. 2009;21(12):1303–9.
192. Kishimoto T. IL-6: from its discovery to clinical applications. Int Immunol. 2010;22(5):347–52.
193. Gu GM, et al. Oral and serum IL-6 levels in oral lichen planus patients. Oral Surg Oral Med Oral Pathol Oral Radiol Endod. 2004;98(6):673–8.
194. Kho H-S, et al. MUC1 and Toll-like receptor-2 expression in burning mouth syndrome and oral lichen planus. Arch Oral Biol. 2013;58(7):837–42.
195. Fayyazi A, et al. T lymphocytes and altered keratinocytes express interferon-gamma and interleukin 6 in lichen planus. Arch Dermatol Res. 1999;291(9):485–90.
196. Goel S, et al. Role of serum interleukin-6 in deciding therapy for multidrug resistant oral lichen planus. J Clin Exp Dent. 2015;7(4):e477–82.
197. Matsushima K, et al. Molecular cloning of a human monocyte-derived neutrophil chemotactic factor (MDNCF) and the induction of MDNCF mRNA by interleukin 1 and tumor necrosis factor. J Exp Med. 1988;167(6):1883–93.
198. Trompezinski S, et al. Comparative effects of polyphenols from green tea (EGCG) and soybean (genistein) on VEGF and IL-8 release from normal human keratinocytes stimulated with the proinflammatory cytokine TNFalpha. Arch Dermatol Res. 2003;295(3):112–6.
199. Simone RE, et al. Lycopene inhibits NF-kB-mediated IL-8 expression and changes redox and PPARγ signalling in cigarette smoke-stimulated macrophages. PLoS One. 2011;6(5):e19652.
200. Waugh DJ, Wilson C. The interleukin-8 pathway in cancer. Clin Cancer Res. 2008;14(21):6735–41.
201. Little MC, et al. Oral mucosal keratinocytes express RANTES and ICAM-1, but not interleukin-8, in oral lichen planus and oral lichenoid reactions induced by amalgam fillings. Clin Exp Dermatol. 2003;28(1):64–9.
202. Mahmoud MM, Afifi MM. Anti-angiogenic therapy (bevacizumab) in the management of oral lichen planus. Eur J Oral Sci. 2016;124(2):119–26.
203. Dan H, et al. Association of interleukin-8 gene polymorphisms and haplotypes with oral lichen planus in a Chinese population. Inflammation. 2010;33(2):76–81.
204. Ouyang W, et al. Regulation and functions of the IL-10 family of cytokines in inflammation and disease. Annu Rev Immunol. 2011;29:71–109.
205. Sabat R, et al. Biology of interleukin-10. Cytokine Growth Factor Rev. 2010;21(5):331–44.
206. Saraiva M, O'Garra A. The regulation of IL-10 production by immune cells. Nat Rev Immunol. 2010;10(3):170–81.
207. Lavaee F, et al. The evaluation of the serum level of IL-10 in OLP patients. Comp Clin Pathol. 2018;27(1):131–4.
208. Stephens JC, et al. Haplotype variation and linkage disequilibrium in 313 human genes. Science. 2001;293(5529):489–93.
209. Del Vecchio M, et al. Interleukin-12: biological properties and clinical application. Clin Cancer Res. 2007;13(16):4677–85.
210. Constant SL, Bottomly K. Induction of Th1 and Th2 CD4+ T cell responses: the alternative approaches. Annu Rev Immunol. 1997;15:297–322.
211. Kang K, et al. IL-12 synthesis by human Langerhans cells. J Immunol. 1996;156(4):1402–7.
212. Jiang C, et al. Association of interleukin 12A gene polymorphisms with oral lichen planus in Chinese population. J Oral Pathol Med. 2015;44(8):602–6.
213. Onishi RM, Gaffen SL. Interleukin-17 and its target genes: mechanisms of interleukin-17 function in disease. Immunology. 2010;129(3):311–21.
214. Yu JJ, Gaffen SL. Interleukin-17: a novel inflammatory cytokine that bridges innate and adaptive immunity. Front Biosci. 2008;13:170–7.
215. Cosmi L, et al. Evidence of the transient nature of the Th17 phenotype of CD4+CD161+ T cells in the synovial fluid of patients with juvenile idiopathic arthritis. Arthritis Rheum. 2011;63(8):2504–15.
216. Lee YK, et al. Late developmental plasticity in the T helper 17 lineage. Immunity. 2009;30(1):92–107.
217. Cosmi L, et al. Human interleukin 17-producing cells originate from a CD161+CD4+ T cell precursor. J Exp Med. 2008;205(8):1903–16.
218. Shen Z, et al. Expression of Foxp3 and interleukin-17 in lichen planus lesions with emphasis on difference in oral and cutaneous variants. Arch Dermatol Res. 2014;306(5):441–6.
219. Firth FA, et al. Regulation of immune cells in oral lichen planus. Arch Dermatol Res. 2015;307(4):333–9.
220. Wang J, et al. Long non-coding RNA DQ786243 modulates the induction and function of CD4(+) Treg cells through Foxp3-miR-146a-NF-κB axis: implications for alleviating oral lichen planus. Int Immunopharmacol. 2019;75:105761.
221. Ge X, et al. Renin promotes STAT4 phosphorylation to induce IL-17 production in keratinocytes of oral lichen planus. iScience. 2020;23(4):100983.
222. Liang J, et al. Correlation of miRNA-155 and IL-17 mRNA expression in peripheral blood of female patients with oral lichen planus. Int J Clin Exp Med. 2016;9(10):10569–74.
223. Hussine AA, et al. EVALUATION OF THE POSSIBLE ROLE OF IL-17 AND ITS RECEPTOR IL-17R IN THE PATHOGENESIS OF ORAL LICHEN PLANUS. Al-Azhar J Dental Sci. 2016;19(1):1–8.
224. Liu J, et al. Association of IL-17A and IL-17F polymorphisms with gastric cancer risk in Asians: a meta-analysis. Hum Immunol. 2015;76(1):6–12.
225. Zhang X, et al. Genetic polymorphisms of interleukin 17A and interleukin 17F and their association with inflammatory bowel disease in a Chinese Han population. Inflamm Res. 2013;62(8):743–50.
226. Hammad A, et al. Interleukin-17A rs2275913, Interleukin-17F rs763780 and rs2397084 gene polymorphisms as possible risk factors in Juvenile

lupus and lupus related nephritis. Autoimmunity. 2016;49(1):31–40.
227. Shi G, Zhang L. Influence of interleukin-17 gene polymorphisms on the development of pulmonary tuberculosis. Genet Mol Res. 2015;14(3):8526–31.
228. Smith DE. The biological paths of IL-1 family members IL-18 and IL-33. J Leukoc Biol. 2011;89(3):383–92.
229. Orozco A, et al. Interleukin 18 and periodontal disease. J Dent Res. 2007;86(7):586–93.
230. Bai J, et al. Interleukin-18 gene polymorphisms and haplotypes in patients with oral lichen planus: a study in an ethnic Chinese cohort. Tissue Antigens. 2007;70(5):390–7.
231. Perusina Lanfranca M, et al. Biological and pathological activities of interleukin-22. J Mol Med. 2016;94(5):523–34.
232. Eyerich S, et al. Th22 cells represent a distinct human T cell subset involved in epidermal immunity and remodeling. J Clin Invest. 2009;119(12):3573–85.
233. Zhu J, Yamane H, Paul WE. Differentiation of effector CD4 T cell populations. Annu Rev Immunol. 2010;28:445.
234. Ghoreschi K, et al. Generation of pathogenic TH17 cells in the absence of TGF-β signalling. Nature. 2010;467(7318):967–71.
235. Parks OB, et al. Interleukin-22 signaling in the regulation of intestinal health and disease. Front Cell Dev Biol. 2016;3:85.
236. Lu Z, et al. MicroRNAs: new regulators of IL-22. Cell Immunol. 2016;304:1–8.
237. Yu R, et al. IL-22 mediates the oral mucosal wound healing via STAT3 in keratinocytes. Arch Oral Biol. 2016;72:14–20.
238. Van Belle AB, et al. IL-22 is required for imiquimod-induced psoriasiform skin inflammation in mice. J Immunol. 2012;188(1):462–9.
239. Fujita H. The role of IL-22 and Th22 cells in human skin diseases. J Dermatol Sci. 2013;72(1):3–8.
240. Kim C, et al. A role for mucosal IL-22 production and Th22 cells in HIV-associated mucosal immunopathogenesis. Mucosal Immunol. 2012;5(6):670–80.
241. Radaeva S, et al. Interleukin 22 (IL-22) plays a protective role in T cell-mediated murine hepatitis: IL-22 is a survival factor for hepatocytes via STAT3 activation. Hepatology. 2004;39(5):1332–42.
242. De Luca A, et al. IL-22 defines a novel immune pathway of antifungal resistance. Mucosal Immunol. 2010;3(4):361–73.
243. Yang X, Zheng SG. Interleukin-22: a likely target for treatment of autoimmune diseases. Autoimmun Rev. 2014;13(6):615–20.
244. Pan H-F, et al. Emerging role of interleukin-22 in autoimmune diseases. Cytokine Growth Factor Rev. 2013;24(1):51–7.
245. Zhao M, Li Y, Xiao W. Anti-apoptotic effect of interleukin-22 on fibroblast-like synoviocytes in patients with rheumatoid arthritis is mediated via the signal transducer and activator of transcription 3 signaling pathway. Int J Rheum Dis. 2017;20(2):214–24.
246. Pennino D, et al. IL-22 suppresses IFN-γ–mediated lung inflammation in asthmatic patients. J Allergy Clin Immunol. 2013;131(2):562–70.
247. Basu R, et al. Th22 cells are an important source of IL-22 for host protection against enteropathogenic bacteria. Immunity. 2012;37(6):1061–75.
248. Croxford AL, Mair F, Becher B. IL-23: one cytokine in control of autoimmunity. Eur J Immunol. 2012;42(9):2263–73.
249. Chen J, et al. Immunoexpression of interleukin-22 and interleukin-23 in oral and cutaneous lichen planus lesions: a preliminary study. Mediat Inflamm. 2013;2013:801974.
250. Dong C. TH17 cells in development: an updated view of their molecular identity and genetic programming. Nat Rev Immunol. 2008;8(5):337–48.
251. McGeachy MJ, et al. The interleukin 23 receptor is essential for the terminal differentiation of interleukin 17–producing effector T helper cells in vivo. Nat Immunol. 2009;10(3):314–24.
252. Toussirot É. The IL23/Th17 pathway as a therapeutic target in chronic inflammatory diseases. Inflamm Allergy Drug Targets. 2012;11(2):159–68.
253. Hillyer P, et al. Investigating the role of the interleukin-23/-17A axis in rheumatoid arthritis. Rheumatology. 2009;48(12):1581–9.
254. Kryczek I, et al. Induction of IL-17+ T cell trafficking and development by IFN-γ: mechanism and pathological relevance in psoriasis. J Immunol. 2008;181(7):4733–41.
255. Larsen JM, et al. IL-23 and TH17-mediated inflammation in human allergic contact dermatitis. J Allergy Clin Immunol. 2009;123(2):486–492.e1.
256. Geremia A, Jewell DP. The IL-23/IL-17 pathway in inflammatory bowel disease. Expert Rev Gastroenterol Hepatol. 2012;6(2):223–37.
257. Yen D, et al. IL-23 is essential for T cell–mediated colitis and promotes inflammation via IL-17 and IL-6. J Clin Invest. 2006;116(5):1310–6.
258. Hölttä V, et al. IL-23/IL-17 immunity as a hallmark of Crohn's disease. Inflamm Bowel Dis. 2008;14(9):1175–84.
259. Ohyama H, et al. The involvement of IL-23 and the Th17 pathway in periodontitis. J Dent Res. 2009;88(7):633–8.
260. Lester SR, et al. Gingival concentrations of interleukin-23 and-17 at healthy sites and at sites of clinical attachment loss. J Periodontol. 2007;78(8):1545–50.
261. Zheng Y, et al. Interleukin-22 mediates early host defense against attaching and effacing bacterial pathogens. Nat Med. 2008;14(3):282–9.
262. Silva LC, Ortigosa LC, Benard G. Anti-TNF-α agents in the treatment of immune-mediated inflammatory diseases: mechanisms of action and pitfalls. Immunotherapy. 2010;2(6):817–33.

263. Parameswaran N, Patial S. Tumor necrosis factor-α signaling in macrophages. Crit Rev Eukaryot Gene Expr. 2010;20(2):87–103.
264. Postal M, Appenzeller S. The role of tumor necrosis factor-alpha (TNF-α) in the pathogenesis of systemic lupus erythematosus. Cytokine. 2011;56(3):537–43.
265. Schottelius AJ, et al. Biology of tumor necrosis factor-α–implications for psoriasis. Exp Dermatol. 2004;13(4):193–222.
266. Younes F, et al. Expression of TNF and the 55-kDa TNF receptor in epidermis, oral mucosa, lichen planus and squamous cell carcinoma. Oral Dis. 1996;2(1):25–31.
267. Sklavounou-Andrikopoulou A, et al. Elevated serum levels of the apoptosis related molecules TNF-α, Fas/Apo-1 and Bcl-2 in oral lichen planus. J Oral Pathol Med. 2004;33(7):386–90.
268. Karatsaidis A, et al. Survival signalling in keratinocytes of erythematous oral lichen planus. J Oral Pathol Med. 2007;36(4):215–22.
269. Zhou G, et al. Activation of nuclear factor-kappa B correlates with tumor necrosis factor-alpha in oral lichen planus: a clinicopathologic study in atrophic-erosive and reticular form. J Oral Pathol Med. 2009;38(7):559–64.
270. Pezelj-Ribaric S, et al. Salivary levels of tumor necrosis factor-α in oral lichen planus. Mediat Inflamm. 2004;13(2):131–3.
271. Ghallab NA, El-Wakeel N, Shaker OG. Levels of salivary IFN-gamma, TNF-alfa, and TNF receptor-2 as prognostic markers in (erosive) oral lichen planus. Mediat Inflamm. 2010;2010:847632.
272. Zhou ZT, Wei BJ, Shi P. Osteopontin expression in oral lichen planus. J Oral Pathol Med. 2008;37(2):94–8.
273. Yamamoto T, et al. Serum cytokine levels in patients with oral mucous membrane disorders. J Oral Pathol Med. 1991;20(6):275–9.
274. Yamamoto T, et al. Serum cytokines, interleukin-2 receptor, and soluble intercellular adhesion molecule-1 in oral disorders. Oral Surg Oral Med Oral Pathol. 1994;78(6):727–35.
275. Sun A, et al. Levamisole can reduce the high serum tumour necrosis factor-α level to a normal level in patients with erosive oral lichen planus. Clin Exp Dermatol. 2007;32(3):308–10.
276. Akpınar Kara Y. The measurement of serum TNF-α levels in patients with lichen planus. Acta Dermatovenerol Alp Pannonica Adriat. 2017;26(4):85–8.
277. Simark-Mattsson C, Eklund C. Reduced immune responses to purified protein derivative and C andida albicans in oral lichen planus. J Oral Pathol Med. 2013;42(9):691–7.
278. Mozaffari HR, et al. Salivary and serum levels of tumor necrosis factor-alpha in oral lichen planus: a systematic review and meta-analysis study. Oral Surg Oral Med Oral Pathol Oral Radiol. 2017;124(3):e183–9.
279. Chauhan I, et al. Association of cytokine gene polymorphisms with oral lichen planus in Malayalam-speaking ethnicity from South India (Kerala). J Interf Cytokine Res. 2013;33(8):420–7.
280. Carrozzo M, et al. Cytokine gene polymorphisms in hepatitis C virus-related oral lichen planus. Exp Dermatol. 2007;16(9):730–6.
281. Jin X, et al. Association between-308 G/A polymorphism in TNF-α gene and lichen planus: a meta-analysis. J Dermatol Sci. 2012;68(3):127–34.
282. Zhou Y, Vieira AR. Association between TNFα-308 G/A polymorphism and oral lichen planus (OLP): a meta-analysis. J Appl Oral Sci. 2018;26:e20170184.
283. Zhang J, et al. Biologics, an alternative therapeutic approach for oral lichen planus. J Oral Pathol Med. 2011;40(7):521–4.
284. Worsnop F, et al. Reaction to biological drugs: infliximab for the treatment of toxic epidermal necrolysis subsequently triggering erosive lichen planus. Clin Exp Dermatol. 2012;37(8):879–81.
285. Schroder K, et al. Interferon-γ: an overview of signals, mechanisms and functions. J Leukoc Biol. 2004;75(2):163–89.
286. Hu X, Ivashkiv LB. Cross-regulation of signaling pathways by interferon-γ: implications for immune responses and autoimmune diseases. Immunity. 2009;31(4):539–50.
287. Szabo SJ, et al. Molecular mechanisms regulating Th1 immune responses. Annu Rev Immunol. 2003;21:713.
288. Hwang ES, et al. T helper cell fate specified by kinase-mediated interaction of T-bet with GATA-3. Science. 2005;307(5708):430–3.
289. Kelchtermans H, et al. Effector mechanisms of interleukin-17 in collagen-induced arthritis in the absence of interferon-γ and counteraction by interferon-γ. Arthritis Res Ther. 2009;11(4):1–13.
290. Kelchtermans H, Billiau A, Matthys P. How interferon-γ keeps autoimmune diseases in check. Trends Immunol. 2008;29(10):479–86.
291. Mattsson CS, et al. Distribution of interferon-γ mRNA-positive cells in oral lichen planus lesions. J Oral Pathol Med. 1998;27(10):483–8.
292. Youngnak-Piboonratanakit P, et al. Expression of IFN-γ before and after treatment of oral lichen planus with 0.1% fluocinolone acetonide in orabase. J Oral Pathol Med. 2009;38(9):689–94.
293. Colobran R, et al. The chemokine network. II. On how polymorphisms and alternative splicing increase the number of molecular species and configure intricate patterns of disease susceptibility. Clin Exp Immunol. 2007;150(1):1–12.
294. Kimkong I, et al. Association of interferon-gamma gene polymorphisms with susceptibility to oral lichen planus in the Thai population. Arch Oral Biol. 2012;57(5):491–4.
295. Akhurst RJ, Hata A. Targeting the TGFβ signalling pathway in disease. Nat Rev Drug Discov. 2012;11(10):790–811.
296. Kubiczkova L, et al. TGF-β–an excellent servant but a bad master. J Transl Med. 2012;10(1):1–24.

297. Simark-Mattsson C, et al. Distribution of interleukin-2, -4, -10, tumour necrosis factor-alpha and transforming growth factor-beta mRNAs in oral lichen planus. Arch Oral Biol. 1999;44(6):499–507.
298. Zhang J, Zhou G. Green tea consumption: an alternative approach to managing oral lichen planus. Inflamm Res. 2012;61(6):535–9.
299. Chen Y, et al. MMPs, TIMP-2, and TGF-β1 in the cancerization of oral lichen planus. Head Neck. 2008;30(9):1237–45.
300. Taghavi ZA, et al. Evaluation of serum TNF-α and TGF-β in patients with oral lichen planus: serum markers in oral lichen planus. J Dental Res Dental Clin Dent Prospects. 2012;6(4):143–7.
301. Tan YQ, et al. Increased circulating CXCR 5+ CD 4+ T follicular helper-like cells in oral lichen planus. J Oral Pathol Med. 2017;46(9):803–9.
302. Wang H, et al. IL-25 promotes Th2-type reactions and correlates with disease severity in the pathogenesis of oral lichen planus. Arch Oral Biol. 2019;98:115–21.
303. Javvadi L, et al. Expression of IL33 and IL35 in oral lichen planus. Arch Dermatol Res. 2018;310(5):431–41.
304. De Carvalho MFMS, et al. Cytokines levels and salivary microbiome play a potential role in oral lichen planus diagnosis. Sci Rep. 2019;9(1):1–10.
305. Messer G, et al. Polymorphic structure of the tumor necrosis factor (TNF) locus: an NcoI polymorphism in the first intron of the human TNF-beta gene correlates with a variant amino acid in position 26 and a reduced level of TNF-beta production. J Exp Med. 1991;173(1):209–19.
306. Godessart N, Kunkel SL. Chemokines in autoimmune disease. Curr Opin Immunol. 2001;13(6):670–5.
307. Bombeccari GP, et al. Ruolo delle epatopatie nella fase acuta del lichen planus orale. Dental Cadmos. 2012;80(4):171–81.
308. Lebre MC, et al. Differential expression of inflammatory chemokines by Th1-and Th2-cell promoting dendritic cells: a role for different mature dendritic cell populations in attracting appropriate effector cells to peripheral sites of inflammation. Immunol Cell Biol. 2005;83(5):525–35.
309. Iijima W, et al. Infiltrating CD8+ T cells in oral lichen planus predominantly express CCR5 and CXCR3 and carry respective chemokine ligands RANTES/CCL5 and IP-10/CXCL10 in their cytolytic granules: a potential self-recruiting mechanism. Am J Pathol. 2003;163(1):261–8.
310. Vu TH, Werb Z. Matrix metalloproteinases: effectors of development and normal physiology. Genes Dev. 2000;14(17):2123–33.
311. Bode W, et al. Insights into MMP-TIMP interactions. Ann N Y Acad Sci. 1999;878(1):73–91.
312. Saklatvala J, et al. Structural basis of matrix metalloproteinase function. In: Biochemical society symposia. Cambridge: Portland Press; 2003.
313. Sutinen M, et al. Expression of matrix metalloproteinases (MMP-1 and-2) and their inhibitors (TIMP-1,-2 and-3) in oral lichen planus, dysplasia, squamous cell carcinoma and lymph node metastasis. Br J Cancer. 1998;77(12):2239–45.
314. Rubaci AH, et al. The roles of matrix metalloproteinases-2,-7,-10 and tissue inhibitor of metalloproteinase-1 in the pathogenesis of oral lichen planus. J Oral Pathol Med. 2012;41(9):689–96.
315. Mazzarella N, et al. Matrix metalloproteinase gene expression in oral lichen planus: erosive vs. reticular forms. J Eur Acad Dermatol Venereol. 2006;20(8):953–7.
316. De Iudicibus S, et al. Molecular mechanism of glucocorticoid resistance in inflammatory bowel disease. World J Gastroenterol: WJG. 2011;17(9):1095.
317. Li CC, et al. Suppression of dendritic cell-derived IL-12 by endogenous glucocorticoids is protective in LPS-induced sepsis. PLoS Biol. 2015;13(10):e1002269.
318. Galon J, et al. Gene profiling reveals unknown enhancing and suppressive actions of glucocorticoids on immune cells. FASEB J. 2002;16(1):61–71.
319. Nicolaides NC, et al. Recent advances in the molecular mechanisms determining tissue sensitivity to glucocorticoids: novel mutations, circadian rhythm and ligand-induced repression of the human glucocorticoid receptor. BMC Endocr Disord. 2014;14(1):1–12.
320. Hearing SD, et al. Wide variation in lymphocyte steroid sensitivity among healthy human volunteers. J Clin Endocrinol Metab. 1999;84(11):4149–54.
321. Creed TJ, et al. The effects of cytokines on suppression of lymphocyte proliferation by dexamethasone. J Immunol. 2009;183(1):164–71.
322. Wang L, et al. MicroRNA microarray-based identification of involvement of miR-155 and miR-19a in development of oral lichen planus (OLP) by modulating Th1/Th2 balance via targeting eNOS and toll-like receptor 2 (TLR2). Med Sci Monit. 2018;24:3591.
323. Ma F, et al. The microRNA miR-29 controls innate and adaptive immune responses to intracellular bacterial infection by targeting interferon-γ. Nat Immunol. 2011;12(9):861–9.
324. Urbanek MO, Nawrocka AU, Krzyzosiak WJ. Small RNA detection by in situ hybridization methods. Int J Mol Sci. 2015;16(6):13259–86.
325. Liu M, et al. TNF-α is a novel target of miR-19a. Int J Oncol. 2011;38(4):1013–22.
326. Stanczyk J, et al. Altered expression of microRNA-203 in rheumatoid arthritis synovial fibroblasts and its role in fibroblast activation. Arthritis Rheum. 2011;63(2):373–81.
327. Cui Y. In silico mapping of polymorphic miRNA–mRNA interactions in autoimmune thyroid diseases. Autoimmunity. 2014;47(5):327–33.
328. Wu D, et al. Association of single nucleotide polymorphisms in MPO and COX genes with oral lichen planus. Int J Immunogenet. 2015;42(3):161–7.
329. Zhou Q, et al. Decreased expression of miR-146a and miR-155 contributes to an abnormal Treg phe-

notype in patients with rheumatoid arthritis. Ann Rheum Dis. 2015;74(6):1265–74.
330. Banerjee A, et al. Micro-RNA-155 inhibits IFN-γ signaling in CD4+ T cells. Eur J Immunol. 2010;40(1):225–31.
331. Gassling V, et al. Disease-associated miRNA-mRNA networks in oral lichen planus. PLoS One. 2013;8(5):e63015.
332. Liu F, Wu J, Ye F. Expression of miRNA-155 and miRNA-146a in peripheral blood mononuclear cells and plasma of oral lichen planus patients. Zhonghua Kou Qiang Yi Xue Za Zhi=Chinese J Stomatol. 2015;50(1):23–7.
333. Arão TC, et al. Increased miRNA-146a and miRNA-155 expressions in oral lichen planus. Arch Dermatol Res. 2012;304(5):371–5.
334. Ma H, et al. MicroRNAs in oral lichen planus and potential miRNA–mRNA pathogenesis with essential cytokines: a review. Oral Surg Oral Med Oral Pathol Oral Radiol. 2016;122(2):164–73.
335. Fritzsche C, Schleicher U, Bogdan C. Endothelial nitric oxide synthase limits the inflammatory response in mouse cutaneous leishmaniasis. Immunobiology. 2010;215(9–10):826–32.
336. Shah SM, et al. Differential expression of Th1-and Th2-type cytokines in peripheral blood mononuclear cells of murrah buffalo (*Bubalus bubalis*) on TLR2 induction by *B. Subtilis* peptidoglycan. Asian-Australasian J Anim Sci. 2012;25(7):1021.
337. Fukushima A, et al. TLR2 agonist ameliorates murine experimental allergic conjunctivitis by inducing CD4 positive T-cell apoptosis rather than by affecting the Th1/Th2 balance. Biochem Biophys Res Commun. 2006;339(4):1048–55.
338. Thacher TD, Clarke BL. Vitamin D insufficiency. In: Mayo clinic proceedings. London: Elsevier; 2011.
339. Holick MF. Vitamin D deficiency. N Engl J Med. 2007;357(3):266–81.
340. Liu W, et al. Intestinal epithelial vitamin D receptor signaling inhibits experimental colitis. J Clin Invest. 2013;123(9):3983–96.
341. Haussler MR, et al. The nuclear vitamin D receptor: biological and molecular regulatory properties revealed. J Bone Miner Res. 1998;13(3):325–49.
342. Gupta J, et al. Vitamin D in the treatment of oral lichen planus: a pilot clinical study. J Indian Acad Oral Med Radiol. 2019;31(3):222.
343. Aranow C. Vitamin D and the immune system. J Investig Med. 2011;59(6):881–6.
344. Steinman L. A brief history of TH17, the first major revision in the TH1/TH2 hypothesis of T cell–mediated tissue damage. Nat Med. 2007;13(2):139–45.
345. D'Aurizio F, et al. Is vitamin D a player or not in the pathophysiology of autoimmune thyroid diseases? Autoimmun Rev. 2015;14(5):363–9.
346. Kriegel MA, Manson JE, Costenbader KH. Does vitamin D affect risk of developing autoimmune disease? A systematic review. in Seminars in arthritis and rheumatism. London: Elsevier; 2011.
347. Du J, et al. Experimental study on 1, 25 (OH) 2D3 amelioration of oral lichen planus through regulating NF-κB signaling pathway. Oral Dis. 2017;23(6):770–8.
348. Marzano A, et al. Evidence for vitamin D deficiency and increased prevalence of fractures in autoimmune bullous skin diseases. Br J Dermatol. 2012;167(3):688–91.
349. Marzano AV, et al. Vitamin D and skeletal health in autoimmune bullous skin diseases: a case control study. Orphanet J Rare Dis. 2015;10(1):1–7.
350. EL-Komy M, Samir N, Shaker O. Estimation of vitamin D levels in patients with pemphigus vulgaris. J Eur Acad Dermatol Venereol. 2014;28(7):859–63.
351. Alshouibi E, et al. Vitamin D and periodontal health in older men. J Dent Res. 2013;92(8):689–93.
352. Garcia MN, et al. One-year effects of vitamin D and calcium supplementation on chronic periodontitis. J Periodontol. 2011;82(1):25–32.
353. Dietrich T, et al. Association between serum concentrations of 25-hydroxyvitamin D and gingival inflammation. Am J Clin Nutr. 2005;82(3):575–80.
354. Dietrich T, et al. Association between serum concentrations of 25-hydroxyvitamin D3 and periodontal disease in the US population. Am J Clin Nutr. 2004;80(1):108–13.
355. De Filippis A, et al. Vitamin D reduces the inflammatory response by *Porphyromonas gingivalis* infection by modulating human β-defensin-3 in human gingival epithelium and periodontal ligament cells. Int Immunopharmacol. 2017;47:106–17.
356. McMahon L, et al. Vitamin D-mediated induction of innate immunity in gingival epithelial cells. Infect Immun. 2011;79(6):2250–6.
357. Oh C, Kim HJ, Kim H-M. Vitamin D maintains E-cadherin intercellular junctions by downregulating MMP-9 production in human gingival keratinocytes treated by TNF-α. J Periodontal Implant Sci. 2019;49(5):270–86.
358. Bosshardt D, Lang N. The junctional epithelium: from health to disease. J Dent Res. 2005;84(1):9–20.
359. Du J, et al. 1, 25-Dihydroxyvitamin D protects intestinal epithelial barrier by regulating the myosin light chain kinase signaling pathway. Inflamm Bowel Dis. 2015;21(11):2495–506.
360. Nakano K, Vousden KH. PUMA, a novel proapoptotic gene, is induced by p53. Mol Cell. 2001;7(3):683–94.
361. Han J-W, et al. Expression of bbc3, a pro-apoptotic BH3-only gene, is regulated by diverse cell death and survival signals. Proc Natl Acad Sci. 2001;98(20):11318–23.
362. Ahmed SA. The role of serum vitamin D deficency in oral lichen planus case control study. Diyala J Med. 2019;17(2):189–98.
363. Ge X, et al. Vitamin D/VDR signaling induces miR-27a/b expression in oral lichen planus. Sci Rep. 2020;10(1):1–10.

364. Shen H, et al. Vitamin D receptor genetic polymorphisms are associated with oral lichen planus susceptibility in a Chinese Han population. BMC Oral Health. 2020;20(1):1–7.
365. Alalwani MS, Kharma MY, Aws G. Profound study for functions of antimicrobial peptides in prevention of oral disease. Br J Med Med Res. 2016;14(5):1.
366. Fábián TK, Fejérdy P, Csermely P. Saliva in health and disease, chemical biology of. In: Wiley encyclopedia of chemical biology, vol. 4. Hoboken: Wiley; 2008. p. 1–9.
367. Brandtzaeg P. Do salivary antibodies reliably reflect both mucosal and systemic immunity? Ann N Y Acad Sci. 2007;1098(1):288–311.
368. Khurshid Z, et al. Oral antimicrobial peptides: types and role in the oral cavity. Saudi Pharm J. 2016;24(5):515–24.
369. Yang D, et al. Mammalian defensins in immunity: more than just microbicidal. Trends Immunol. 2002;23(6):291–6.
370. Yang D, et al. Multiple roles of antimicrobial defensins, cathelicidins, and eosinophil-derived neurotoxin in host defense. Annu Rev Immunol. 2004;22:181.
371. Koczulla AR, Bals R. Antimicrobial peptides. Drugs. 2003;63(4):389–406.
372. Mookherjee N, Hancock R. Cationic host defence peptides: innate immune regulatory peptides as a novel approach for treating infections. Cell Mol Life Sci. 2007;64(7):922–33.
373. Ganz T. Defensins: antimicrobial peptides of innate immunity. Nat Rev Immunol. 2003;3(9):710–20.
374. Wang W, et al. Activity of α-and θ-defensins against primary isolates of HIV-1. J Immunol. 2004;173(1):515–20.
375. Diamond G, Ryan L. Beta-defensins: what are they REALLY doing in the oral cavity? Oral Dis. 2011;17(7):628–35.
376. MacKay B, et al. Isolation of milligram quantities of a group of histidine-rich polypeptides from human parotid saliva. Infect Immun. 1984;44(3):688–94.
377. Troxler R, et al. Structural relationship between human salivary histatins. J Dent Res. 1990;69(1):2–6.
378. Bercier JG, et al. Salivary histatins in patients with recurrent oral candidiasis. J Oral Pathol Med. 1999;28(1):26–9.
379. Oudhoff M, et al. Histatins enhance wound closure with oral and non-oral cells. J Dent Res. 2009;88(9):846–50.
380. Larrick JW, et al. Human CAP18: a novel antimicrobial lipopolysaccharide-binding protein. Infect Immun. 1995;63(4):1291–7.
381. Nishikimi T, et al. Adrenomedullin. In: Endocrinology of the heart in health and disease. London: Elsevier; 2017. p. 41–58.
382. Lundy FT, et al. Radioimmunoassay quantification of adrenomedullin in human gingival crevicular fluid. Arch Oral Biol. 2006;51(4):334–8.
383. Vitorino R, et al. Identification of human whole saliva protein components using proteomics. Proteomics. 2004;4(4):1109–15.
384. Wilmarth PA, et al. Two-dimensional liquid chromatography study of the human whole saliva proteome. J Proteome Res. 2004;3(5):1017–23.
385. Denny P, et al. The proteomes of human parotid and submandibular/sublingual gland salivas collected as the ductal secretions. J Proteome Res. 2008;7(5):1994–2006.
386. Gorr S-U. Antimicrobial peptides of the oral cavity. Periodontol 2000. 2009;51(1):152–80.
387. Dhaifalah I, et al. Azurocidin levels in maternal serum in the first trimester can predict preterm prelabor rupture of membranes. J Matern Fetal Neonatal Med. 2014;27(5):511–5.
388. El Karim IA, et al. Antimicrobial activity of neuropeptides against a range of micro-organisms from skin, oral, respiratory and gastrointestinal tract sites. J Neuroimmunol. 2008;200(1–2):11–6.
389. Salem A. Histamine H4 receptor: a potential novel therapeutic target in oral lichen planus and oral tongue cancer. DSHealth Dissertation Series; 2019.
390. Joly S, et al. Loss of human β-defensin 1, 2, and 3 expression in oral squamous cell carcinoma. Oral Microbiol Immunol. 2009;24(5):353–60.
391. Abiko Y, et al. Differential expression of human beta-defensin 2 in keratinized and non-keratinized oral epithelial lesions; immunohistochemistry and in situ hybridization. Virchows Arch. 2001;438(3):248–53.
392. Augustine J, et al. Epithelial loss correlated with decreased beta defensins and increased risk of candida infections in oral lichen planus. Oral Surg Oral Med Oral Pathol Oral Radiol. 2015;119(3):e111.
393. Kucukkolbasi H, et al. Evaluation of hβD-1 and hβD-2 levels in saliva of patients with oral mucosal diseases. West Indian Med J. 2013;62(3):230–8.
394. Azzi L, et al. Human β2-defensin in oral lichen planus expresses the degree of inflammation. J Biol Regul Homeost Agents. 2017;31(2 Suppl 1):77–87.
395. Polesello V, et al. DEFB1 polymorphisms and salivary hBD-1 concentration in Oral Lichen Planus patients and healthy subjects. Arch Oral Biol. 2017;73:161–5.
396. Shi N, et al. Overexpression of human β-defensin 2 promotes growth and invasion during esophageal carcinogenesis. Oncotarget. 2014;5(22):11333.
397. Verma C, et al. Defensins: antimicrobial peptides for therapeutic development. Biotechnol J. 2007;2(11):1353–9.
398. Kanda N, Watanabe S. Histamine enhances the production of human β-defensin-2 in human keratinocytes. Am J Phys Cell Phys. 2007;293(6):C1916–23.
399. Niyonsaba F, et al. Evaluation of the effects of peptide antibiotics human β-defensins-1/-2 and LL-37 on histamine release and prostaglandin D2 production from mast cells. Eur J Immunol. 2001;31(4):1066–75.

400. Subramanian H, et al. β-Defensins activate human mast cells via Mas-related gene X2. J Immunol. 2013;191(1):345–52.
401. Mineshiba J, et al. Transcriptional regulation of β-defensin-2 by lipopolysaccharide in cultured human cervical carcinoma (HeLa) cells. FEMS Immunol Med Microbiol. 2005;45(1):37–44.
402. Horr B, et al. STAT1 phosphorylation and cleavage is regulated by the histamine (H4) receptor in human atopic and non-atopic lymphocytes. Int Immunopharmacol. 2006;6(10):1577–85.
403. Salem A, et al. Human β-defensin 2 expression in oral epithelium: potential therapeutic targets in oral lichen planus. Int J Mol Sci. 2019;20(7):1780.
404. Rivera ES, et al. Histamine as an autocrine growth factor: an unusual role for a widespread mediator. Semin Cancer Biol. 2000;10(1):15–23.
405. Darvas Z, et al. Autonomous histamine metabolism in human melanoma cells. Melanoma Res. 2003;13(3):239–46.
406. Dy M, Schneider E. Histamine–cytokine connection in immunity and hematopoiesis. Cytokine Growth Factor Rev. 2004;15(5):393–410.
407. Medina VA, Rivera ES. Histamine receptors and cancer pharmacology. Br J Pharmacol. 2010;161(4):755–67.
408. Maintz L, Novak N. Histamine and histamine intolerance. Am J Clin Nutr. 2007;85(5):1185–96.
409. Thangam EB, et al. The role of histamine and histamine receptors in mast cell-mediated allergy and inflammation: the hunt for new therapeutic targets. Front Immunol. 2018;9:1873.
410. Walter M, Stark H. Histamine receptor subtypes: a century of rational drug design. Front Biosci. 2012;4(2):461–88.
411. Konttinen YT, et al. Non-professional histamine producing cells, immune responses and autoimmunity. Histamine H4 receptor: a novel drug target in immunoregulation and inflammation. London: Versita; 2013. p. 201–38.
412. Panula P, et al. International union of basic and clinical pharmacology. XCVIII. Histamine receptors. Pharmacol Rev. 2015;67(3):601–55.
413. Smolinska S, et al. Histamine and gut mucosal immune regulation. Allergy. 2014;69(3):273–81.
414. Klocker J, et al. Expression of histamine degrading enzymes in porcine tissues. Inflamm Res. 2005;54:S54–7.
415. Massari NA, Nicoud MB, Medina VA. Histamine receptors and cancer pharmacology: an update. Br J Pharmacol. 2020;177(3):516–38.
416. Nakamura T, et al. Molecular cloning and characterization of a new human histamine receptor, HH4R. Biochem Biophys Res Commun. 2000;279(2):615–20.
417. Akdis CA, Simons FER. Histamine receptors are hot in immunopharmacology. Eur J Pharmacol. 2006;533(1–3):69–76.
418. Kubo Y, Nakano K. Regulation of histamine synthesis in mouse CD4+ and CD8+ T lymphocytes. Inflamm Res. 1999;48(3):149–53.
419. Szeberényi JB, et al. Inhibition of effects of endogenously synthesized histamine disturbs in vitro human dendritic cell differentiation. Immunol Lett. 2001;76(3):175–82.
420. Dib K, et al. The histamine H4 receptor is a potent inhibitor of adhesion-dependent degranulation in human neutrophils. Wiley Online Library; 2014.
421. Thurmond RL. The histamine H4 receptor: from orphan to the clinic. Front Pharmacol. 2015;6:65.
422. Garcia-Pola MJ, Huerta G. Ansiety as an etiologic factor in oral lichen planus. Med Oral. 2000;5(1):7–13.
423. Falus A, et al. Paracrine and autocrine interactions in melanoma: histamine is a relevant player in local regulation. Trends Immunol. 2001;22(12):648–52.
424. Faustino-Rocha AI, et al. Antihistamines as promising drugs in cancer therapy. Life Sci. 2017;172:27–41.
425. Johnson C, et al. Inhibition of mast cell-derived histamine decreases human cholangiocarcinoma growth and differentiation via c-kit/stem cell factor–dependent signaling. Am J Pathol. 2016;186(1):123–33.
426. Grimm M, et al. Prognostic value of histamine H1 receptor expression in oral squamous cell carcinoma. Clin Oral Investig. 2013;17(3):949–55.
427. Martinel Lamas DJ, Rivera ES, Medina VA. Histamine H4 receptor: insights into a potential therapeutic target in breast cancer. Front Biosci. 2015;7(1):1–9.
428. Medina VA, et al. Histamine in cancer. Histamine H4 receptor: a novel drug target in immunoregulatory and inflammatory diseases; 2013.
429. Khazaie K, et al. The significant role of mast cells in cancer. Cancer Metastasis Rev. 2011;30(1):45–60.
430. Wei T, et al. Interleukin-17A promotes tongue squamous cell carcinoma metastasis through activating miR-23b/versican pathway. Oncotarget. 2017;8(4):6663.
431. Lodi G, et al. Interventions for treating oral lichen planus: a systematic review. Br J Dermatol. 2012;166(5):938–47.
432. Oda T, et al. Molecular cloning and characterization of a novel type of histamine receptor preferentially expressed in leukocytes. J Biol Chem. 2000;275(47):36781–6.
433. Yamaura K, et al. Expression of the histamine H4 receptor in dermal and articular tissues. Life Sci. 2013;92(2):108–13.
434. Inami Y, Andoh T, Kuraishi Y. Prevention of topical surfactant–induced itch-related responses by chlorogenic acid through the inhibition of increased histamine production in the epidermis. J Pharmacol Sci. 2013;121(3):242–5.
435. Hämäläinen L, et al. Alterations in the expression of EMT-related proteins claudin-1, clau-

din-4 and claudin-7, E-cadherin, TWIST1 and ZEB1 in oral lichen planus. J Oral Pathol Med. 2019;48(8):735–44.
436. Bussink AP, et al. Evolution of mammalian chitinase (-like) members of family 18 glycosyl hydrolases. Genetics. 2007;177(2):959–70.
437. Kawai T, Akira S. Toll-like receptors and their crosstalk with other innate receptors in infection and immunity. Immunity. 2011;34(5):637–50.
438. Tampa M, et al. Markers of oral lichen planus malignant transformation. Dis Markers. 2018;2018:1959506.
439. Poon IK, et al. Apoptotic cell clearance: basic biology and therapeutic potential. Nat Rev Immunol. 2014;14(3):166–80.
440. Lee CG, et al. Role of chitin and chitinase/chitinase-like proteins in inflammation, tissue remodeling, and injury. Annu Rev Physiol. 2011;73:479–501.
441. Johansen JS, et al. Serum YKL-40, a new prognostic biomarker in cancer patients? Cancer Epidemiol Biomark Prev. 2006;15(2):194–202.
442. Imai Y, et al. YKL-40 is a serum biomarker reflecting the severity of cutaneous lesions in psoriatic arthritis. J Dermatol. 2013;40(4):294–6.
443. Imai Y, et al. YKL-40 (chitinase 3-like-1) as a biomarker for psoriasis vulgaris and pustular psoriasis. J Dermatol Sci. 2011;64(1):75–7.
444. Alpsoy S, et al. Atherosclerosis, some serum inflammatory markers in psoriasis. G Ital Dermatol Venereol. 2014;149(2):167–75.
445. Erfan G, et al. Serum YKL-40: a potential biomarker for psoriasis or endothelial dysfunction in psoriasis? Mol Cell Biochem. 2015;400(1):207–12.
446. Salomon J, et al. Chitinase-3-like protein 1 (YKL-40) Is expressed in lesional skin in hidradenitis suppurativa. In Vivo. 2019;33(1):141–3.
447. Salomon J, et al. Chitinase-3-like protein 1 (YKL-40) is a new biomarker of inflammation in psoriasis. Mediat Inflamm. 2017;2017:9538451.
448. Abu El-Hamd M, et al. Serum YKL-40 in patients with psoriasis vulgaris treated by narrow-band UVB phototherapy. J Dermatolog Treat. 2019;30(6):545–8.
449. Khattab FM, Said NM. Chitinase-3-like protein 1 (YKL-40): novel biomarker of lichen planus. Int J Dermatol. 2019;58(9):993–6.
450. Humberto JSM, et al. Cytokines, cortisol, and nitric oxide as salivary biomarkers in oral lichen planus: a systematic review. Braz Oral Res. 2018;32:e82.
451. Monaco C, et al. T-cell-mediated signalling in immune, inflammatory and angiogenic processes: the cascade of events leading to inflammatory diseases. Curr Drug Targets Inflamm Allergy. 2004;3(1):35–42.
452. Christopoulos A, et al. Biology of vascular endothelial growth factor and its receptors in head and neck cancer: beyond angiogenesis. Head Neck. 2011;33(8):1220–9.
453. Li Y, et al. Salivary mycobiome dysbiosis and its potential impact on bacteriome shifts and host immunity in oral lichen planus. Int J Oral Sci. 2019;11(2):1–10.
454. Rios H, et al. Periostin null mice exhibit dwarfism, incisor enamel defects, and an early-onset periodontal disease-like phenotype. Mol Cell Biol. 2005;25(24):11131–44.
455. Ruan K, Bao S, Ouyang G. The multifaceted role of periostin in tumorigenesis. Cell Mol Life Sci. 2009;66(14):2219–30.
456. Zhang ZR, et al. Expression and clinical significance of periostin in oral lichen planus. Exp Therap Med. 2018;15(6):5141–7.
457. Barnes L, et al. Pathology and genetics of head and neck tumours, vol. 9. IARC; 2005.
458. Rode M, Kogoj-Rode M. Malignant potential of the reticular form of oral lichen planus over a 25-year observation period in 55 patients from Slovenia. J Oral Sci. 2002;44(2):109–11.
459. van der Meij EH, Mast H, van der Waal I. The possible premalignant character of oral lichen planus and oral lichenoid lesions: a prospective five-year follow-up study of 192 patients. Oral Oncol. 2007;43(8):742–8.
460. Oliveira Alves MG, et al. Oral lichen planus: a retrospective study of 110 Brazilian patients. BMC Res Notes. 2010;3:157.
461. Radochová V, Dřízhal I, Slezák R. A retrospective study of 171 patients with oral lichen planus in the East Bohemia-Czech Republic–single center experience. J Clin Exp Dent. 2014;6(5):e556.
462. Georgakopoulou EA, et al. Oral lichen planus as a preneoplastic inflammatory model. J Biomed Biotechnol. 2012;2012:759626.
463. Lodi G, et al. Current controversies in oral lichen planus: report of an international consensus meeting. Part 2. Clinical management and malignant transformation. Oral Surg Oral Med Oral Pathol Oral Radiol Endod. 2005;100(2):164–78.
464. van der Meij EH, et al. A review of the recent literature regarding malignant transformation of oral lichen planus. Oral Surg Oral Med Oral Pathol Oral Radiol Endod. 1999;88(3):307–10.
465. Mattsson U, Jontell M, Holmstrup P. Oral lichen planus and malignant transformation: is a recall of patients justified? Crit Rev Oral Biol Med. 2002;13(5):390–6.
466. Larsson A, Warfvinge G. Malignant transformation of oral lichen planus. Oral Oncol. 2003;39(6):630–1.
467. Gonzalez-Moles MA, Scully C, Gil-Montoya JA. Oral lichen planus: controversies surrounding malignant transformation. Oral Dis. 2008;14(3):229–43.
468. Fitzpatrick SG, Hirsch SA, Gordon SC. The malignant transformation of oral lichen planus and oral lichenoid lesions: a systematic review. J Am Dent Assoc. 2014;145(1):45–56.
469. Ingafou M, et al. Oral lichen planus: a retrospective study of 690 British patients. Oral Dis. 2006;12(5):463–8.

470. Pakfetrat A, et al. Oral Lichen Planus: a retrospective study of 420 Iranian patients. Med Oral Patol Oral Cir Bucal. 2009;14(7):E315–8.
471. Kaplan I, et al. The dynamics of oral lichen planus: a retrospective clinicopathological study. Head Neck Pathol. 2012;6(2):178–83.
472. Bermejo-Fenoll A, et al. A retrospective clinicopathological study of 550 patients with oral lichen planus in south-eastern Spain. J Oral Pathol Med. 2010;39(6):491–6.
473. Torrente-Castells E, et al. Clinical features of oral lichen planus. A retrospective study of 65 cases. Med Oral Patol Oral Cir Bucal. 2010;15(5):e685–90.
474. Shen ZY, et al. A retrospective clinicopathological study on oral lichen planus and malignant transformation: analysis of 518 cases. Med Oral Patol Oral Cir Bucal. 2012;17(6):e943–7.
475. Aghbari SMH, et al. Malignant transformation of oral lichen planus and oral lichenoid lesions: a meta-analysis of 20095 patient data. Oral Oncol. 2017;68:92–102.
476. Krutchkoff DJ, Cutler L, Laskowski S. Oral lichen planus: the evidence regarding potential malignant transformation. J Oral Pathol. 1978;7(1):1–7.
477. Rad M, et al. Correlation between clinical and histopathologic diagnoses of oral lichen planus based on modified WHO diagnostic criteria. Oral Surg Oral Med Oral Pathol Oral Radiol Endod. 2009;107(6):796–800.
478. van der Meij EH, Schepman KP, van der Waal I. The possible premalignant character of oral lichen planus and oral lichenoid lesions: a prospective study. Oral Surg Oral Med Oral Pathol Oral Radiol Endod. 2003;96(2):164–71.
479. van der Meij EH, van der Waal I. Lack of clinicopathologic correlation in the diagnosis of oral lichen planus based on the presently available diagnostic criteria and suggestions for modifications. J Oral Pathol Med. 2003;32(9):507–12.
480. Giuliani M, et al. Rate of malignant transformation of oral lichen planus: a systematic review. Oral Dis. 2019;25(3):693–709.
481. González-Moles M, et al. Malignant transformation risk of oral lichen planus: a systematic review and comprehensive meta-analysis. Oral Oncol. 2019;96:121–30.
482. Gandolfo S, et al. Risk of oral squamous cell carcinoma in 402 patients with oral lichen planus: a follow-up study in an Italian population. Oral Oncol. 2004;40(1):77–83.
483. Lozada-Nur F. Oral lichen planus and oral cancer: is there enough epidemiologic evidence? Oral Surg Oral Med Oral Pathol Oral Radiol Endod. 2000;89(3):265–6.
484. Ma J, et al. The magnitude of the association between human papillomavirus and oral lichen planus: a meta-analysis. PLoS One. 2016;11(8):e0161339.
485. Liu T, et al. Study on expression of p16 and human papillomavirus 16 and 18 (E6) in OLP and its malignant transformation. Pathol Res Pract. 2018;214(2):296–302.
486. Ismail SB, Kumar SK, Zain RB. Oral lichen planus and lichenoid reactions: etiopathogenesis, diagnosis, management and malignant transformation. J Oral Sci. 2007;49(2):89–106.
487. Eisenberg E. Oral lichen planus: a benign lesion. J Oral Maxillofac Surg. 2000;58(11):1278–85.
488. Mignogna MD, Fedele S, Lo Russo L. Dysplasia/neoplasia surveillance in oral lichen planus patients: a description of clinical criteria adopted at a single centre and their impact on prognosis. Oral Oncol. 2006;42(8):819–24.
489. Mignogna MD, et al. Field cancerization in oral lichen planus. Eur J Surg Oncol. 2007;33(3):383–9.
490. Mignogna MD, et al. Clinical guidelines in early detection of oral squamous cell carcinoma arising in oral lichen planus: a 5-year experience. Oral Oncol. 2001;37(3):262–7.
491. Slaughter DP, Southwick HW, Smejkal W. Field cancerization in oral stratified squamous epithelium; clinical implications of multicentric origin. Cancer. 1953;6(5):963–8.
492. Braakhuis BJ, et al. A genetic explanation of Slaughter's concept of field cancerization: evidence and clinical implications. Cancer Res. 2003;63(8):1727–30.
493. Cheng YS, et al. Diagnosis of oral lichen planus: a position paper of the American Academy of Oral and Maxillofacial Pathology. Oral Surg Oral Med Oral Pathol Oral Radiol. 2016;122(3):332–54.
494. Kramer IR, et al. Definition of leukoplakia and related lesions: an aid to studies on oral precancer. Oral Surg Oral Med Oral Pathol. 1978;46(4):518–39.
495. van der Meij EH, et al. Interobserver and intraobserver variability in the clinical assessment of oral lichen planus. J Oral Pathol Med. 2002;31(2):95–8.
496. Choi S, Myers JN. Molecular pathogenesis of oral squamous cell carcinoma: implications for therapy. J Dent Res. 2008;87(1):14–32.
497. Fatahzadeh M, Rinaggio J, Chiodo T. Squamous cell carcinoma arising in an oral lichenoid lesion. J Am Dent Assoc. 2004;135(6):754–9. quiz 796
498. Lo Muzio L, et al. The possible association between oral lichen planus and oral squamous cell carcinoma: a clinical evaluation on 14 cases and a review of the literature. Oral Oncol. 1998;34(4):239–46.
499. Hande AH, et al. Evidence based demonstration of the concept of 'field cancerization' by p53 expression in mirror image biopsies of patients with oral squamous cell carcinoma—an immunohistochemical study. Romanian J Morphol Embryol. 2015;56(3):1027–33.
500. Mignogna MD, et al. Clinical behaviour of malignant transforming oral lichen planus. Eur J Surg Oncol. 2002;28(8):838–43.
501. Markopoulos AK, et al. Malignant potential of oral lichen planus; a follow-up study of 326 patients. Oral Oncol. 1997;33(4):263–9.

502. Mignogna MD, et al. Immune activation and chronic inflammation as the cause of malignancy in oral lichen planus: is there any evidence ? Oral Oncol. 2004;40(2):120–30.
503. Grivennikov SI, Greten FR, Karin M. Immunity, inflammation, and cancer. Cell. 2010;140(6):883–99.
504. Zamarron BF, Chen W. Dual roles of immune cells and their factors in cancer development and progression. Int J Biol Sci. 2011;7(5):651–8.
505. Rich J, Borton A, Wang X. Transforming growth factor-beta signaling in cancer. Microsc Res Tech. 2001;52(4):363–73.
506. Xia J, et al. Expressions of CXCR7/ligands may be involved in oral carcinogenesis. J Mol Histol. 2011;42(2):175–80.
507. Kane LP, et al. Induction of NF-kappaB by the Akt/PKB kinase. Curr Biol. 1999;9(11):601–4.
508. Kane LP, et al. Akt-dependent phosphorylation specifically regulates Cot induction of NF-kappa B-dependent transcription. Mol Cell Biol. 2002;22(16):5962–74.
509. Chan G, et al. Cyclooxygenase-2 expression is up-regulated in squamous cell carcinoma of the head and neck. Cancer Res. 1999;59(5):991–4.
510. Yao L, et al. The function and mechanism of COX-2 in angiogenesis of gastric cancer cells. J Exp Clin Cancer Res. 2011;30(1):13.
511. Wang D, Dubois RN. Prostaglandins and cancer. Gut. 2006;55(1):115–22.
512. Lysitsa S, et al. COX-2 expression in oral lichen planus. Dermatology. 2008;217(2):150–5.
513. Battino M, et al. Oxidative stress markers in oral lichen planus. Biofactors. 2008;33(4):301–10.
514. Ergun S, et al. Evaluation of oxidative stress and antioxidant profile in patients with oral lichen planus. J Oral Pathol Med. 2011;40(4):286–93.
515. Kawanishi S, et al. Oxidative and nitrative DNA damage in animals and patients with inflammatory diseases in relation to inflammation-related carcinogenesis. Biol Chem. 2006;387(4):365–72.
516. Zhang L, et al. Molecular analysis of oral lichen planus. A premalignant lesion? Am J Pathol. 1997;151(2):323–7.
517. Kim J, et al. Evaluation of premalignant potential in oral lichen planus using interphase cytogenetics. J Oral Pathol Med. 2001;30(2):65–72.
518. Mithani SK, et al. Molecular genetics of premalignant oral lesions. Oral Dis. 2007;13(2):126–33.
519. Zhang L, et al. High frequency of allelic loss in dysplastic lichenoid lesions. Lab Investig. 2000;80(2):233–7.
520. Accurso BT, et al. Allelic imbalance in oral lichen planus and assessment of its classification as a premalignant condition. Oral Surg Oral Med Oral Pathol Oral Radiol Endod. 2011;112(3):359–66.
521. Sudbø J, et al. DNA content as a prognostic marker in patients with oral leukoplakia. N Engl J Med. 2001;344(17):1270–8.
522. Sudbø J, et al. The influence of resection and aneuploidy on mortality in oral leukoplakia. N Engl J Med. 2004;350(14):1405–13.
523. Girod SC, Pape HD, Krueger GR. p53 and PCNA expression in carcinogenesis of the oropharyngeal mucosa. Eur J Cancer B Oral Oncol. 1994;30b(6):419–23.
524. O'Flatharta C, et al. Telomerase activity detected in oral lichen planus by RNA in situ hybridisation: not a marker for malignant transformation. J Clin Pathol. 2002;55(8):602–7.
525. Valente G, et al. Sequential immunohistochemical p53 expression in biopsies of oral lichen planus undergoing malignant evolution. J Oral Pathol Med. 2001;30(3):135–40.
526. Kilpi A, et al. Expression of c-erbB-2 protein in keratinocytes of oral mucosal lichen planus and subsequent squamous cell carcinoma. Eur J Oral Sci. 1996;104(3):278–84.
527. Parise Junior O, et al. Prognostic impact of p53, c-erbB-2 and epidermal growth factor receptor on head and neck carcinoma. Sao Paulo Med J. 2004;122(6):264–8.
528. Acay RR, et al. Evaluation of proliferative potential in oral lichen planus and oral lichenoid lesions using immunohistochemical expression of p53 and Ki67. Oral Oncol. 2006;42(5):475–80.
529. Zargaran M, et al. Suitability/unsuitability of cell proliferation as an indicator of malignant potential in oral lichen planus: an immunohistochemical study. Asian Pac J Cancer Prev. 2013;14(11):6979–83.
530. Nankivell P, et al. Investigation of p16(INK4a) as a prognostic biomarker in oral epithelial dysplasia. J Oral Pathol Med. 2014;43(4):245–9.
531. Han JS, et al. Bimodal activation of BubR1 by Bub3 sustains mitotic checkpoint signaling. Proc Natl Acad Sci U S A. 2014;111(40):E4185–93.
532. Mukherjee A, et al. The role of BUB and CDC proteins in low-grade breast cancers. Lancet. 2015;385(Suppl 1):S72.
533. Bangur CS, et al. Identification of genes over-expressed in small cell lung carcinoma using suppression subtractive hybridization and cDNA microarray expression analysis. Oncogene. 2002;21(23):3814–25.
534. Friedman RS, et al. Molecular and immunological evaluation of the transcription factor SOX-4 as a lung tumor vaccine antigen. J Immunol. 2004;172(5):3319–27.
535. Rosa EA, et al. Oral lichen planus and malignant transformation: the role of p16, Ki-67, Bub-3 and SOX4 in assessing precancerous potential. Exp Ther Med. 2018;15(5):4157–66.
536. van der Waal I. Oral potentially malignant disorders: is malignant transformation predictable and preventable? Med Oral Patol Oral Cir Bucal. 2014;19(4):e386–90.

5 Diagnosis

5.1 Clinical Classification of OLP Lesions

The most frequent LP lesions arise in the skin and/or oral mucosa but can also occur in the skin appendages (nails and hair) and external genitalia (more frequently in women) [1]. Rarely the larynx, esophagus, and conjunctiva may be involved [2]. Usually LP lesions (cutaneous, OLP, or genital) remain confined to the single affected organ, but sometimes it is possible to observe an association of multiple clinical forms, especially in young female patients [1]. The anatomical district where LP lesions are most frequently localized is the mucous membrane of the oral cavity. Twenty percent of women and 15% of men with OLP also have genital and skin involvement. Furthermore, as already mentioned in *Chap. 2*, it is estimated that 70–77% of cases of cutaneous LP are concomitant with OLP [3–5].

Cutaneous LP lesions present as flat and itchy purplish papules and plaques, located mainly on the flexor surface of the wrists and/or ankles, the extensor surface of the lower legs, the lower mid-back, and the intergluteal fissure [6]. These flat papules may have a reticulum of white fine lines called *Wickham's striae*, which may develop several months after OLP lesions appear [2].

LP of the skin appendages, when it affects the scalp, called *lichen planopilaris* (Fig. 5.1), causes purplish, scaly, and itchy papular lesions in the follicular and perifollicular sites, follicular plugging, bottle-brush hair formation (multiple bundles of hair emerging from a single follicular orifice), and up to the appearance of atrophic scarring lesions and patchy alopecia. Nail involvement causes pitting, subungual hyperkeratosis, longitudinal melanonychia (a brownish vertical streak), onychorrhexis (longitudinal ridging and grooving), onychoschizia (distal splitting), and onycholysis (separation of the nail plate from the nail bed). Permanent nail matrix damage can lead to the formation of pterygium (raised central ridge) and anonychia (permanent nail loss) [6]. Nail LP is rare in OLP patients and it affects 10% of individuals with cutaneous LP [7].

Genital LP is characterized by lesions similar to cutaneous LP [6]. Since 1982 [8] cases of *vulvovaginal-gingival syndrome* have been

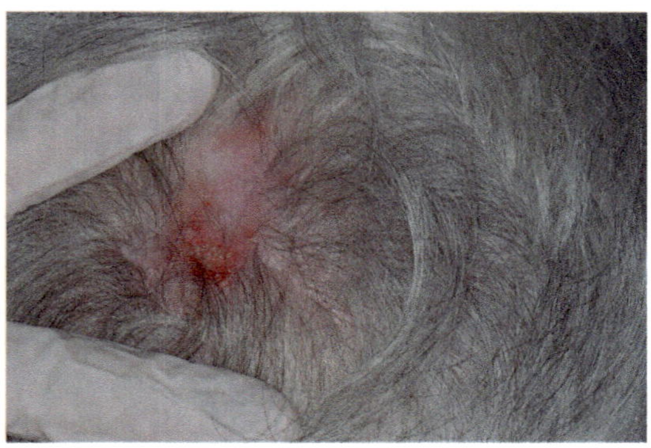

Fig. 5.1 Lichen planopilaris with purplish scaly and erosive lesions with the appearance of scarring alopecia

G. Isola et al., *Oral Lichen Planus and Lichenoid Lesions*,
https://doi.org/10.1007/978-3-031-29765-6_5

described, which develop in 20% of women with OLP [9, 10] and are characterized by the presence of burning, pain, secretion, dyspareunia, and the possibility of malignant degeneration [11, 12]. The vulva may be affected by white reticular/plaque or erythematous and erosive lesions, agglutination, and scarring which may cause urogenital stenosis and dysfunction, rarely needing surgical interventions [13]. Vulvovaginal-gingival syndrome may be due to a genetic predisposition, since 80% of these patients showed positivity of the HLA-II DQB1*0201 versus 42% in controls [14]. *Peno-gingival syndrome*, the male equivalent first described in 1993 [15], manifests as reticular, annular, or papular, sometimes erosive and painful, lesions, and they can also develop into carcinoma; scarring is rare [13, 16]. These female and male patients show gingival involvement with reticular and atrophic-erythematous lesions and desquamative gingivitis. Oral and genital lesions appear simultaneously in about 50% of patients, while in 30% of cases, the oral manifestations appear prematurely [13]. Vulvovaginal-gingival syndrome and peno-gingival syndrome have a chronic course and the treatment is challenging [13].

Other forms of *LP of the extraoral mucous membranes* are *esophageal LP*, and, even more rarely, it can assist in the involvement of the ocular, urinary, nasal, laryngeal, optic, gastric, or anal mucosa [5, 17–20]. Unlike cutaneous LP, esophageal LP almost exclusively affects middle-aged or older women who also have oral involvement [21] (Fig. 5.2) and is associated with a significant increase in the risk of squamous carcinoma [22]. Therefore, this category of patients should be well looked after, especially if they have a history of esophageal disorders, weight loss, and dysphagia [23]. In addition to the mechanical dilation of the esophagus to prevent weight loss (an intervention that can cause damage due to the Koebner phenomenon or reactive isomorphism), various therapeutic approaches have been proposed including systemic cyclosporine [24], oral tacrolimus, local injections of triamcinolone acetonide [25, 26], and topical budesonide (1 mg twice a day for 8 weeks or 2–3 mg twice a day mixed with 8 mL honey) [23, 27].

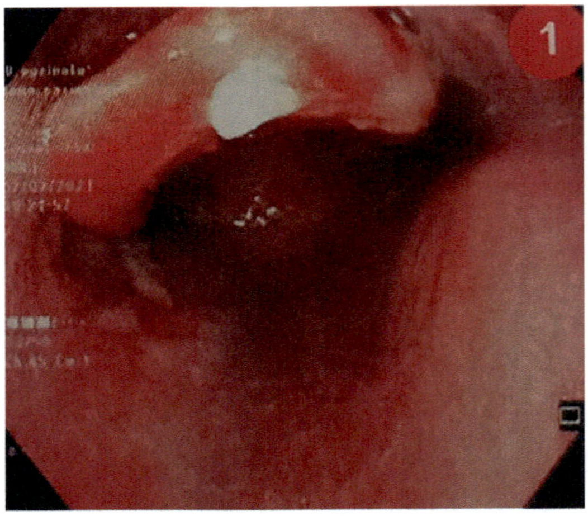

Fig. 5.2 Erosive esophageal LP involving the epiglottis in a 78-year-old nonsmoking woman

Recently, the World Health Organization (WHO) defined *OLP* as "a chronic inflammatory disorder of unknown etiology with characteristic relapses and remissions, displaying white reticular lesions, accompanied or not by atrophic, erosive and ulcerative and/or plaque-type areas. Lesions are frequently bilaterally symmetrical. Desquamative gingivitis may be a feature" [28]. One of the most relevant clinical features of OLP is in fact the frequent bilateral expression and the spread of the lesions in multiple oral districts. This factor can be of great help to the clinician in suspecting OLP and being able to make a differential diagnosis with other white lesions characterized by a unilateral distribution. All the districts of the oral cavity can potentially be affected by the lesions and multiple regions can be involved at the same time. The most affected area is that of the buccal mucous membranes with a frequency of 82–85% of cases: the lesions are mainly localized in the middle and posterior-inferior part, in correspondence with the vestibular fornix and the retromolar region. The tongue is involved, especially on the dorsal surface and rarely in the ventral one, in 35–40% of cases, the gingival and alveolar mucous membranes in 10–15% of cases, the palate in 8–10% of cases, and the lips in 15–20% of cases. However, the lesions remain usually confined to the buccal mucous membranes, gums, and lingual dorsum [1].

There are two types of OLP lesions, *white* (papular, reticular, plaque subtype) and *red* (atrophic-erythematous, erosive or ulcer-erosive, and bullous), for a total of *six clinical forms* [1, 29]. These clinical subtypes sometimes appear in the oral mucosa mixed together [6, 29]. White lesions are characterized by moderate mucous thickening (therefore a hyper-parakeratosis of the oral epithelium involved) and often organize themselves in white or gray striae that can form a reticular pattern on a diffuse erythematous background [1, 6, 29]. On the dorsal surface of the tongue, sometimes, the striae are organized into annular lesions characterized by keratotic lines that form circles of varying sizes [6]. Red lesions are characterized by a marked epithelial atrophy and superficial erosion. The deeper loss of the epithelial matrix leads to ulceration's onset [1] with a yellowish surface (due to the fibrinous exudate) surrounded by an area of erythema [30]. The vacuolation of the epithelial layers close to the basement membrane, on the other hand, leads to the formation of bullous OLP lesions [1]. In addition, OLP lesions can be associated with deposits of melanin (inflammatory melanosis) which give a brown pigmentation to the affected mucous membranes, although this is rarely the case in light-skinned people [30–32].

The group with red lesions is also associated with greater local symptoms exacerbating during food and drink intake, but, in severe cases, patients may report spontaneous symptoms [1]. About two-thirds of patients with OLP are estimated to experience some form of oral discomfort [33]. Symptoms, when present, can range from mild mucosal sensitivity to continual debilitating pain and burning [30]. As mentioned, OLP lesions can persist for many years with periods of exacerbation and quiescence (Sect. 4.5.5). During periods of quiescence, erythema/ulceration decreases and pain or sensitivity is attenuated [30]. Instead, during exacerbations (related, e.g., to an imbalance of the immune system in periods of psychological stress and anxiety), there are a worsening of erythema/ulceration and an increase in pain or sensitivity [30, 34].

In this regard many *scoring systems* for OLP severity have been developed. About OLP signs, Thongprasom et al. proposed a direct measurement of OLP lesions elaborating a scale that ranges from 0 to 5: absence of lesions (0), hyperkeratotic striae (1), atrophic area < 1 cm^2 (2), atrophic area > 1 cm^2 (3), erosive area < 1 cm^2 (4), and erosive area > 1 cm^2 (5) [35]. Kaliakatsou et al. elaborated another scale obtained from direct measurements: absence of lesions (0), white striae only (1), white striae plus erosion <1 cm^2 (2), white striae plus erosion >1 cm^2 (3), white striae plus ulceration <1 cm^2 (4), and white striae plus ulceration >1 cm^2 (5) [36]. Malhotra et al. [37] elaborated a scoring system based on the site involvement (< or > 50% site), whereas Escudier et al. [38] assigned a score based on the clinical OLP subtype severity (reticular, atrophic-erythematous, and erosive/ulcerative). In some of these studies, the disease severity was also influenced by the different subsites involved in the oral cavity [38, 39]. Scoring OLP signs may give an objective, but incomplete, measure of disease activity. The effort in several researches has also been to develop subjective scores for symptom severity related to OLP. Raj et al. scored disease severity with a scale ranging from 0 to 4: 0, no symptoms; 1, mild (occasional symptoms); 2, moderate (e.g., while eating spicy food); 3, severe (i.e., while eating any food); and 4, intolerable (always present) [40]. Numerical Rating Scale (NRS) for pain has also been employed as OLP scoring system: 0 (no pain), 1–3 (mild pain), 4–6 (moderate pain), 7–9 (severe pain), and 10 (very severe pain) [41]. To improve OLP grading systems, some authors combined signs and symptoms scores proposed in the literature in order to obtain a final disease score useful for the evaluation of downstaging after treatment [42–44]. Wang et al. [45] critically reviewed many of these OLP scoring systems, and the authors concluded that "because of the natural course of OLP characterized by remissions and exacerbations and also due to the varying distribution pattern and the varying clinical types, e.g. reticular and erosive, the relevance of a disease scoring system based on morphologic parameters is somewhat questionable. Instead, one may consider to only look for a quality of life scoring system adapted for use in OLP patients." To date, there is no universally accepted scale.

As mentioned before, it is possible to distinguish six clinical forms of OLP: papular, reticular, plaque, atrophic-erythematous, erosive or ulcer-erosive, and bullous subtype.

5.1.1 Papular OLP

The *papular form* is characterized by the presence of raised papules of white-pearly color and with dimensions of about 1–2 mm. The papule is a primitive elementary lesion of the epithelia characterized by small dimensions. However, in this case the oral papules have very small dimensions, and, developing on a soft and distensible mucous surface, they are difficult to appreciate on digital palpation. Papular OLP usually does not cause symptoms and is the simplest clinical form with a usually benign course. In the more extensive and pronounced forms, the patient may experience a sensation of roughness of the buccal mucosa, where this type of lesions is more frequently localized bilaterally [1]. The "pure" papular OLP form is observed when the papules appear side by side, but this pattern is rarely observed [1, 29] (Fig. 5.3). In fact, usually these papules tend to merge forming a more extensive reticular model of the lesion [1].

5.1.2 Reticular OLP

Reticular OLP is the most common clinical pattern [29]; it is mainly localized in the buccal mucous membranes and is characterized by a weaving of white keratotic striae, Wickham's striae, given by the confluence of papular lesions, thus forming a pattern that resembles a grid or a spider web (Fig. 5.4). The pattern of these striae often follows the morphology of the affected oral areas and, above all, the movement capacity and extension of the oral mucosa [1].

The reticular form is also observable on the lingual dorsum, in the lingual marginal borders and ventral portion bordering on the oral floor, on the lips, and, rarely, on the gingival mucosa. The papules can also merge forming an annular pattern, in which the lesions appear as whitish rings approximately 8–15 mm in diameter, with a central area of apparently normal or variably erythematous mucosa [1].

5.1.3 Plaque OLP

Hyperkeratotic papules can aggregate, forming another elementary lesion called plaque which, in OLP disease, appears always white and variable in extension. Plaque can be distinguished from healthy oral mucosa on palpation and this clinical subtype may also be completely asymptomatic. *Plaque OLP* is mainly localized on the lingual dorsum (Fig. 5.5), the gums (Fig. 5.6), and buccal mucous membranes [1]. White OLP

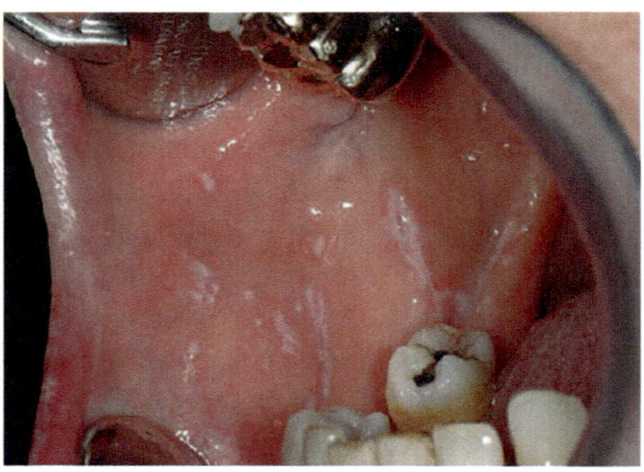

Fig. 5.3 Papular OLP lesions. Note the small size of the oral papules. From [5] with permission

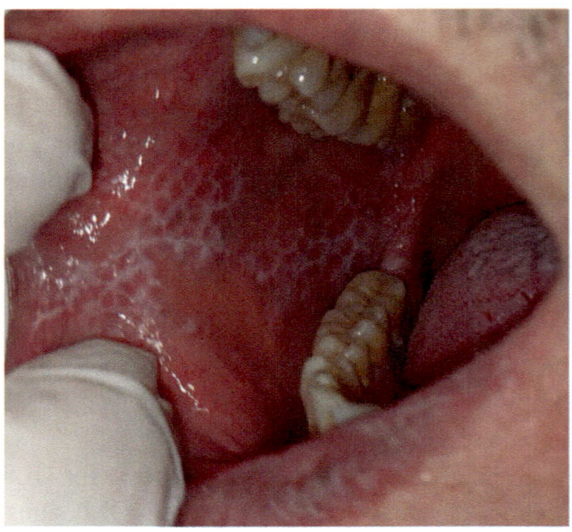

Fig. 5.4 Reticular OLP in a patient with no symptoms

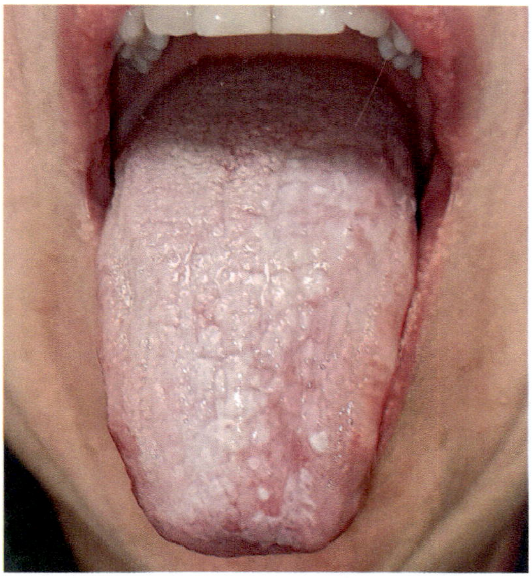

Fig. 5.5 Plaque OLP on the lingual dorsum. The patient did not report any symptoms

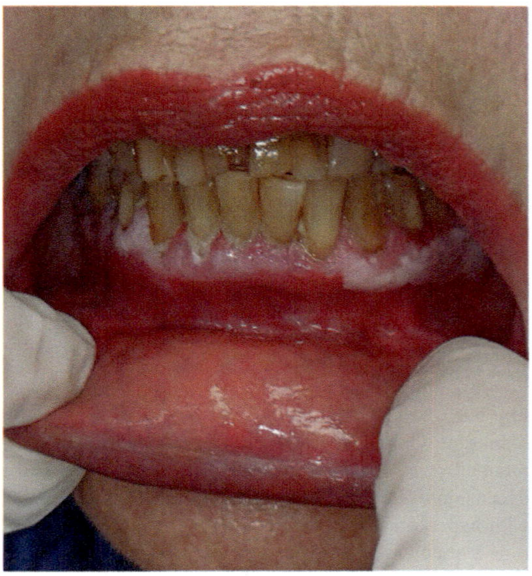

Fig. 5.6 Plaque OLP affecting the gums. The patient reported modest and occasional symptoms

plaques may resemble leukoplakia lesions: the presence of striae can help distinguish OLP plaque from leukoplakia [29].

5.1.4 Atrophic-Erythematous OLP

The *atrophic and erythematous OLP form* is characterized by suffering and a reduction in the epithelium thickness. The atrophic mucous membranes appear more or less bright red in color and entail a certain suffering for patients, due to greater sensitivity and pain of the mucous membranes when consuming solid foods and drinks. Atrophic lesions, almost always bilateral, may be variable in extension. The typical localization of atrophic OLP is at the attached gingiva which appears erythematous and opaque [1] (Fig. 5.7).

5.1.5 Erosive and Ulcer-Erosive OLP

A chronic suffering of the tissues and a trauma related to normal chewing frictions can lead to an aggravation of a simple atrophic form that can turn into an *erosive OLP* (*EOLP*) [1] (Fig. 5.8), one of the most common forms of OLP [29].

Erosion is an elementary lesion characterized by a superficial epithelial loss confined to the epithelium itself (i.e., that does not exceed the basement membrane). Given that, despite the redness and reduction of epithelial thickness, the basal membrane and therefore the epithelial-connective border are preserved, there is no possibility of spontaneous bleeding in erosive OLP [1]. Patients affected by EOLP often report more or less intense symptoms characterized by burning and pain during oral functions [46] (Fig. 5.9).

In the context of the most affected atrophic-erosive areas and not subjected to frictional self-cleaning during oral functions, superficial pseudomembranes are often observed that can be removed with a gauze, usually causing small bleeding. Sometimes even simple clinical palpation, functional movement, or superficial trauma can cause them [1].

If the erosive forms of OLP are confined to the gingival mucosa, the condition is generally referred to as desquamative gingivitis [9, 47–49]. These lesions are often accompanied by plaque

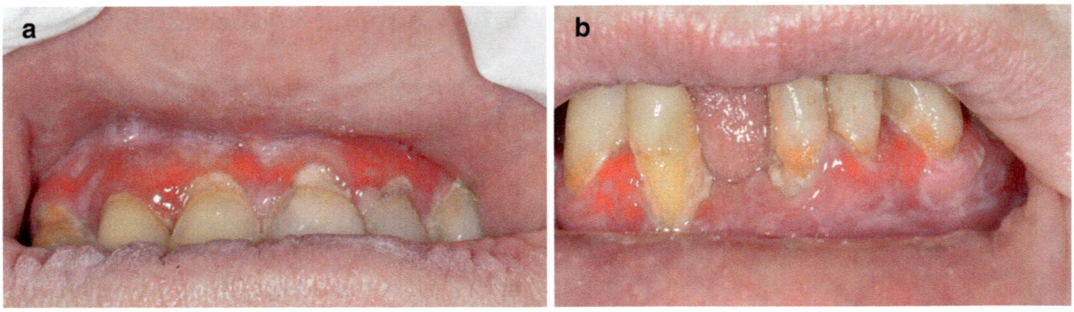

Fig. 5.7 Atrophic gingival lichen in a patient affected by periodontal disease. The gums (**a–b**) appear erythematous and painful to normal masticatory frictions. Note the reticular pattern mixed with atrophic areas

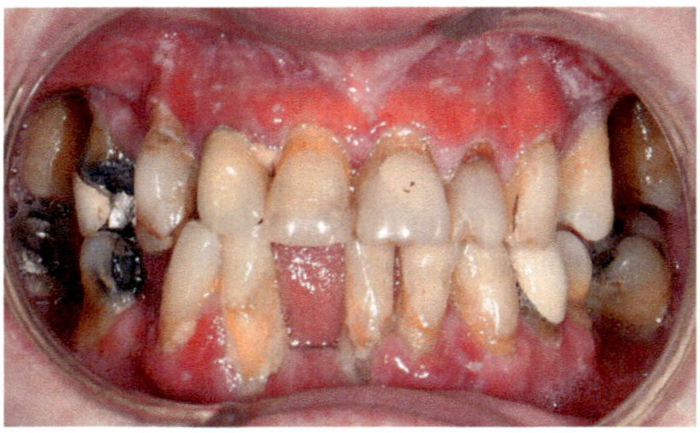

Fig. 5.8 The same patient of Fig. 5.7. After therapy suspension of a few months, the lesions worsened assuming an erosive aspect. The intense painful symptoms, exacerbated by mechanical friction (feeding and toothbrushing), made oral hygiene difficult with a consequent considerable accumulation of plaque 1 month after nonsurgical periodontal therapy

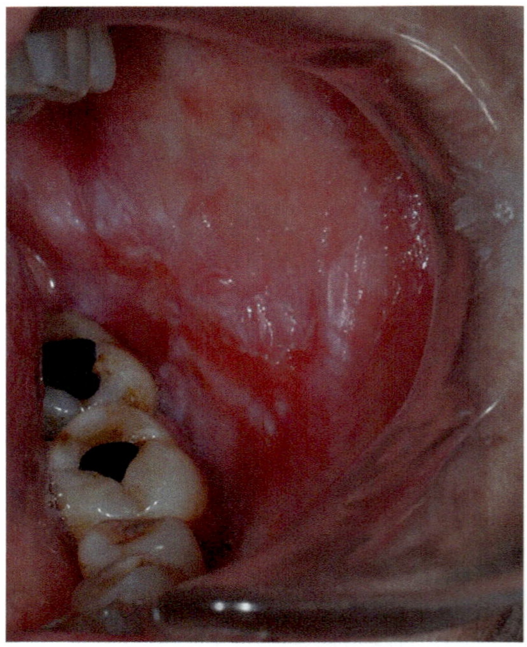

Fig. 5.9 Atrophic-erosive OLP of buccal mucous membranes. It should be noted that the main lesion is surrounded by a substantial reticular/plaque border, as if the expansion of the process entailed an initial inflammation with hyperkeratotic reaction of the epithelium, followed, as it worsens, by atrophy and erosion of the more superficial layers. The patient referred symptoms to the intake of hot, acidic, and spicy foods

accumulation which causes a progressive attachment loss and a severe progression of periodontal disease [50] (Fig. 5.8). In fact, plaque and tartar accumulation could exacerbate OLP, probably due to the Koebner phenomenon [49]. Desquamative gingivitis clinically presents with a fiery red erythematous aspect that affects the entire height of the attached gingiva [6]. The attached gingiva of the vestibular side is more frequently involved (more rarely there is a lingual or palatal involvement) which assumes an opaque appearance and bleeds easily. The marginal gingiva is usually spared [1].

Superficial erosive lesions can extend deeper (beyond the basement membrane), leading to the formation of *ulcerative OLP*. The more eroded areas of mucosa have the greatest ulceration risk. Clinically, ulcerative OLP is distinguished from a pure erosive form by the color of the lesion: the erosion appears intensely erythematous and red, while the ulceration is characterized by a more variegated appearance with different colors that describe the tissue suffering and the reparative reactions of the underlying connective tissue [1] (Fig. 5.10). Furthermore, the ulcerated tissue

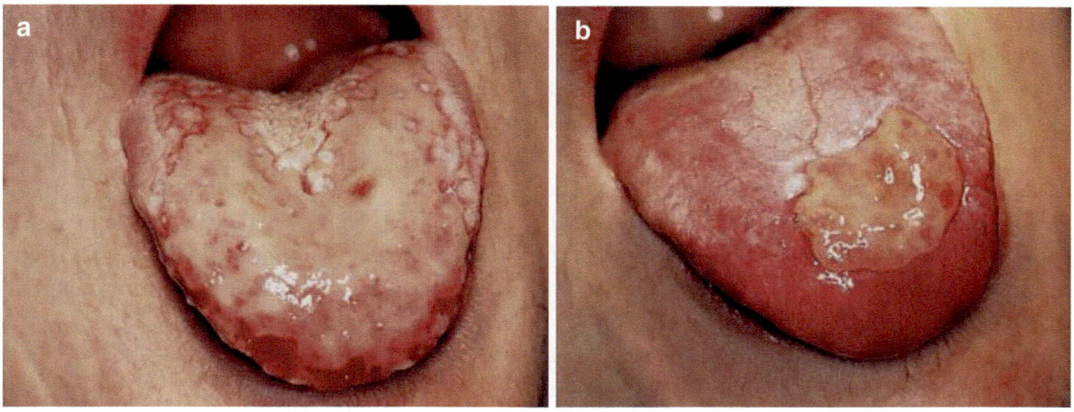

Fig. 5.10 (**a**) Oral lichen planus-related ulceration on the dorsum of the tongue. (**b**) The dorsum of the tongue after 8 weeks of topical tacrolimus therapy. From [36] with permission

tends to bleed spontaneously and is subject to contamination by the oral microbial flora [46, 50].

5.1.6 Bullous OLP

Bullous OLP is the less frequent variant and is characterized by the presence of vesiculo-bullous formations [1] (Fig. 5.11) which tend to enlarge and break [51]. These lesions can vary in diameter from a few millimeters to a few centimeters, and, if subjected to trauma, they rupture, exposing an ulcerated, bleeding, and generally very painful tissue. Symptoms are related to the extent of the lesions and the affected areas. Generally, the regions most affected by bullous OLP are the distal sectors of the mucous membranes, the palatine pillars, the soft palate, the fornices, and the adherent gingiva [1].

Nikolsky's sign could be positive [51]. It is defined as a *displacement of the intact superficial epidermis by a shearing force, indicating a plane of cleavage in the epidermis* [52]. From a pathophysiological point of view, it is associated with *acantholysis* [53], that is, the *loss of coherence between the epidermal cells due to the breaking of their intercellular bridges* [54]. In acantholysis, the cells remain intact but are no longer attached to each other; they tend to be distributed along the smallest possible (spherical) surface, causing cracks, vesicles, and intraepidermal blisters [54]. The sign can also be evoked in apparently healthy areas and on the surface of the oral mucosa [53, 55]. However, the identification of intact vesiculo-bullous lesions in the oral cavity is really challenging for the clinician due to the brittle nature of the oral mucosa and also due to its constant exposure to frictional irritation. Furthermore, the rupture of these lesions leads to erosions or ulcerations on the mucosal surface, thus making the diagnosis of these lesions even more difficult because these often resemble each other clinically and it is sometimes difficult to differentiate them [52]. Nikolsky's sign is generally positive in diseases with intraepidermal acantholysis and is typically negative in diseases with dermoepidermal separation [53], helping to distinguish pemphigus vulgaris from bullous pemphigoid [56]. Nikolsky's sign has high specificity (96.3%) in the oral cavity and can be really useful in the diagnosis of bullous diseases of the

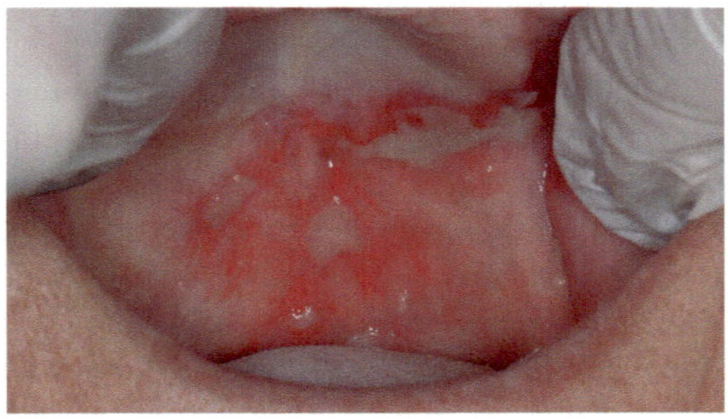

Fig. 5.11 Bullous OLP of the soft palate. Presence of ulceration secondary to blister rupture

oral cavity [57], but it is moderately sensitive for the diagnosis of pemphigus vulgaris [58].

Nikolsky originally described three methods to elicit the sign [58–60]:

1. The stratum corneum can be detached for a long distance, even on apparently normal skin, by pulling a residue of the broken wall of the blister.
2. The stratum corneum can be removed on visibly normal areas of the skin on the periphery of existing lesions by lateral pressure with a finger.
3. Normal-appearing skin can be denuded by exposing the humid surface of the granular layer by rubbing the epidermis.

Nikolsky's sign can also be useful on a prognostic level in indicating the active phase of pemphigus [55]. If, after exerting pressure on the skin or oral mucosa, the eroded blister becomes wet and shiny, Nikolsky's sign is considered "wet," while if the surface appears dry, then Nikolsky's sign is considered "dry" [54, 56]. In patients with active pemphigus vulgaris, a wet sign is expected, while the dry sign indicates reepithelialization under a pemphigus blister which would mean healing and therefore a favorable detection [61]. Similar considerations could also be valid for bullous OLP, which however is a rarer finding; therefore Nikolsky's sign should be indicative, in the first instance, of other vesiculo-bullous diseases, such as pemphigus vulgaris.

Nikolsky's false sign, also known as *Sheklakov's sign*, consists of pulling the residual roof of a ruptured blister, thereby extending the erosion onto the surrounding normal skin. In this case, the induced erosion is limited in size, there is no tendency to spread spontaneously, and it heals quickly [54, 62]. It is defined as "false" because it consists of a subepidermal cleavage that occurs in the perilesional area [63]. Nikolsky's false sign is positive in subepidermal vesiculo-bullous disorders such as bullous pemphigoid, cicatricial pemphigoid, gestational pemphigoid, dermatitis herpetiformis, linear IgA disease, epidermolysis bullosa acquisita, junctional and dystrophic epidermolysis bullosa, porphyrias, and systemic lupus erythematosus (SLE) [62].

Nikolsky's pseudo-sign or *epidermal peeling sign* can instead be elicited in the same way as the Nikolsky's true sign, but this could only be evoked in the erythematous areas involved. In this case the underlying mechanism is epidermal cell necrosis in contrast to acantholysis in Nikolsky's true sign [54, 55, 62]. Nikolsky's pseudo-sign is positive in Stevens-Johnson syndrome, toxic epidermal necrolysis, some cases of burns, and bullous ichthyosiform erythroderma [62].

5.1.7 Mixed and Atypical OLP

The most frequent findings are *mixed OLP* variants in which, in a variable way, the various clinical forms of OLP are associated. From a prognostic point of view, the white forms of OLP (papular, reticular, annular, and plaque) should be considered as quiescent variants of the disease, while the red forms of OLP (atrophic, erosive or ulcer-erosive, and bullous) are considered clinical evolutionary variants [1]. The *Koebner phenomenon* (*reactive isomorphism*), for which inflammatory processes, typical of the dermatosis in progress (OLP in this case), could develop following mechanical trauma (even mild), could partially explain the common appearance of the most severe lesions at more traumatized sites, for example, the buccal mucosa or the lateral surfaces of the tongue [50] (Sect. 3.1.3).

In addition to these, there are also *atypical OLP* forms which are distinguished by the different clinical-morphological characteristics. Among these, for example, there is a form of *pigmented OLP* in which the mucous membranes involved in the pathological process, even in the post-inflammatory period of the acute phases [64], take on a characteristic melanic pigmentation [1].

5.2 Histopathology of OLP Lesions

OLP and LP can be considered, respectively, a form of mucositis/dermatitis of the interface, intended as the basal portion of the epithelium in contact with the basement membrane [1]. Interface mucositis is a hallmark of OLP [65], but it is also found in other oral lesions such as OLL and systemic lupus erythematosus (SLE) [66, 67]. Typical histopathological features of OLP lesions (Fig. 5.12) could be:

1) *Superficial hyperkeratosis* [68]. White OLP variants only (papular, reticular, and especially plaque) present an increased thickness of the various epithelial components with *acanthosis* (epithelium hyperplasia), *hypergranulosis* (increase in the number of cells in the granular layer), and *hyperkeratosis* (para- or orthokeratosis). In this regard, parakeratosis, or the nuclei maintenance in the most superficial layer of the epithelium, is normal in the oral mucosa, unlike for orthokeratosis in which the cells in the stratum corneum do not maintain the nucleus. It is also possible to observe *spongiosis* (accumulation of fluids within the epidermis which causes cell detachment) of the intermediate layers of the Malpighian epithelium (stratum basale and stratum spinosum), with variable intensity based on the inflammatory aggressiveness of the disease [1]. The focal areas of hyperkeratinization are those that clinically originate Wickham's striae, while the atrophic epithelium presents histologically with rete pegs (or

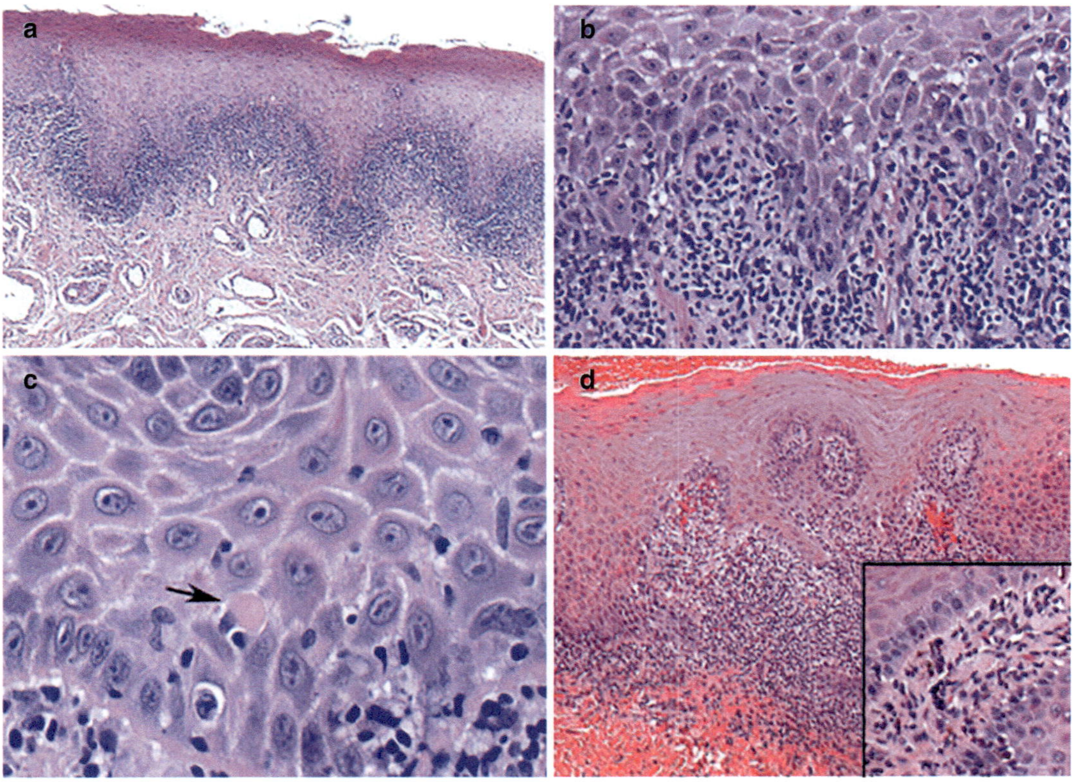

Fig. 5.12 Histopathological features of the reticular form of OLP. (**a**) Oral mucosal stratified squamous epithelium exhibits a thickened surface layer of parakeratin, sawtooth rete ridge morphology, a thin eosinophilic band adjacent to the basal cell layer, and a dense band-like chronic inflammatory cell infiltrate in the superficial lamina propria (H&E stain, original magnification ×100). (**b**) A dense predominantly lymphocytic infiltrate is situated in the lamina propria abutting oral mucosal stratified squamous epithelium. Hydropic degeneration in basal cells is apparent. Dissolution of the basement membrane is also seen (H&E stain, original magnification ×250). (**c**) Lymphocyte-mediated injury of oral mucosal stratified squamous epithelium, with keratinocyte apoptosis represented as a colloid (Civatte) body (arrow, H&E stain, original magnification ×400). (**d**) Melanosis and melanin incontinence with associated melanophages can sometimes be found, especially in biopsies from individuals with dark complexions (insert, H&E stain, original magnification ×250). H&E, hematoxylin and eosin. From [32] with permission

rete ridges that are the epithelial extensions that project into the underlying connective tissue) arranged like a "saw tooth" [51]. In fact, based on the site of the lesion and the clinical subtype (white or red lesions), the histological characteristics of the OLP can vary considerably. Therefore the epithelium may appear acanthotic or atrophic based on the clinical form [65]. Furthermore, compared to cutaneous LP, OLP shows less frequently the sawtooth rete ridges and more frequently the atrophy with lack of the rete ridges [69–71].

2) *Liquefactive or hydropic degeneration of basal keratinocytes with formation of Civatte bodies due to keratinocyte apoptosis* [68]. The initial inflammatory-reactive phases of OLP are characterized by a marked hyperplasia of the Langerhans cells (LCs) which, under normal conditions, would be hardly recognizable under the active microscope, but in this case they appear more voluminous with an optically light cytoplasm and show a pseudo-epithelioid appearance. In the initial inflammatory phases, the oral keratinocytes in the spinous layer often appear edematous within a spongiotic context, while those in the basal layer undergo a process of karyo-cytological suffering (i.e., involving the elements of the nucleoplasm and of the cytoplasm) which subsequently results in a vacuolation or liquefactive/hydropic degeneration that makes the epithelial-connective demarcation difficult to distinguish. In the advanced inflammatory phases, there are gradual trophic-cellular changes, capable of slowing down the keratinocyte turnover, and lymphocyte aggression against the basal keratinocytes is observed. The progress of the hydropic degeneration of the basal layer leads to a focal and gradual regression of this epithelial component, to the point that, at times, the spinous layer appears in direct contact with the submucosal connective [1]. Hydropic degeneration is accompanied by keratinocyte apoptosis [51]. In fact, within the infiltrate, in the basal layer and in the superficial lamina propria, it is possible to identify intensely eosinophilic and homogeneous rounded masses, called Civatte bodies or cytoid or hyaline bodies: these are apoptotic/necrotic and prematurely keratinized basal keratinocytes that collect in the submucosa or dermis, sometimes in small clusters, and in which the presence of DNA fragmentation processes has been demonstrated [1, 66, 72–77]. The erosion of the basal layer causes the rete ridges to show an anomalous and pointed appearance, defined as "saw tooth" [1]. When the damage of the basal layer extends, involving, beyond the degeneration of the basal keratinocytes, a wide interruption of their anchoring elements such as hemidesmosomes, filaments, and fibrils, a weakening of the interface of the epithelial-connective tissue is produced which results in the formation histological fissures (called *Max Joseph spaces*) and, clinically, bullous lesions of the oral cavity (bullous OLP) [1, 6, 78]. Therefore, from a histopathological point of view, during the initial inflammatory-reactive phases and the immunological and phlogistic active phases and, finally, in the periods of regression and quiescence, there are substantially common karyo-cytological manifestations between OLP and cutaneous LP. Similarly, in erosive forms, in the deeper epithelial layers, phenomena of suffering and vacuolation are observed, and moreover in the ulcerated areas, it is possible to observe all those epithelial-mesenchymal inflammatory reactions typical of ulcerative suffering and microbial contamination. In general, in atrophic-erosive OLP, the epithelial thicknesses appear more reduced, with suffering and variable losses of epithelial layers [1].

3) *Lymphocyte inflammatory band below the basement membrane* [68]. The connective lymphocytic infiltrate arranged "in a band" immediately below the basement membrane is also referred to as a *lichenoid infiltrate*. In the initial inflammatory-reactive phases, an initial lymphocytic exocytosis begins to be distinguished in the submucosa, therefore in the context of the subepithelial lamina propria. In the most advanced phases, always at the level of the dermal layer adjacent to the

suffering basement membrane, the typical band of inflammatory lymphocytic infiltrate is characterized, capable of occupying all the superficial connective tissue, the space of the lamina propria, darkening up to cancel the epithelial junction [1]. There may also be an increase in the number of intraepithelial lymphocytes [6]. The inflammatory infiltrate consists mainly of lymphocytes that are optically distinguishable by their intense basophilia and, sometimes, by the presence of a voluminous, rounded, and hyperchromic nucleus. In particular, this lichenoid infiltrate is mainly represented by $CD4^+$ T lymphocytes close to the mesenchymal-connective tissue, while $CD8^+$ T lymphocytes are mainly localized in the portion adjacent to the epithelium, where they express their cytotoxic functions. In the context it is also possible to detect some macrophages, neutrophilic granulocytes, mast cells, and rare plasma cells (recognizable by the basophilic cytoplasm and the eccentric nucleus with heterochromatin arranged in the shape of a *wagon wheel*), while, characteristically, eosinophilic granulocytes are absent [1]. The presence of a mixed and more widespread inflammatory infiltrate should make the suspicion of a lichenoid condition rather than a real idiopathic OLP [6]. In fact, generally, the inflammation in OLP is superficial rather than deep and perivascular inflammation is not usually present [65]. Furthermore, in the erythematous-inflammatory phases, there are a distension and proliferation of the submucosal capillary bed [1].

4) *Absence of maturative disorders of the epithelium* [68]. The various histopathological criteria proposed by van der Meij and van der Waal (2003) and the American Academy of Oral and Maxillofacial Pathology (2016) all agree that it is necessary to exclude the presence of epithelial dysplasia before making a diagnosis of OLP [32]. However, this last element has been much debated, and the most recent diagnostic criteria do not exclude the diagnosis of OLP if epithelial dysplasia is present, given the malignant potential of this disease [79]. Furthermore, the past and present diagnostic WHO criteria (1978 and 2021) do not mention the absence of dysplasia to exclude the diagnosis of OLP [28, 32]. However, this aspect is discussed in depth in Sect. 5.3.

Other histopathological findings may include the presence of melanosis, melanin incontinence with associated melanophages (i.e., macrophages that engulf granules containing melanocytic pigments), particularly in dark-skinned subjects. Melanin incontinence is not specific to OLP as it can be observed in many other oral inflammatory disorders that share a lichenoid inflammatory process [80].

However, it should be noted that the histopathological assessment could be subjective since the OLP appears to have typical but not sufficiently specific characteristics, but a histological examination is always recommended as it allows at least to exclude the presence of foci of dysplasia and oral squamous cell carcinoma (OSCC) [68, 81]. In particular, erosive lesions often lack various histological characteristics of lichen planus; therefore it is not always easy to reach a definitive diagnosis [65]. Inadequate diagnosis is one of the most common causes of nonresponse to treatment [68].

5.3 Diagnostic Criteria and Definitive OLP Diagnosis

The definitive diagnosis of OLP is fundamental for the therapeutic setting and decision-making management in the context of its chronic course. But some difficulties and interpretative perplexities have always emerged in the context of this pathology [1], due to the fact that many oral diseases can have clinical and microscopic characteristics similar to those of OLP, including proliferative verrucous leukoplakia (PVL) [32]. Indeed, not infrequently, microscopic "lichenoid" characteristics are observed in dysplasia and oral squamous cell carcinoma (OSCC) [82, 83]. Therefore, an incorrect diagnosis of OLP may occur, especially when limited clinical information is provided to the pathologist and when atypical cellular changes are accompanied by a lichenoid infiltrate [32]. A correct diagnosis requires knowledge of the clinical and histological characteristics of OLP and a good communication between the clinician and the pathologist. Since the OLP diagnosis requires an assessment of the basement membrane area, biopsies must include the full-thickness intact epithelium [65]. But it must be premised that a definitive OLP diagnosis cannot be based only on clinical criteria or only on histopathological results, as there is risk of reaching misleading conclusions resulting in a misdiagnosis within other potentially malignant disorders similar to OLP but with different behavior (e.g., erythroplakia or PVL) [29, 84]. Therefore, the main challenges in diagnosing OLP are due to the fact that many clinical and microscopic features of OLP are not specific of the disease. Furthermore, the histopathological features of OLP appear to fall into a spectrum, potentially influenced by the stage of disease activity at the time of biopsy, by any recent therapy of the condition, by the clinical subtype (reticular or erosive), and/or by anatomical sites (buccal mucosa or gum). At present, there are still no widely accepted diagnostic criteria for OLP [32].

5.3.1 WHO Criteria (1978)

The first set of diagnostic criteria of OLP was published in 1978 by the WHO Collaborating Center for Oral Precancerous Lesions (Table 5.1) [85].

The 1978 WHO criteria which did not address a way to distinguish or exclude epithelial dysplasia from the OLP diagnosis [85] and their application revealed great interobserver and intraobserver variability [86, 87]. Onofre et al. found clinicopathological discrepancies in the diagnosis of OLP in a quarter of the selected cases [88]. Furthermore, the WHO criteria did not describe the difference between OLP and OLL.

5.3.2 van der Meij and van der Waal Modified Criteria (2003)

In order to reduce this interpretative variability, in 2003, van der Meij and van der Waal proposed changes to the diagnostic criteria postulated by the WHO [89] (Table 5.2). First of all, a differentiation of OLP and OLL criteria is made. From a clinical point of view, the key feature for OLP diagnosing is the presence of bilateral white reticulum, but not necessarily plaque, atrophic, erosive, or bullous lesions. From a histopathological point of view, the absence of dysplasia (i.e., atypical cytomorphologies such as enlargement of the nucleus or hyperchromasia, prevalent dyskeratosis, increase in mitotic figures) is explicitly mentioned in order to diagnose OLP. In this way, an attempt was made to exclude lichenoid dysplasia, i.e., lesions characterized by epithelial dysplasia together with a lympho-monocytic band infiltrate. The authors suggested using the terms "histopathologically compatible with" or "clinically compatible with" when microscopic features or clinical features (e.g., lack of bilateral lesion) appeared less obvious. A heterogeneous population of the inflammatory infiltrate, the deeper submucosal extension of the infiltrate beyond the superficial connective tissue, and perivascular infiltration are elements that indicate OLL, rather than OLP. The complete correspondence of the clinical and histopathological criteria of van der Meij and van der Waal (also defined as modified WHO diag-

Table 5.1 WHO OLP diagnostic criteria (1978)

Clinical criteria	Histopathological criteria
Usually multiple and often symmetric in distribution	Orthokeratosis or parakeratosis
White papular, reticular (lace-like network of slightly raised gray-white lines), annular, or plaque-type lesions	Epithelial thickness varies; sawtooth rete ridges sometimes seen
White lines radiating from the papules	Civatte bodies in the basal layer of the epithelium or superficial lamina propria
Atrophic lesions with or without erosion	A narrow band of eosinophilic material in the basement membrane
Bullae are rare	Well-defined band-like zone of cellular infiltration that is confined to the superficial lamina propria, consisting mainly of lymphocytes
	Liquefaction degeneration in the basal cell layer

Table 5.2 van der Meij and van der Waal diagnostic criteria (2003)

Clinical criteria	Histopathological criteria
Bilateral, more or less symmetric lesions	Well-defined, band-like zone of cellular infiltration consisting mainly of lymphocytes and confined to the superficial lamina propria
Erosive, atrophic, bullous, and plaque-type lesions are only accepted as a subtype in the presence of reticular lesions elsewhere in the oral mucosa	Liquefaction degeneration in the basal cell layer
Lace-like network of slightly raised gray-white lines (reticular pattern)	Absence of epithelial dysplasia
In all other lesions that resemble OLP, but do not meet the above criteria, the term "clinically compatible with" should be used	When histopathological features are less evident, the term "histopathologically compatible with" should be used
OLP/OLL Definitive Diagnosis	
OLP: To obtain a definitive OLP diagnosis, the clinical and histopathological criteria should be fully satisfied.	
OLL: The term OLL will be used under the following conditions: 1. Clinically typical of OLP but histopathologically only compatible with OLP 2. Histopathologically typical of OLP but clinically only compatible with OLP 3. Clinically compatible with OLP and histopathologically compatible with OLP	

nostic criteria) is the necessary condition for diagnosing OLP [1, 29, 32, 84].

Rad et al. [90] found greater agreement between clinicians and pathologists in the diagnosis of OLP when the van der Meij and van der Waal criteria were used rather than those of the WHO of 1978. However, as already mentioned, uniformly accepted criteria are lacking and adopted by the entire scientific community. The difficulty in reaching consensus is partly due to variations in the histopathological OLP characteristics. For example, the presence of hyperkeratosis (diagnostic criterion adopted by the WHO) depends on the site involved and OLP variant (frequent in white lesions, but not in red ones). One of the most characteristic histopathological findings of this mucocutaneous pathology is the presence of the predominantly lymphocytic band infiltrate at the level of the lamina propria, but this element is also subject to variations, as its intensity is linked to the activity of the disease and by the implementation of a therapeutic intervention before the biopsy. Furthermore, the subsets of inflammatory cells in the infiltrate can vary according to the clinical subtype (reticular or erosive), the anatomical site (buccal or gingival mucosa), or the presence of another concomitant inflammatory process. In red lesions, the overlap of neutrophilic granulocytes related to the ulcer lesion could alter the microscopic characteristics. In OLP gingival lesions, the inflammatory infiltrate is often mixed with the presence of plasma cells due to gingivitis or periodontitis associated with plaque or tartar. Therefore, tissue samples that do not fully meet the modified WHO criteria should require pathologists to consider some interference factors such as those described above, and this evaluation brings into play the subjectivity factor [32]. In addition, various diagnostic criteria are not exclusive to OLP. For example, the liquefactive degeneration of basal keratinocytes is also found in other conditions such as OLL-GvHD (graft-versus-host disease-induced OLL), lupus erythematosus, OLDRs (oral lichenoid drug reactions—drug-induced OLL), and OLCHR (oral lichenoid contact hypersensitivity reaction—OLL due to contact hypersensitivity) [91]. The presence of Civatte bodies, a histopathological finding in OLP, supports its diagnosis, but these are also found in lupus erythematosus, OLDR, GvHD, and other interface dermatitis [91–93]. The presence of sawtooth epithelial ridges also constitutes a supporting, but not a diagnostic, element of OLP [32]. On the other hand, in recent years, the efforts of researchers have focused on understanding the pathogenesis of OLP and in the search for potential diagnostic, therapeutic, and prognostic markers of this pathology (Sects. 4.3–4.4). Current knowledge of the pathophysiological mechanisms of OLP can help clinicians and pathologists also in the correlation of histopathological characteristics [32]. For example, lymphocyte exocytosis within the epithelium is a recognized feature more in OLP than in other lichenoid conditions such as MMP (mucous membrane pemphigoid) in which the immune response is directed toward adhesion molecules of the basal membrane, while in OLP cytotoxic $CD8^+$ T lymphocytes attack basal keratinocytes [3, 73]. Furthermore, the presence of eosinophilic granulocytes (which have not been related to the pathogenesis of OLP) could be indicative of other disorders such as MMP and OLCHR rather than OLP itself [32]. The absence of eosinophilic granulocytes and the migration of lymphocytes into the epithelium are not part of the WHO criteria of 1978 and of the modified criteria of 2003.

5.3.3 American Academy of Oral and Maxillofacial Pathology Criteria (2016)

In 2005, WHO recommended to develop additional diagnostic criteria to ensure a differential diagnosis between OLP and OLL, despite both showing a risk of neoplastic transformation [84]. For this reason, in 2016, a position paper of the American Academy of Oral and Maxillofacial Pathology proposed new diagnostic criteria [32] (Table 5.3).

OLP diagnosis requires satisfaction of all clinical and histopathological criteria. All conditions characterized by interface chronic mucositis that do not fully meet these diagnostic criteria should be designated as OLL, or the doctor should provide a descriptive diagnosis, such as "lichenoid mucositis" or "chronic mucositis with lichenoid characteristics." Regarding the clinical criteria, the authors specify that, since a pure bullous OLP form has never been reported, if a pure bullous lesion occurs, bullous OLP should not be diagnosed, but other vesiculo-bullous diseases such as MMP should be considered as well as PV (pemphigus vulgaris). Regarding the histopathological aspects, the authors confirmed the need for the absence of dysplasia to diagnose OLP, and furthermore, given the ability of proliferative verrucous leukoplakia (PVL) to present clinical and microscopic characteristics similar to OLP, the authors proposed as a new and additional criterion the absence of a verrucous epithelial architecture for OLP diagnosis. This type of architecture is characterized by a papillary or verrucous configuration of the spinous cell layer accompanied by variable levels of undulation of the mucosal surface. However, the possibility of an emerging PVL cannot be excluded, since the verrucous architectural changes in the epithelium may not yet be evident, while the clinical and histopathological characteristics could meet the new criteria proposed. Furthermore, in some cases OLCHR may show histopathological characteristics that could satisfy all the new criteria proposed, and the cause-effect relationship with an inducing agent may not be clearly indicated clinically; therefore in these cases, the presence of eosinophils and/or a perivascular lymphoplasmacytic infiltrate in the deep lamina propria generally allows to exclude

Table 5.3 American Academy of Oral and Maxillofacial Pathology OLP diagnostic criteria (2016)

Clinical criteria	Histopathological criteria
Multifocal symmetric distribution	Band-like or patchy, predominately lymphocytic infiltrate in the lamina propria confined to the epithelium-lamina propria interface
White and red lesions exhibiting one or more of the following forms: – Reticular/papular – Atrophic (erythematous) – Erosive (ulcerative) – Plaque – Bullous	Basal cell liquefactive (hydropic) degeneration
Lesions are not localized exclusively to the sites of smokeless tobacco placement	Lymphocytic exocytosis
Lesions are not localized exclusively adjacent to and in contact with dental restorations	Absence of epithelial dysplasia
Lesion onset does not correlate with the start of a medication	Absence of verrucous epithelial architectural change
Lesion onset does not correlate with the use of cinnamon-containing products	

the diagnosis of OLP. However, the authors recognized that adherence to these diagnostic criteria could exclude some cases of OLP; but obtaining a population of patients truly affected by OLP, compared to those with OLL, will allow to obtain an improvement in the validity of future investigations which will aim to clarify the pathogenesis, the potential for malignant transformation, and any accessory diagnostic protocols that could improve the diagnostic process. However, strict adherence to these criteria, in any case, cannot exclude some rare cases that mimic OLP, such as LPP (lichen planus pemphigoides), CUS (chronic ulcerative stomatitis), or paraneoplastic pemphigoid without use of further investigations such as DIF (direct immunofluorescence) and IIF (indirect immunofluorescence) [32].

Therefore, the diagnostic process of OLP should not be considered definitive with an initial biopsy. Follow-up clinical evaluation for monitoring the therapeutic response and any changes in the appearance of the lesions and, in some cases, further biopsies and investigations such as immunofluorescence may be necessary (especially in the differential diagnosis of gingival manifestations) to reach a real final diagnosis of OLP [1, 32].

5.3.4 Updated WHO Criteria (2020)

In March 2020, the WHO Collaborating Centre for Oral Cancer in the UK convened a workshop attended by invited experts to discuss the advances in knowledge and recent changes in the understanding of oral potentially malignant disorders (OPMDs) [28]. OLP should be diagnosed basing on both clinical and histopathological criteria (Table 5.4) and should be distinguished from other clinically similar disorders such as OLL [89], OLDR [94], OLCHR [95], LPP, CUS, and acute/chronic GvHD [32, 96].

WHO provided the diagnostic criteria relating only to OLP. About OLL, the Working Group agreed to the van der Meij and van der Waal (2003) consideration: lichenoid lesions are disorders that do not present the clinical and/or histopathological characteristics considered typical

Table 5.4 WHO updated OLP diagnostic criteria (2020)

Clinical criteria	Histopathological criteria
Presence of bilateral, more or less symmetrical white lesions affecting buccal mucosa and/or tongue and/or lip and/or gingiva	Presence of a well-defined band-like predominantly lymphocytic infiltrate that is confined to the superficial part of the connective tissue
Presence of a white papular lesions and lace-like network of slightly raised white lines (reticular, annular, or linear pattern) with or without erosions and ulcerations	Signs of vacuolar degeneration of the basal and/or suprabasal cell layers with keratinocyte apoptosis
Sometimes presents as desquamative gingivitis	In the atrophic type, there are epithelial thinning and sometimes ulceration caused by failure of epithelial regeneration as a result of basal cell destruction. A mixed inflammatory infiltrate may be found

(but compatible) with OLP. Therefore OLLs include [28]:

1. Atypical OLP and unilateral lichenoid lesions [89, 97, 98]
2. OLCHR (lichenoid lesions in close contact relationship to a dental restoration, often amalgam) [95, 99]
3. OLDR [95]
4. Oral lesions following intake of food or some substances, such as cinnamon (cinnamon stomatitis)
5. OLL-GvHD

Furthermore, lichenoid contact reactions to betel quid have been reported among betel quid users [100]. Finally, the Working Group recommended to avoid the use of the term "oral lichenoid dysplasia" to describe an entity among OLP or lichenoid disorders which show dysplastic changes. If dysplasia is present, the diagnosis should be "oral epithelial dysplasia with lichenoid features" (i.e., if the latter features are indeed evident) or "OLP with dysplasia" [28]. It seems that these two terminologies would indicate the same pathological entity. If so, this would not allow to distinguish between a primarily maturative epithelium disorder with an inflammatory-reactive infiltrate and a primarily immune-mediated disorder (OLP or OLL) in which histopathological atypia is present.

5.4 Additional Investigations in the Diagnosis of OLP

Given the difficulties, especially in nontypical forms, in some cases additional investigations may prove useful to confirm the diagnosis of OLP. Among these investigations, the use of immunofluorescence stands out.

Immunofluorescence (direct or indirect) is a test used in particular for the diagnosis of vesiculo-bullous disorders. These methods are used to detect the presence of autoantibodies in the tissue or serum, without however identifying the antigen toward which these antibodies are directed. The presence or absence in the tissue/serum is simply identified. Performing immunofluorescence requires the use of a tissue that should be sent fresh to the laboratory, since the fixatives denature the antibodies. Therefore, it is often chosen to perform immunofluorescence at the same time as the histological examination, so that, during the surgical act, two biopsy samples are taken:

1. For the histological examination, the biopsy must be taken between the lesion and the healthy tissue and tissues must be preserved in formalin.
2. For immunofluorescence, biopsy sampling should be carried out in the adjacent healthy mucosa and stored in Michel's solution or in a sterile saline solution.

To understand how immunofluorescence works, the antibodies' structure should first be known. Antibodies are composed by a fixed region, the same for a single type of antibody, and a variable region that binds to the antigen. In the immunofluorescence test, a fluorescent antibody is used to visualize the autoantibody (in the tissue/serum) by binding to its fixed region which is different for IgA, IgM, and IgG. Direct immunofluorescence may also be employed to identify the presence of complement C3 and fibrinogen [101].

5.4.1 Direct Immunofluorescence (DIF)

Direct immunofluorescence (DIF) is used to directly detect the presence of autoantibodies bound to the cells of the collected tissue. It is one of the most widely used additional diagnostic procedures for mucocutaneous disorders and can help support a diagnosis of OLP [32, 46]. DIF employment is justifiable in the presence of ambiguous clinical and histopathological characteristics of other diseases (such as lupus erythematosus [LE] [102]) and not particularly conclusive of OLP, in clinical situations where a bullous and intensely erythematous component prevails or where lesions are mainly ulcer-erosive and exclusively involving the gums [5, 68]. This test may be useful to differentiate OLP from other vesiculo-bullous diseases that typically present as desquamative gingivitis, such as mucous membrane pemphigoid (MMP) and chronic ulcerative stomatitis (CUS) [103, 104].

DIF in OLP patients is generally negative or may produce particular alterations [105]. The most typical feature in the DIF examination of OLP tissues is the detection of fibrinogen and fibrin (best indicator in the diagnosis of OLP [105]) in the form of linear, granular, or shaggy deposits, usually singularly or sometimes in combination with other immunoreagents such as complement C3 and immunoglobulins IgG, IgM, and IgA [105, 106] (only Civatte bodies are coated with immunoglobulins [107]), along the basement membrane and/or the superficial lamina propria [68, 72, 103, 104, 108–114]. It should be specified that, when present, the deposition of IgM, and less often of IgA, IgG, and complement C3, was found exclusively on the Civatte bodies [46] which can be positive (in addition to fibrin) also for C4 and keratin [6]. However, complement and immunoglobulin deposits are not a consistent feature in OLP. Laminin and fibronectin staining may be absent precisely in the areas of heavy fibrin deposition and formation of Civatte bodies, suggesting damage to the basement membrane in these areas [6]. DIF shows that in OLP the Civatte bodies tend to group in clusters of ten or more elements, and this characteristic could be useful to distinguish LP from LE since, in the latter condition, the Ig deposits show a more linear arrangement [115]. The combination of the presence of fibrin deposits and fluorescent cytoid bodies is more characteristic of OLP rather than LE, although in both conditions identical deposits of Ig could be found in the bodies of Civatte, C3, or linear fibrin in the basement membrane [116]. However, C3 complement deposition occurs more frequently in LE than in LP where anti-C3 can be observed with a weak linear, fine, granular, or discontinuous appearance and the presence of IgM is more suggestive of LE than LP [72]. However, this DIF pattern can also be observed, as just mentioned, in other inflammatory conditions, as well as in potentially malignant and malignant oral disorders [117], and therefore cannot be considered specific for OLP [32]. Furthermore, DIF detections of tissues with idiopathic OLP appear to be identical to those of drug-related OLL (OLDR) [118].

As already mentioned, DIF requires the use of fresh tissue for frozen sections or tissue stored in a suitable means of transport (Michel's solution). Therefore, this diagnostic procedure adds costs to the diagnostic process but may be considered necessary in some situations in which the available clinical and histopathological information is insufficient to support a definitive diagnosis of OLP [32].

5.4.2 Indirect Immunofluorescence (IIF)

Indirect immunofluorescence (IIF) is employed to detect the presence of serum autoantibodies in vesiculo-bullous diseases. In this test, the patient's serum is incubated with the normal oral mucosa/skin or monkey esophagus. During this time, serum autoantibodies bind to the appropriate antigen of the oral mucosa/skin of the patient or monkey esophagus and will be detected through fluorescent secondary antihuman antibodies, similar to DIF [101, 119]. However, for subepithelial bullous disorders (such as MMP and bullous pemphigoids), IIF has low sensitivity that may be enhanced though a variant of this method called "salt split skin" (IIF-SSS). This test involves the use of 1 M NaCl solution tissue pre-treatment. Through this technique the skin undergoes a separation at the level of the basement membrane with the consequent formation of two layers (epidermal and dermal side) [101, 120]. This determines a better exposure of the antigens, on the epidermal and dermal side in a differentiated way. For example, the autoantibodies bind the epidermal side of the split in MMP/bullous pemphigoid, whereas in epidermolysis bullosa acquisita, they bind to the dermal side [121].

Here are some patterns that can be observed in vesiculo-bullous disorders through DIF and IIF:

- Pemphigus vulgaris (PV): IgG (anti-desmoglein 3 [Dsg3]) and C3 deposits around the surface of the keratinocytes in the prickle cell layer resulting in a "fish-scale" appearance [122]
- Pemphigus foliaceus (PF; rare in the oral cavity): IgG (anti-desmoglein 1 [Dsg1]) and C3 deposits with a similar appearance to the PV but to a higher level in the prickle cell layer [122]
- Bullous pemphigoid (BP) or mucous membrane pemphigoid (MMP): autoantibody deposits (usually IgG or C3, sometimes IgA and/or IgM in addition) at the basement membrane zone [123]
- Linear IgA disease: linear IgA (sometimes also IgM) deposits [124]

Therefore, IIF is a test employed for the detection of circulating antibodies in the bloodstream. However, this technique is not useful alone or in addition to the clinical diagnosis of OLP/OLL [46]. Several authors report that the IIF is negative and useless in the diagnosis of OLP [32, 65]. Using this test, Lin S-C et al. detected anti-basal cell antibodies in the serum of 54% of the 63 examined OLP patients [125]. According to Mutafchieva et al. [81], DIF and IIF would be mandatory in patients with bullous OLP and manifestations of desquamative gingivitis in order to distinguish it from PV, MMP, dermatitis herpetiformis, and other similar disorders. There are studies that have indicated the use of IIF in the diagnosis of OLDR. For example, in skin reactions to drugs, reactive circulating antibodies with the basal cells of the skin give rise to a ring-shaped fluorescence pattern, sometimes referred to as a "string of pearls" or BCCA (basal cell cytoplasmic autoantibody), which aids in the diagnosis of these drug reactions [126, 127].

Based on these data, IIF is not suitable for the diagnosis of OLP, but is indicated only when the diagnostic suspicion focuses more on other immune-inflammatory diseases rather than OLP.

Furthermore, as already mentioned, immunofluorescence cannot identify autoantibody type and, consequently, always distinguish between different vesiculo-bullous disorder subtypes. Other tests are required to identify the target-specific autoantibodies. In this regard, in vesiculo-bullous disorders, the enzyme-linked immunosorbent assay (ELISA) method may be useful to identify specific antibodies and/or antigens. In this test a microtiter plate is coated with the appropriate antigen (e.g., BP180, BP230, Dsg1, Dsg3) [101]. ELISA showed to be more sensitive in PV diagnosis compared to IIF [128] but demonstrated similar specificity and sensitivity for pemphigoid diagnosis [129]. ELISA has not been employed in OLP diagnosis; however it may be useful to differentiate bullous OLP from PV and MMP or other vesiculo-bullous oral disorders.

5.4.3 Other Investigations and Biomarkers

Over the years, there have been numerous efforts by scientists in the search for diagnostic methods capable of corroborating the diagnosis of OLP as well as providing prognostic, therapeutic response and risk of malignant transformation indications.

First of all it is advisable to perform *complete blood tests* which should be included in the overall patient assessment [51].

Although cytological changes can be detected in the OLP, the use of *exfoliative cytology* is not recommended [130].

Some studies showed a higher incidence of *Candida albicans* infection in patients with OLP, and *PAS* (periodic acid-Schiff) reactive *staining* of biopsy specimens and *Candida* cultures or smears can be performed [131].

It has been proposed that allergy to dental materials is common in patients with OLL. *Skin patch testing* is a recognized and accepted method for identifying allergens responsible for type I and type IV allergic reactions.

Susceptible individuals may be sensitized after long exposure to dental materials in direct contact with the oral mucosa. Basal keratinocytes may be antigenically altered by these contacts for the release of mercury or other products. OLCHR are, in fact, characterized by type IV delayed hypersensitivity reaction which involves sensitized macrophages and T lymphocytes against the antigen (hapten). However it is not known how mercury or other haptens are able to trigger immune reactions. Standardized hapten batteries are commonly used to perform the *dental series epicutaneous patch test* (Trolab). The test substances are applied to the skin of the back and read after 72 h of exposure. Patients are considered to be patch test positive for an allergen if they develop erythematous, edematous (vesicular), or bullous (ulcerative) reactions at the site of contact [46].

Although in the past amalgam was one of the most used restorative materials, reported cases of hypersensitivity to amalgam are relatively rare. Skin patch testing studies investigating contact sensitivity responses to mercury and amalgam have yielded mixed results, with a percentage of patients with OLP between 8% and 78.9% [46].

Lind et al. reported that 34% of patients with OLP (topographically related to amalgam restorations) tested positive for mercury compounds [132]. According to a study by Laine et al. [133], which included 118 patients with OLL topographically related to dental restorations, 67.8%

of these tested positive for the metal patch test of dental filling materials. Positive tested patients more commonly presented contact OLLs with limited extension to the restoration compared to negative tested patients who more often showed lesions that exceeded the adjacent areas, indicating the association of the OLL with the filling material.

Regarding *tissue biomarkers*, alterations in toll-like receptors (TLRs), in histamine HA (and its receptors; Sect. 4.4.4), and also in local tissue levels of IL-22, IL- 23 (distinction between cutaneous LP, OLP, and EOLP), and IFN-γ. The roles of other tissue biomarkers such as the VEGF/EGFR family and periostin are also being investigated (Sect. 4.4.5).

As regards the *neoplastic risk biomarkers* in OLP, these have been described in Sect. 4.5.4. Among these, studies on p53, PCNA, HER2/neu, p16, and Ki-67 stand out. The recent discoveries on the alteration of the expression of H4R and the factors released by mast cells (MCs) are also of interest (Sect. 4.4.4).

As part of the *serological and salivary investigations*, many potential biomarkers of the disease were evaluated, described in Sects. 4.3 and 4.4. Among these markers, in the context of cytokines, the potentially most promising biomarkers for prognostic evaluation (more or less aggressive erosive forms), the therapeutic response and the risk of neoplastic transformation seem to be the serum and especially salivary levels of IL-6, IL-8, IL-17, TNF-α. The levels of some mi-RNAs (including especially miR-146a and miR-155) are also altered, especially in the erosive forms. It has been shown that the levels of human beta-defensin 2 (hBD-2) in oral fluids are higher in the red OLP forms compared to the white ones (Sect. 4.4.3). Salivary nitric oxide (NO) also appears to be a useful diagnostic, therapeutic, and prognostic biomarker of OLP, while studies on serum levels of chitinase-3-like protein 1 (YKL-40), although promising, are only in the initial phase (Sect. 4.4.5). The results on the role of salivary cortisol are conflicting (Sect. 4.4.5). In addition, some authors report an elevation in the serum titer of antinuclear antibodies (ANA) [51]. Studies have also shown the presence of gastric parietal cell serum autoantibodies (GPCA) in different groups of OLP patients [134]. Furthermore, the treatment of OLP patients with levamisole and vitamin B12 (vit B12) showed a significant reduction in the GPCA levels which was associated with a contextual improvement of oral lesions [135]. Therefore, serum levels of GPCA could constitute a potential biomarker for diagnosing OLP, but, for both ANA and GPCA, there is still little evidence to reach definitive conclusions. In completing the diagnostic framework, it is also advisable to evaluate in patients with suspected OLP, through serological investigations, the possible presence of HCV infection [68].

Finally, the possible role of *antioxidant and peroxidation levels* and *immunoglobulins* as potential biomarkers in OLP remains to be mentioned.

1. As regards the first point, low salivary levels of peroxidation products have been reported in oral carcinoma and OLP [136, 137]. Additionally, a decrease in antioxidant activity in cancer has been reported [138] in addition to studies that have shown that the integration of antioxidants such as vitamins C and E (vit C and E) is useful in cancer prevention [139, 140]. As mentioned in Sect. 4.5.3, it has been showed that the total antioxidant activity (TAA) serum level in patients with OLP was significantly lower compared to healthy subjects and that salivary levels of the lipid peroxidation product malondialdehyde (MDA) were significantly higher in the OLP group compared to controls [141]. Rai et al. [142] demonstrated in patients with OLP an increase in the levels of lipid peroxidation products, including malondialdehyde (MDA) and 8-hydroxydeoxyguanosine (8-OHdG), and a decrease in the levels of some antioxidants such as vit C and vit E, compared to healthy subjects. After treatment with curcumin for over 200 days, the level of lipid peroxidation products (oxidants) decreased and that of antioxidants increased. Therefore, levels of vit C and E, as antioxidants, could be useful biomarkers suitable for predicting potentially malignant conditions such as OLP.

2. Regarding immunoglobulins, Sistig et al. [143] reported increased levels of IgG and IgA in patients with OLP. Ghalayani et al. [144] also observed an increase in IgA and IgG levels in patients with OLP and OLL compared to healthy subjects. An increase in salivary IgA levels was also observed in patients with oral leukoplakia, OLP, and oral cancer [143, 145]. However, some authors report that these values, although higher than in healthy subjects, do not show a statistically significant difference [146].

5.5 Differential Diagnosis

More than 40 years ago, the concept of interface dermatitis/lichenoid tissue reaction (IFD/LTR) was introduced in dermatology to define a series of inflammatory skin diseases that share common histopathological characteristics, including liquefactive/vacuolar changes of the basal keratinocytes and a "band" of subepithelial concentration of inflammatory mononuclear cells, including activated T lymphocytes, macrophages, and dendritic cells (DCs) [67, 147, 148].

Traditionally, cutaneous IFD/LTR have been divided into two subgroups: "IFD/LTR or lymphocyte-rich disorders," including lichen planus (LP), discoid lupus erythematosus (DLE), chronic graft-versus-host disease (cGvHD), and lichenoid drug reactions, and "IFD/LTR or lymphocyte-poor disorders," including acute and subacute cutaneous LE, dermatomyositis, acute graft-versus-host disease (aGvHD), and the spectrum of erythema multiforme (EM) [147].

Similar to the skin, the oral mucosa is affected by a variety of lesions with lichenoid features such as OLP and OLL, which include a group of disorders of the oral mucosa that probably represent a common pattern of reaction in response to extrinsic antigens, altered autoantigens, or superantigens [67]. Historically, there have been unresolved debates and controversies around the terminology of oral lichen and lichenoid lesions [96], and there are still no definitive diagnostic and histological criteria capable of distinguishing OLP and OLL [67]. Furthermore, there is still no consensus on the possible different clinical behavior of the disorders of the OLP and OLL group with respect to the development of oral cancer [96]. During the World Workshop in Oral Medicine IV in 2006, it was proposed to classify the OLP and OLL group into four distinct disorders: idiopathic OLP, OLDR (oral lichenoid drug reaction) or oral lichenoid reactions caused by exposure systemic to drugs, OLCHR (oral lichenoid contact hypersensitivity reaction) or OLCLs (oral lichenoid contact lesions) or those triggered by the local hypersensitive reaction to dental materials, and OLL from GvHD (graft-versus-host disease) or oral lichenoid lesions triggered by the GvHD [95]. Although this was a step forward, this classification did not provide clear and reliable clinical and histological criteria to differentiate these three types of OLL from OLP and excluded several other pathological entities with clinical-histological characteristics from IFD/LTR [96]. In fact, OLLs are not always more localized than OLP lesions, there is no clear evidence that OLCLs are only in topographical relationship with amalgam fillings, and also the temporal association of OLDRs with the intake of certain drugs (with mechanisms of action among the most disparate) is highly variable [67].

OLLs have already been mentioned in Sect. 3.1.2, but in this chapter the diagnostic aspects and management will be studied in depth. The elements of differential diagnosis of OLP with OLL and other disorders that show clinical-histological elements of IFD/LTR in the oral cavity (OIFD or OLTR) will also be investigated.

5.5.1 Specific and Non-specific OLP Characteristics

Idiopathic OLP is characterized by a genetically induced increase in the production of Th1 cytokines (in particular IFN-γ and TNF-α) [96], although a recent study has suggested a possible contributing role of Th2-mediated inflammation and its progression induced by myeloid DCs which, in turn, are activated by thymic stromal lymphopoietin secreted by epithelial cells [149].

The progressive characterization of the pathogenesis of OLP (Chap. 4) will contribute to the identification of new markers having a differentiating diagnostic role, but, to date, the diagnosis is mainly clinical and histological (although many markers seem to constitute potential diagnostic elements; see Sect. 5.4.3). As already mentioned in the previous paragraphs, the clinical manifestations alone can sometimes be sufficiently diagnostic, in particular when they occur in the bilateral or papular reticular keratotic pattern, but given the chronic and variable course, the risk of cancerization, and the possible presence of dysplasia, it is always advisable to perform a biopsy examination before starting active treatment, as the inappropriate diagnosis is a common cause of therapy failure [150]. Regarding differential diagnosis, when ulcer-erosive lesions are predominant, it is possible to confuse OLP with other diseases such as pemphigus vulgaris (PV), mucous membrane pemphigoid (MMP), and persistent erythema multiforme (EM) [5, 150, 151], while the presence of reticular lesions accompanying erosive ones can help in the diagnosis of OLP [68]. The DIF can be diagnostically helpful in patients who have predominantly ulcer-erosive lesions, in order to exclude other vesiculo-ulcerative autoimmune diseases [96]. Sometimes, to obtain a definitive diagnosis and differentiate OLP from other vesiculo-bullous disorders (in particular MMP), additional immunological tests are required such as salt split skin, IIF, immunoprecipitation/immunoblotting (Western blotting or immunofixation), and ELISAs [152]; however, these techniques are expensive, time-consuming, and not widely available [153]. Persistent plaque OLP lesions, particularly in smokers, and in the absence of reticulo-papular lesions typical of the disease, may be difficult to distinguish from other lesions such as oral leukoplakia [68, 96]. Furthermore, even congenital dyskeratosis can sometimes present with lichenoid characteristics [154], and therefore all pediatric cases of suspected OLP must be carefully studied to evaluate the presence or absence of nail dystrophies, abnormal skin pigmentation of the reticles, and hematological abnormalities [96].

5.5.2 Oral Lichenoid Contact Lesions (OLCLs or OLCHR)

In Sect. 3.1.2 it has already been explained what OLCLs are and what they are caused by. In this paragraph, the diagnostic aspects and therapeutic management are explored. The OLCLs could be clinically and histologically indistinguishable from OLP, but usually this kind of lesions is observed in direct topographical relationship with the offending agent [95] (usually amalgam restorations), while OLP may also have extraoral manifestations. From a clinical point of view, it is believed that OLCLs are more commonly asymmetrical and unilateral than OLP, but the evidence to support this is still scarce [32, 96]. Furthermore, the close proximity of OLCLs to amalgam restorations (Fig. 5.13), while common, has not been invariably reported [96]. In addition, OLCLs may not assume the typical reticular appearance of OLP but more commonly present in the form of plaque or atrophic lesions, usually located on the posterior mucous membranes and lingual lateral edges [65, 96].

From a histopathological point of view, the microscopic characteristics of OLCL often overlap with those of OLP and other lichenoid reactions [32, 96]; however histological analysis could help in the differential diagnosis in case it should show an inflammatory subepithelial infiltrate with mixed cells characterized by a diffuse and deeper distribution in the lamina propria [96], although these findings are relatively nonspecific [65]. In addition, histological examination may show the formation of tertiary lymphoid follicles composed of B lymphocytes and containing follicular DCs surrounded by T lymphocytes and macrophages, like the tonsils [156–159].

As mentioned in Sect. 3.1.2, several flavoring agents such as cinnamon, menthol, eugenol, and peppermint have also been associated with OLCL, with lesions occurring at the site of contact, or more often on the lingual lateral border and buccal mucosa [67]. In particular, cinnamon and products containing cinnamic aldehyde may induce in predisposed subjects a “cinnamon stomatitis” which has typical histopathological

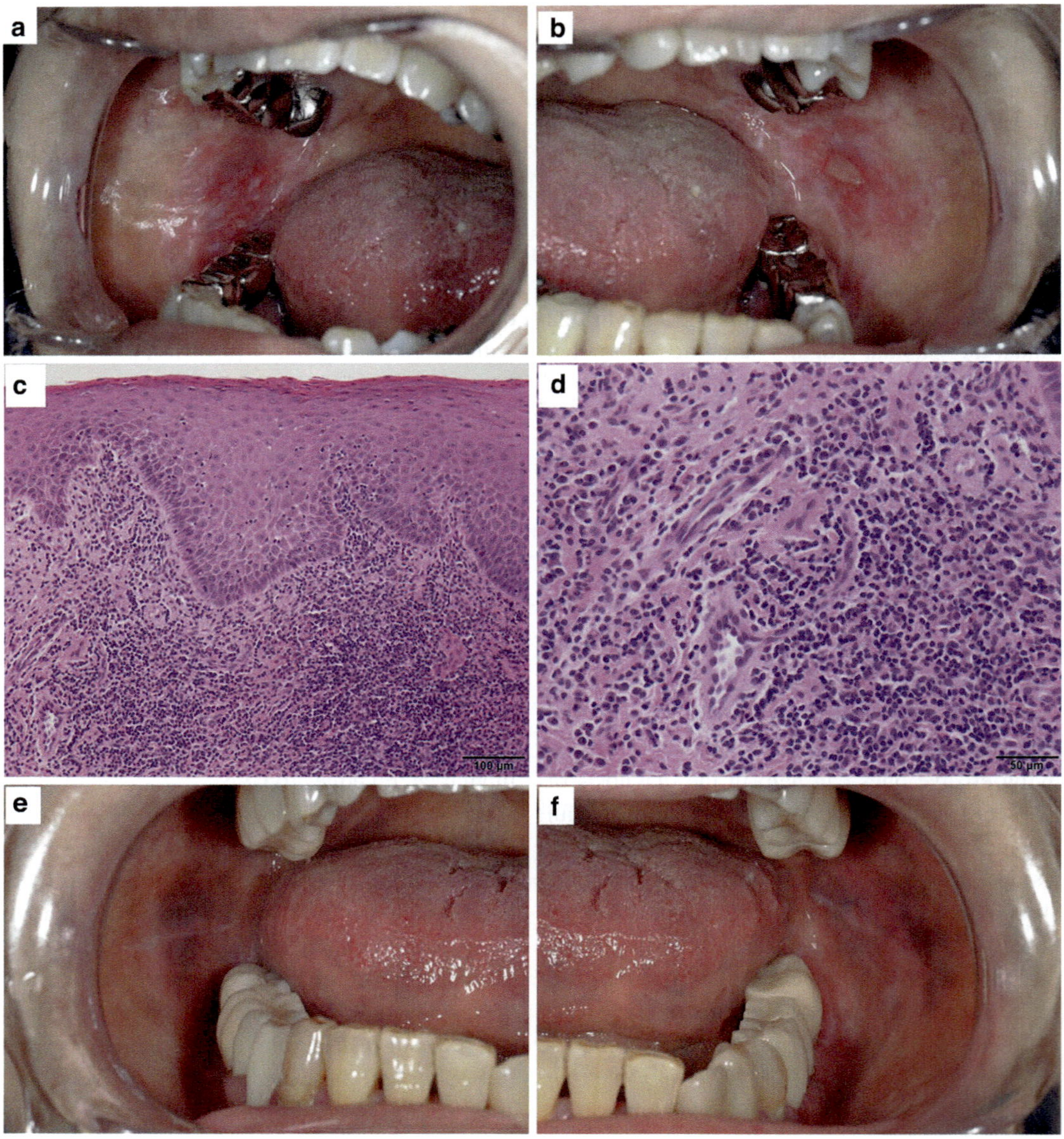

Fig. 5.13 Oral lichenoid contact lesions (OLCLs) related to Au-Ag-Pd alloy in the right buccal mucosa with atrophic lesions (**a**) and atrophic lesions with erosion on the left buccal mucosa (**b**), patch test positive to Au and Pd. Biopsy of (**a**) showed absence of a basal cell liquefaction, an inflammatory infiltrate located deep to superficial infiltrate (**c**), and a substantial number of plasma cells—neutrophils infiltrate in connective tissue (**d**) (H&E stain). The all Au-Ag-Pd alloy was replaced by a ceramic prosthesis, and there was marked improvement of the OLCLs on the right buccal mucosa (**e**) and the left buccal mucosa (**f**). From [155] with permission

characteristics given by a marked epithelial acanthosis with elongated epithelial crests, by a mixed inflammatory infiltrate containing lymphocytes, plasma cells, histiocytes and eosinophils, and a deep perivascular infiltrate. In addition to eating cinnamon, subjects may have been exposed to this agent in everyday products including mouthwash, toothpaste, cinnamon chewing gum, and other products. Most of the reported cases of cinnamon stomatitis come from toothpaste and chewing gum [160, 161].

As discussed in Sect. 5.4.3, the skin patch test of a battery of dental materials (dental screening series) conducted on the back or on the forearm could help in the diagnosis of OLCL [29], although the results on the validity of this test are contrasting [46, 95]. Skin tests are to be preferred over those on the mucosa as they have greater sensitivity and specificity and as the concentration of allergens on the mucous membranes is 5–12 higher than the skin, exposing patients to potential toxic reactions [96]. However, uncertainties remain, as well as in the validity of the patch test in identifying real OLCLs, regarding which compounds or mercury salts/amalgam to use, the distinction of sensitivity from irritant responses, and the ideal contact time of the test materials with the skin (72 h, 96 h, 7 days, 14 days, or even more). And the validity of the extrapolation of skin reactions to evaluate mucosal responses is also questionable. Nonetheless, the skin patch test may still be useful for the clinician to identify suitable restorative replacement material (those to which the patient has not shown any adverse reactions) [95].

DIF in OLCLs may be similar to OLP and the IIF test is negative [162].

In vitro lymphocyte proliferation can be used as an additional tool in the diagnosis of allergies to various drugs [163] and metals [164], in order to restimulate the antigen-specific lymphocytes (memory lymphocytes) of peripheral blood [96]. This test has undergone various modifications and has several names, such as lymphocyte transformation test, lymphocyte stimulation test, lymphocyte proliferation test, or Memory Lymphocyte ImmunoStimulation Assay (MELISA®) test [96]. However, this test appears to be of limited use in OLCLs [165].

The duration of contact between the oral mucosa and the offending material is probably an important factor in the development of OLCL [95]. Some scholars believe that OLCLs resolve spontaneously sometimes without interruption of contact, more often after the interruption of the offensive agent (e.g., restoration in amalgam, food additive, flavor, etc.) in a manner more or less rapid (from a few days to a few months) [32, 65, 95]. However, the evidence is still insufficient to support the routine removal of all amalgam restorations in patients with OLP/OLCL [166], although some authors have reported a 90% improvement in lesions after replacing amalgam restorations in patch test-positive subjects with OLL in close contact with the fillings themselves [167].

In rare cases, OLCLs can be inherently precancerous [168].

5.5.3 Oral Lichenoid Drug Reactions (OLDRs)

In Sect. 3.1.2 it has already been explained what OLDRs are and by which drugs they are caused. Recently, in addition to conventional drugs, some biological drugs have also been reported in association with OLDR including, in particular, TNF-α inhibitors (infliximab, adalimumab, and others) [65, 169]. In this paragraph, the diagnostic aspects and therapeutic management are explored. OLDRs are believed to be unusual compared to skin lichenoid drug reactions; however the incidence of OLDRs is probably underestimated [96]. These lesions are reported more in adults and rarely in the pediatric population [170], as is the case of OLP. Furthermore, this data appears logical given that children use less drugs than adults. Establishing a relationship with the offensive drug can be difficult, since the time interval between the start of a drug treatment and the onset of OLDR lesions is highly variable (up to over a year) [32, 65], although in most cases there appears to be a relatively clear temporal association between use of the suspect drug and the onset of oral lesions [95]. The pathogenesis of OLDR is unknown [65]. It has been hypothesized that predisposed patients may have polymorphisms of CYP450 enzymes with consequent alteration of the metabolism of some drugs [171].

There is currently no specific test for OLDRs [172], and it is often not easy to distinguish them clinically from idiopathic OLP [29] and other oral lichenoid reactions, although the one-sided distribution may facilitate diagnosis [173] (Fig. 5.14). But this is not a constant feature [67]. Furthermore, there are no clear and distinct clinical and histological features that allow a clear differential diagnosis [32, 95]. OLDRs often involve

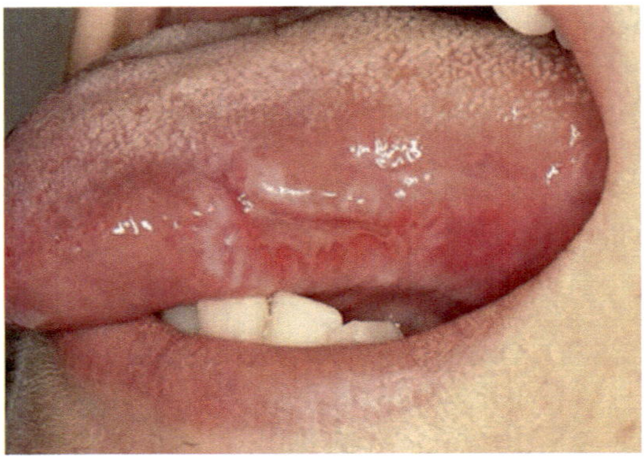

Fig. 5.14 Lichenoid tissue reaction related to rituximab. From [171]

the lip and have an asymmetrical distribution and the contextual cutaneous rash could suggest a drug-related reaction [29].

From a histopathological point of view, the OLDRs share many similarities with OLP [32], but there may also be some differences. The epithelium in OLDRs may be characterized by a greater number of Civatte bodies compared to OLP [95, 174]. Furthermore, the inflammatory infiltrate may be mixed (with also plasma cells and eosinophils) and can extend deeper into the lamina propria, unlike the superficial infiltrate similar to a band typical of OLP; it is often possible to find a chronic inflammatory perivascular infiltrate in OLDRs [32]. However these characteristics cannot be considered specific to the OLDR (in fact they are typically observed also in the DLE [175]); therefore, the most reliable means of diagnosing OLDR is by observing the resolution of the reaction after the suspected drug has been discontinued and the eventual reappearance of the reaction when the patient is given the same drug again. This is both impractical (since the reactions may take a few weeks or several months to resolve) and potentially dangerous (as some drugs are necessary for sick patients) [32, 95]. Therefore, confirming the diagnosis of OLDRs remains problematic [95].

The DIF of the periwound tissue of OLDRs, as well as in OLP, shows a deposition of fibrin with a "shaggy" appearance in the basement membrane and the presence of positive IgM cytoid bodies [118]. Instead, the IIF, unlike OLP, may detect circulating antibodies directed against the basal cells with an annular fluorescence distribution, often referred to as a "string of pearls" model, and this finding can help in the diagnosis of OLDRs [127]. In fact, it has been known for some time that cytoplasmic antibodies circulating against the basal cells appear in drug eruptions, and these have been studied in OLDRs [173], but some scholars still debate the real validity of this kind of investigation [96]. In fact, about 20 years ago, the execution of a modified immunofluorescence test was studied through the use of autologous or allogeneic serum which did not prove useful to distinguish idiopathic OLP from OLDRs through the use of the LPSA (lichen planus-specific antigen) as a marker, and this finding contrasted with previous studies of cytoplasmic autoantibodies against basal cells [176]. A skin explant model originally developed for the assessment of GvHD [177, 178] has been modified for drug reaction assessment (Skimune™ Mab test). In particular, the compound of interest is incubated with PBMCs and skin tissue from the same donor, and the model can predict allergic responses or adverse reactions caused by the compound under examination; this model could be adapted to oral use and possibly help in OLDR diagnosis [67].

5.5.4 OLL Related to Graft-Versus-Host Disease (OLL-GvHD)

In Sect. 3.1.2 it was mentioned what oral lichenoid lesions associated with GvHD (OLL-GvHD) are. In this paragraph all the known aspects will be examined in depth.

GvHD (graft-versus-host disease) is a major complication in people receiving hematopoietic (bone marrow) stem cell transplants and tends to occur quite frequently despite aggressive prophylaxis [95]. In fact, up to 80% of these bone marrow transplant recipients may develop chronic GvHD (cGvHD), usually within the first 6–24 months after the transplant [179]. Although the etiopathogenesis of GvHD is not fully understood, it appears to be due to the reaction of the donor's T lymphocytes against the expression of the minor histocompatibility antigens (mHag) of the recipient's cells [95]. mHag are small peptides found on the cell surface in association with MHC-I and MHC-II molecules. The mHag correspond to polymorphic structures and are therefore instrumental in the molecular definition of the self for the immune system [180]. In fact, T lymphocytes are able to detect differences even in single amino acids and consequently to become immunoreactive causing GvHD in the context of hematopoietic stem cell transplants [181]. Minor histocompatibility antigens have long been known to be responsible for adverse events resulting from the exchange of organs and tissues between individuals identical in the MHC system. Contrary to major compatibility antigens (MHC system), mHag result in relatively slower and more chronic graft rejection reactions [182]. More than 100 mHag has been identified and sequenced to date [180].

GvHD can be distinguished into acute (aGvHD) if it develops within the first 100 days after transplantation and chronic (cGvHD) if it begins or lasts after 100 days [67]. However, the latest consensus criteria from the National Institutes of Health recommend that classification should be based on characteristic symptoms and signs rather than a rigid temporal definition [183]. aGvHD primarily affects three specific organ systems: the skin, liver, and gastrointestinal tract, including the oral cavity [95]. cGvHD represents one of the main causes of morbidity and mortality in this patient population; on average it shows an onset after 6 months from the moment of transplantation [32]. A greater number of organs (including eyes and respiratory tract) tend to be involved in cGvHD, and oral involvement (OLL-GvHD), including salivary glands, is more frequent (up to 80% of total cases) compared to aGvHD [95, 184]. In some cases of cGvHD, the oral cavity may be the only anatomical site involved [184].

OLL-GvHD can be clinically and histologically indistinguishable from OLP [185, 186]. OLL-aGvHD are often painful, being usually characterized by erythematous and ulcerated lesions with marked desquamation [95]. Manifestations of OLL-cGvHD include three distinct disease patterns that may also coexist with each other: (1) oral lichenoid manifestations including white reticular or plaque lesions and red ulcer-erosive and atrophic mucosal lesions; (2) salivary gland dysfunction characterized by hyposalivation and persistent dry mouth (xerostomia); and (3) orofacial fibrosis with limited degree of mouth opening [183, 186].

Therefore, intraoral lesions are very similar to those found in OLP, but the presence of a history of bone marrow transplantation, the presence of marked and persistent dry eye, xerostomia, and/or orofacial fibrosis are important elements that may aid in the differential diagnosis. It is interesting to note that the infiltrates in the salivary glands are similar to those found in Sjögren's syndrome, while orofacial fibrosis with limited mouth opening is a manifestation similar to those of scleroderma, also classified as IFD/LTR [184]. Intraoral GvHD lesions can involve all areas of the oral cavity and tend to cover entire areas such as the buccal mucosa, tongue, lips, palate, and gums, and patients may complain of a burning sensation in the mouth [29, 32].

Although the etiology is probably different, histologically OLL-GvHD and OLP are similar [67]. Despite the difference in antigen specificity, OLL-cGvHD and OLP share similar immunological mechanisms, characterized by infiltration of T lymphocytes, basement membrane damage, and apoptosis of basal keratinocytes [184]. Numerous cytoid bodies can also be observed [32, 65] (Fig. 5.15). The lymphocyte infiltrate may be less intense than that found in OLP and may also be mixed (containing some plasma cells and eosinophils) [32, 65].

Clinical features alone, provided they are present in an anamnestic context of allogeneic hematopoietic stem cell transplantation, are usually sufficiently diagnostic. Histological confirmation of OLL-GvHD is indicated (1) in the absence of signs and symptoms of other organs' or systems' involvement or when investigations on such other sites provide only negative or nonspecific results and (2) in case of atypical clinical presentation to rule out the presence of dysplasia or malignancy, particularly in the context of clinical monitoring of patients with long-standing

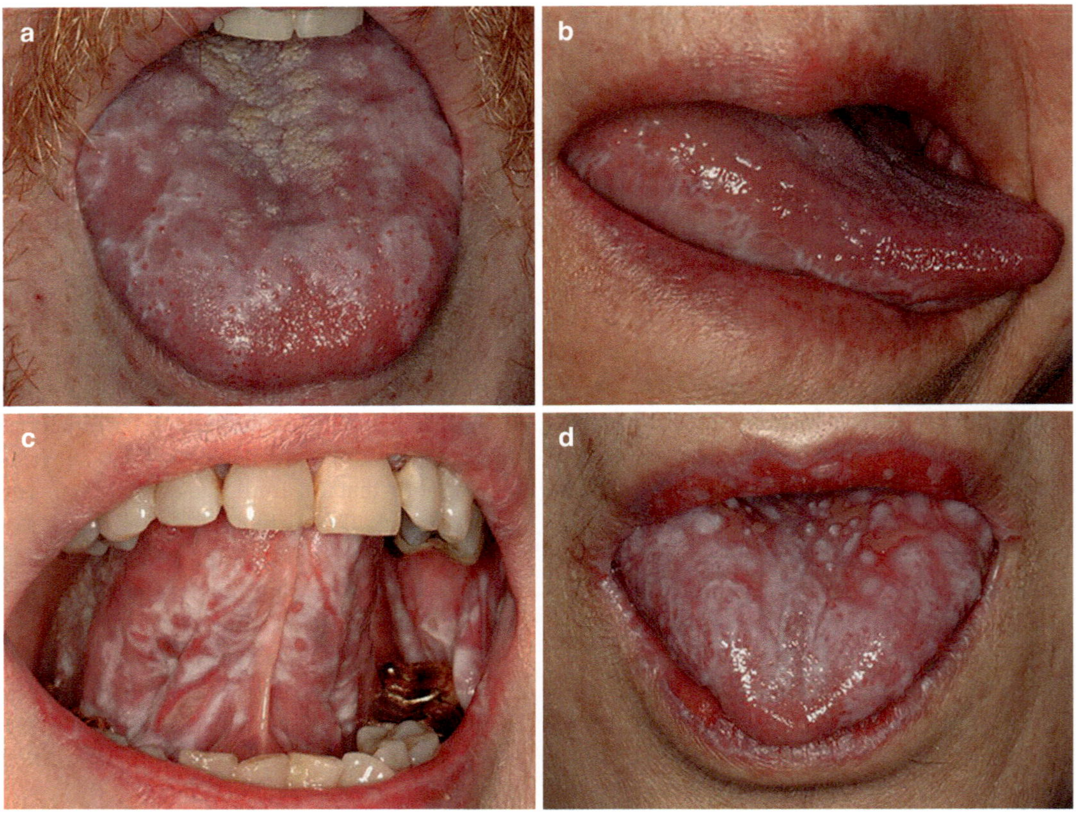

Fig. 5.15 cGvHD lichenoid features of the tongue. Reticular cGvHD of the (**a**) tongue dorsum and (**b**) ventrolateral tongue demonstrating typical hyperkeratotic striations and plaque-like changes. More extensive involvement with heavy reticulation and associated ulcerations of the (**c**) ventral tongue and (**d**) tongue dorsum, with various degrees of erythema. There is prominent involvement of the lips in panel D, which stops abruptly at the vermillion border. From [189] with permission

chronic disease. Patients diagnosed with cGvHD have a higher risk of developing oral cancer and should undergo annual screening [95, 187, 188].

The results of DIF may be similar to those of OLP and the IIF is negative [162].

A review by Imanguli et al. [190] highlighted the problems in attempting to use an evidence-based approach for the management of OLL-GvHD. Since GvHD is often a multiorgan disease, systemic therapy is indicated in the first instance, but few studies have evaluated its effects on oral lesions. The gold standard in the treatment of GvHD is high-dose systemic corticosteroids. These are usually supplemented with a calcineurin inhibitor, traditionally cyclosporine, but more recent studies have been reported on the systemic administration of tacrolimus or sirolimus [95] (the latter is not a calcineurin inhibitor unlike tacrolimus). For example, Johnston et al. reported that out of 8 patients with OLL-cGvHD (out of a total of 19), 3 experienced complete resolution and 5 partial resolution following systemic treatment with sirolimus [191]. The particular effectiveness of extracorporeal photopheresis (ECP) has been demonstrated in the treatment of mucocutaneous lesions from cGvHD, where 63% of 59 patients with OLL-cGvHD responded [192]. The ECP consists of the external sampling of the patient's mononuclear cells (thus including the highly reactive T lymphocytes) which are sensitized to UVA light by adding a photoactive compound (8-methoxypsoralen) and then returned to the patient [95]. A study performed on 15 patients with only manifestations of OLL-cGvHD evaluated the activity of thalidomide (a sedative and immunosuppressive drug), but its side effects frequently required discontinuation of the drug, and the overall response was only 24% [193]. Local therapies for OLL-cGvHD are mainly based on the topical application of corticosteroids [95]. The efficacy of topical budesonide has been demonstrated [194] and dexamethasone in mouthwash [195] but also of other categories of molecules such as cyclosporine [196] and azathioprine [197, 198]. Topical tacrolimus is the most promising [199], but concerns have been raised about its oncogenic potential, which could limit its future use [95]. Local phototherapy with UVA light (PUVA) associated with the topical or systemic use of psoralen sensitizing leukocytes is of concern due to the oncogenic potential of ultraviolet light [195, 200–203]. Low-intensity laser therapy or LLLT (CO_2 laser, 1 W for 2–3 s/1 mm2) has been shown to be effective in reducing pain in severe forms of OLL-GvHD [204]. LLLT, also known as photobiomodulation (PBM), has also been observed to be useful by more recent studies in achieving improvement in oral pain and dryness, but further controlled studies will need to be conducted to confirm the efficacy and safety of PBM, in the therapy of OLL-GvHD, and to create an optimal protocol [205]. Furthermore Picardi et al. [206] observed through the repeated application of platelet gel (PLT-gel) a complete response in seven out of ten patients.

It should also be considered that, given that GvHD often involves several organs or systems, the treatment of OLL-GvHD is usually an integral part of systemic management and specific treatment of oral lesions is indicated as support for systemic immunosuppressive therapy, especially if it has been possible to avoid the intensification of the latter. In general, the information regarding the therapeutic options of OLP is also applicable in OLL-GvHD lesions. In addition to long-term monitoring of oral lesions to avoid the risk of undiagnosed OSCC lesions, careful surveillance for opportunistic infections that may occur in the oral cavity of these patients undergoing strong immunosuppressive therapy is also important [95].

5.5.5 Dental and Pharmacological Management of OLL/OLP

In individuals with potential OLDRs, trigger drugs should be discontinued wherever possible. But this is often difficult because the drug in question may be important to the patient's health and effective alternative drugs may not be available [96]. Also, the lesions can persist for several months after stopping the drug [175]. Patients with suspected OLCL could benefit from targeted replacement of the amalgam restoration, although simple polishing of the restorations and improvement of the patient's oral hygiene can minimize plaque buildup and frictional trauma to the mucosa, thereby leading to an improvement of the OLCL. It will be necessary to adequately inform patients about the benefits and risks of amalgam removal but also about the cyclical nature of the disease characterized by periods of spontaneous remission and exacerbation and the limited evidence to support the effectiveness of amalgam replacement [96]. Risks that will need to be known include potential iatrogenic damage to the teeth, the possibility of worsening of the lesions immediately after amalgam replacement (especially if a rubber dam has not been used), a shorter life span of some alternative materials, and possible further contact reactions generated by the newly placed restorative materials [166].

The primary goal of any OLP/OLL therapy is symptomatic control [150, 207]. Generally, patients with reticular lesions and other asymptomatic lesions do not require active treatment, but the elimination of potential precipitating or provoking factors (sharp or fractured teeth, incongruous dental prostheses, alcohol and tobacco consumption) is fundamental [96]. Patients should be recommended good oral hygiene at home associated with the use of chlorhexidine, since the reduction of plaque can have beneficial effects on lesions [208].

Although there is no permanent cure therapy, various treatment regimens have been introduced to reduce and control the painful symptoms of OLP/OLL [96] (these aspects will be explored in detail in Chap. 6). Curiously, it is also suspected that several suggested treatment modalities may induce OLL [96]:

- Griseofulvin (antifungal)
- Hydroxychloroquine sulfate (antimalarial and immunosuppressant)
- Mesalamine (NSAID)
- Phenytoin (antiepileptic)
- Thalidomide (sedative-hypnotic and immunosuppressant)
- Interferon
- Psychotherapy
- Surgery

The first-line therapy is usually represented by topical agents given the minor side effects; however, when the lesions are widespread, involving the skin or other mucous membranes, and recalcitrant, systemic agents may be necessary. In fact, among the various immunosuppressive drugs commonly used for OLP/OLL, few have been developed specifically for oral disease; consequently there are no adequate studies to determine their efficacy [207]. Furthermore, many aspects of therapy such as the optimal dose, duration of treatment, safety, and true efficacy remain largely unknown [201]. Patients must be warned about the off-label use (administration outside the conditions authorized by the appropriate entities) of the drugs used in the treatment of OLP/OLL [96]. Usually off-label use concerns molecules already known and used for some time, for which there is considerable scientific evidence that would allow their rational use even in clinical situations and in ways not provided for in the technical data sheet and in the package leaflet.

5.5.6 Pemphigus Vulgaris

The term "pemphigus" identifies a group of autoimmune bullous diseases mediated by immunological mechanisms characterized by the formation of circulating autoantibodies directed against particular components of the desmosome (desmogleins; see Fig. 5.16), the most important element of intercellular adhesion in epithelia [209], resulting in loss of cell-to-cell adhesion [210], formation of intraepithelial acantholytic vesicles [211], and erosions of the skin and/or mucous membranes [212]. Currently, several varieties of pemphigus are recognized: pemphigus vulgaris (PV), pemphigus vegetans, pemphigus foliaceus, pemphigus erythematosus, pemphigus herpetiformis, IgA pemphigus, and paraneoplastic pemphigus. Of these, only pemphigus vulgaris and paraneoplastic pemphigus affect the oral cavity [209].

It is a rare disorder with an incidence of 0.5–3.2 cases per 100,000 population/year (it is more common in Ashkenazi Jews) and occurs mainly in female adults, usually between the ages of 30 and 60, more frequently in the fifth and sixth decade of life, especially in the Mediterranean area, due to an immunogenetic association with the HLA-DR4 and HLA-DR6 alleles [209, 210, 212]. The HLA-II alleles are critical for antigen recognition by T lymphocytes [211]; therefore these data suggest that

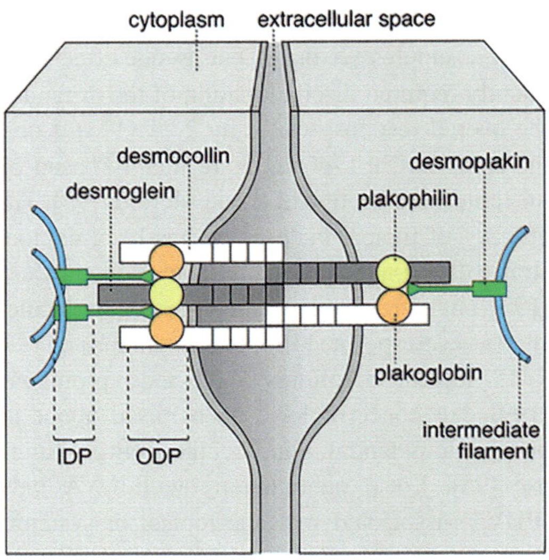

Fig. 5.16 Molecular model of the desmosome. The desmosomal cadherins desmoglein and desmocollin undergo homophilic and heterophilic binding via interaction with the amino-terminal extracellular (*EC*) 1 domain of partner molecules on the same (*cis*) as well as on the neighboring cell (*trans*). The cytoplasmic domains are largely embedded in the outer dense plaque (ODP) where they are associated with plakoglobin and plakophilin. In the inner dense plaque (*IDP*), desmoplakin links these adaptor molecules to the intermediate filament cytoskeleton. From [213] with permission

patients who develop the disease must have HLA-II molecules capable of presenting Dsg3 peptides to T cells [210]. The HLA-I alleles may also play a role in the development of PV [214]. PV can also occur, albeit rarely, in children and adolescents, so it should be considered in the differential diagnosis at these ages [215, 216]. Despite being a rare disorder, PV is the most common form of pemphigus (90%–95%) [217]. It is a chronic bullous dermatosis, with progressive increase in severity, and is potentially life-threatening [212]. The morbidity and mortality of PV are related to the extent of the disease (initial severity and extent of the lesions), the precocity of the treatment, the drug dose necessary for the eradication of the lesions, the patient's age, the antibody titer (when it is high, the prognosis worsens), and the presence of comorbidities [211, 218, 219]. Prior to the introduction of corticosteroids, approximately 75% of patients died within the first year (from sepsis, cachexia, protein loss, or fluid and electrolyte imbalances) [209]. Currently, less than 10% of patients die, usually due to side effects of the treatment [214, 220–222]. Various authors have reported that oral lesions can disappear after 2 months to a year [216, 220].

The etiopathogenesis of PV is autoimmune and consists in the production of serum IgG antibodies directed against the normal molecules of desmosomal adhesion on the cell membrane of keratinocytes, namely, desmogleins (Dsg), especially against Dsg1 (more represented in the skin) and especially against Dsg3 (the most involved especially in forms with only oral localization) [209, 223]. The oral mucosa mainly expresses Dsg3, while the skin expresses Dsg3 and Dsg1 [211] (Fig. 5.17). In fact, the early stages of pemphigus, associated with anti-Dsg3 antibodies, are mainly localized in the mucous membranes (there are no skin lesions due to the presence of Dsg1 throughout the thickness of the skin epithelium, which would thus compensate for the loss of Dsg3 [209]), while in the advanced forms, in which there is also the expression of anti-Dsg1 antibodies, skin lesions appear [214, 219, 223] (Fig. 5.18). Oral lesions are the first manifestation of the disease in 50–90% of cases and are the only signs of the disease for a period of 2–6 months until the appearance of skin lesions [211]. Some studies have found substantial differences in the prevalence of oral lesions as the first manifestation of PV between distinct geographic areas, such as 66% in Bulgaria, 83% in Italy, and 92% in Israel [214]. The binding of antibodies to Dsgs at the oral and cutaneous level causes the loss of cell adhesion, with separation of the epithelial layers (acantholysis) and consequent appearance of blisters on the skin and mucous membranes [214, 223]. Although the antibodies present in the intercellular spaces of the epithelial tissue are generally the IgG type,

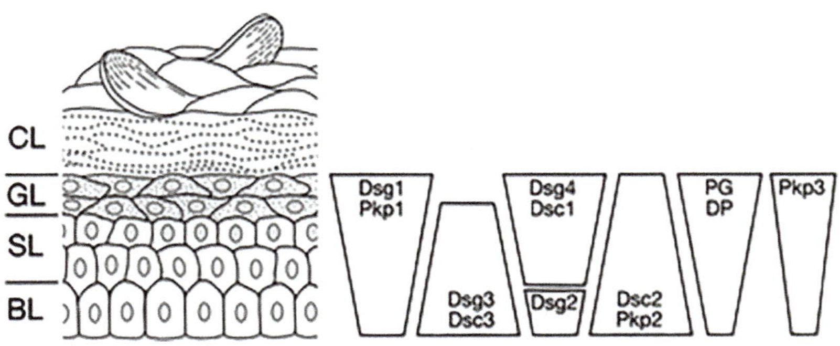

Fig. 5.17 Expression patterns of desmosomal components in the epidermis. The schematic drawing of the epidermis (*left*) indicates the basal (*BL*), spinous (*SL*), granular (*GL*), and corneal (*CL*) layer of the epidermis. On the right, the expression patterns of desmosomal components in the specific epidermal layers are illustrated. For instance, Dsg1 and Pkp 1 are most prominent in the superficial layers, whereas expression of Dsg3 and Dsc 3 is strongest in the deep epidermis. *Dsg* desmoglein, *Dsc* desmocollin, *Pkp* plakophilin, *PG* plakoglobin, *DP* desmoplakin. From [213] with permission

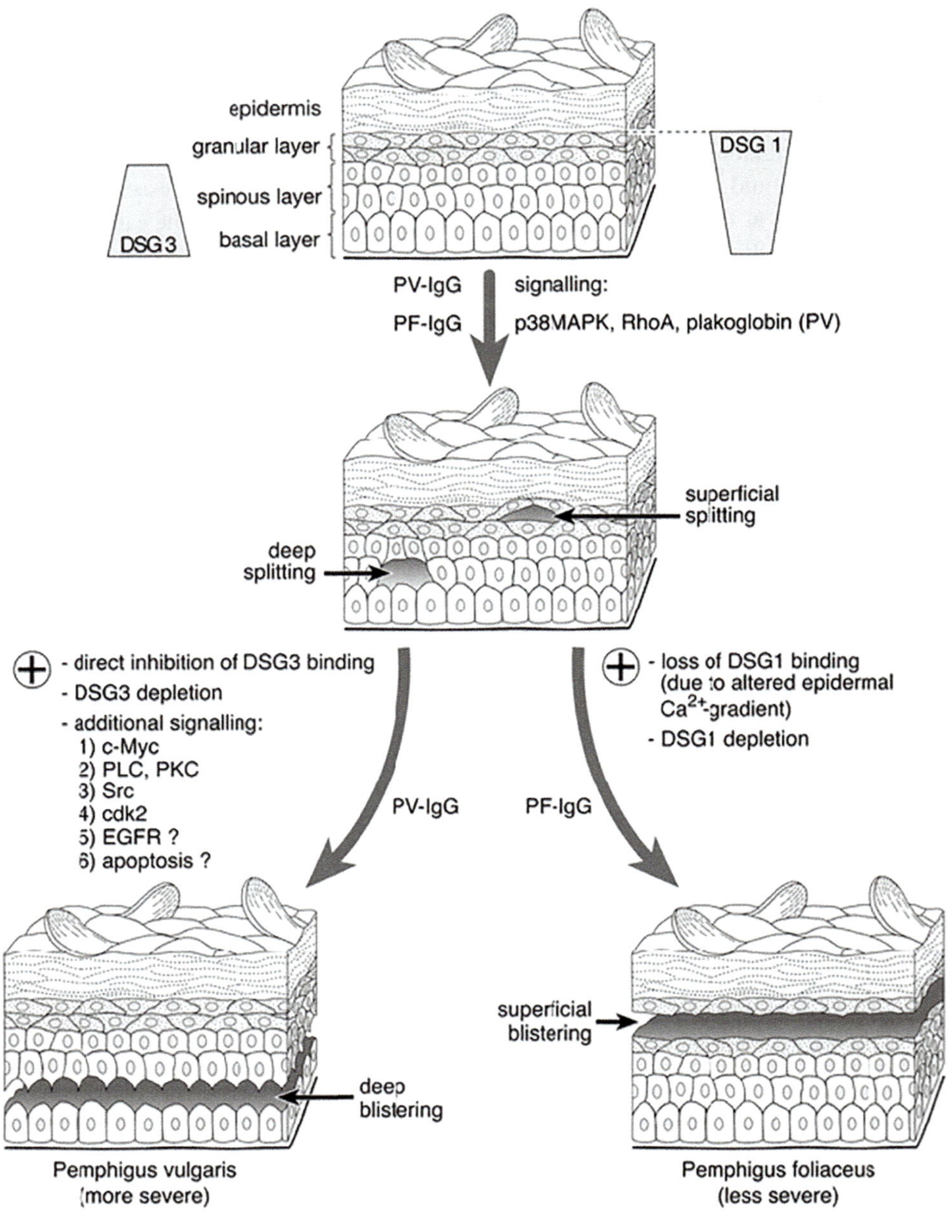

Fig. 5.18 The mechanisms involved in pemphigus acantholysis. Accumulating evidence indicates that PV-IgG and PF-IgG initiate keratinocyte dissociation via intracellular signalling pathways including p38 MAPK, Rho A, and plakoglobin (PV only). In addition, other mechanisms such as direct inhibition of Dsg3 binding and Dsg3 depletion from desmosomes as well as other signalling events seem to contribute to PV pathogenesis, whereas their role for acantholysis in PF is unclear. These mechanisms may account for the more severe clinical phenotype of PV compared to PF. *PLC* phospholipase C, *PKC* protein kinase C, *cdk 2* cyclin-dependent kinase 2, *EGFR* epidermal growth factor receptor. From [213] with permission

they can also be the IgM or IgA type, and complement protein C3 can even be observed [224]. Although PV is considered to be idiopathic, a number of environmental factors that can trigger the disease have been identified, including drugs (particularly penicillin, pyrazolones, thiol-containing drugs, e.g., penicillamine and ACE inhibitors), hormones (in pregnancy), diet (garlic, leeks), physical agents (ionizing radiation), or viruses (especially herpesvirus) [209, 214, 223–226]. Although these are rare causes, they should be studied in patients with a recent diagnosis of PV [224].

Given the primary oral manifestation of the disease, the dentist plays a fundamental role in the early diagnosis of PV. In fact, it has been shown that, with early diagnosis and aggressive therapy, 50–80% of patients can achieve complete remission; moreover, mortality from the disease confined to the oral cavity is estimated at around 6%, while for the cutaneous mucus form, it reaches 20–30% [209]. For this reason, differential diagnosis is of fundamental importance, especially from other clinically similar pathologies, but with a different prognostic significance, such as OLP precisely.

As regards the clinical diagnosis, it is therefore possible to find:

- *Oral lesions*: These consist mainly of multiple vesiculo-bullous lesions that easily rupture (due to the thin roof of the oral vesicles and due to trauma within the oral cavity) with the formation of bleeding and painful ulcers and erythematous erosions with irregular edges that heal with difficulty [209, 211]. These erythematous erosions of PV can be distinguished from the yellow erosions of the MMP (mucous membrane pemphigoid) due to the accumulation of fibrin [209]. Patients report intense oral symptoms due to pain and burning sensation, especially when consuming acidic or spicy foods [216, 220, 227]. The lesions can involve any site of the oral cavity, but the most involved sites are those subjected to friction, such as the soft palate, the buccal mucosa, the lingual belly, the gum, and the lower lip [218, 223, 228, 229] (Fig. 5.19). In the early stages of the disease, multiple and persistent erosions

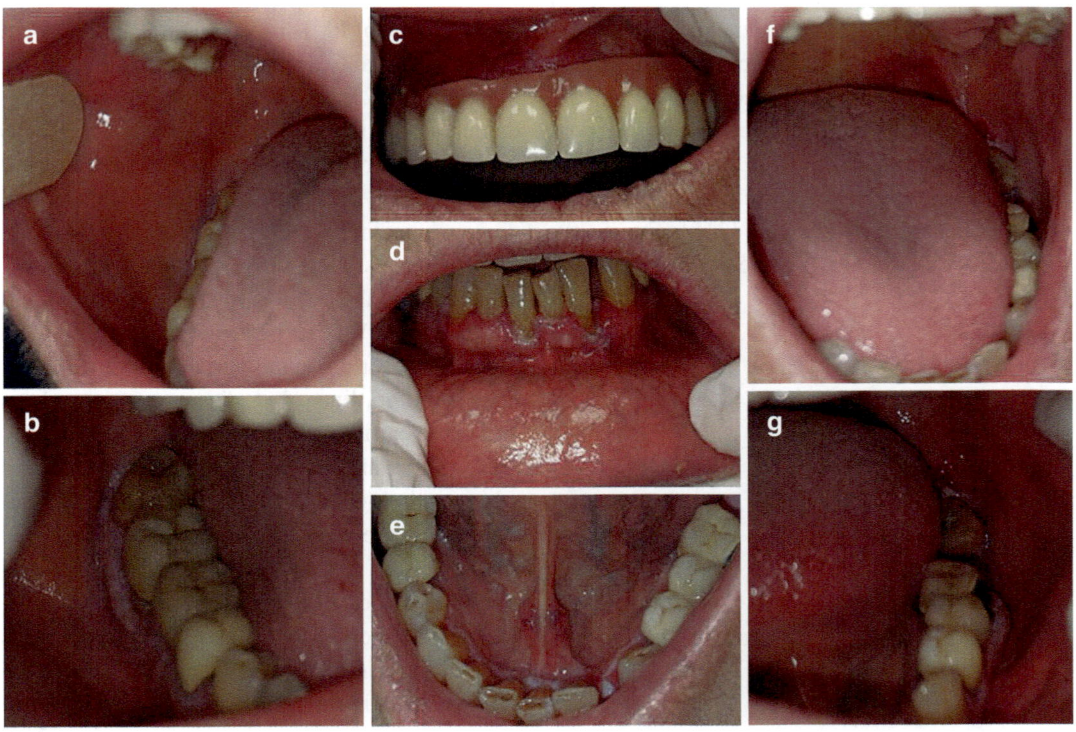

Fig. 5.19 PV oral lesions. (**a**) Left buccal mucosa without lesions, (**b**) left mandibular gingiva, (**c**) maxillary frontal gingiva, (**d**) mandibular frontal gingiva and (**e**) mandibular lingual gingiva with keratotic and erosive lesions, (**f**) right soft palate, and (**g**) right mandibular retromolar and vestibular gingiva with keratotic, atrophic-erythematous, and erosive lesions

appear on the oral mucosa, while in the advanced stages of PV, desquamative gingivitis can develop [214, 219]. Therefore desquamative gingivitis is not exclusive to the erosive forms of OLP, but can also concern other immune-inflammatory diseases, including PV. A useful diagnostic approach may be to traction the unaffected mucosa which (in the case of positive Nikolsky's sign) will tend to tear [209] in case of an active phase of the disease [210]. Nikolsky's sign appears to be highly specific in oral district (96.3%) and can be very useful in the preliminary diagnosis of oral vesiculo-bullous diseases [57]. On the oral mucosa the detection of intact vesiculo-bullous lesions is rarer compared to the skin, in contrast to erosions because of the trauma [218, 223]. Other oral manifestations include sialorrhea, halitosis, and continuous brown or blackish crusting at the vermilion border [223, 230].

- *Skin lesions*: Large flaccid blisters develop on non-erythematous skin, especially in conjunction with trauma [209]. Intact vesiculo-bullous lesions can be detected more easily on the skin, but since they are flaccid blisters (intraepidermal with a thin roof), they easily erode even on the skin where it is possible to observe scabs and erosions [210] (Fig. 5.20). Nikolsky's sign can also be evaluated on the skin. Skin blisters may be asymptomatic and are usually not itchy [211]. Skin blisters in PV can vary in diameter, tension, and brittleness, can be full with clear or hemorrhagic fluid, and can rupture easily due to the thin roof: as a result, lesions erode easily but heal without scarring, through the epithelialization process coming from the edges of erosion (unless secondary infection occurs) [231].
- *Other lesions*: In 13% of cases, PV can also involve the conjunctival, nasal, pharyngeal, laryngeal, esophageal, genital, anal, and even bronchi and stomach mucous membranes [217]. The clinical characteristics of PV suggest a subdivision into two subtypes: a variety with predominantly mucosal localization (extensive oral erosions, nasal, esophageal, and ocular involvement) and a mucus-cutaneous variety (with blisters and erosions at the cutaneous level in addition to mucosal involvement) [209].

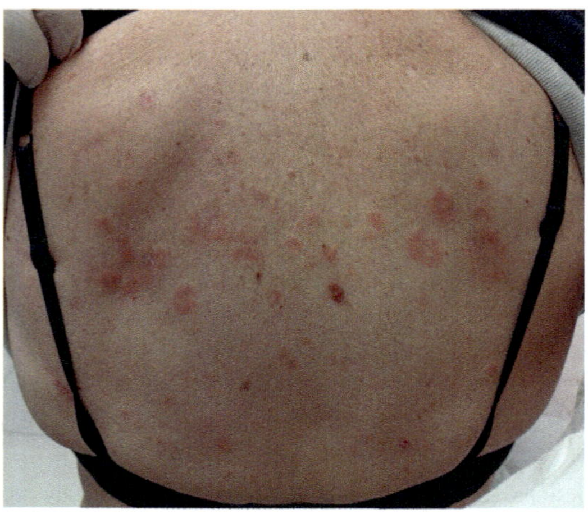

Fig. 5.20 Clinical image of initial cutaneous PV with diffuse erythematous areas and small erosions. Same patient in Fig. 5.23

Diagnosis of PV is based on three independent criteria: clinical features, histology, and immunological tests [216, 220]. These elements are fundamental for the differential diagnosis, and as mentioned earlier, early treatment can improve the prognosis of PV. PV goes into differential diagnosis mainly with recurrent aphthous stomatitis, Behcet's disease, erythema multiforme, EOLP, and oral candidiasis [218]. In children and adolescents, PV must be differentiated from erythema multiforme, acute herpetic gingivostomatitis, impetigo, linear IgA disease, epidermolysis bullosa, cicatricial pemphigoid, bullous pemphigoid, and paraneoplastic pemphigus [215]. From a histopathological point of view, PV is characterized by the loss of keratinocyte cell-to-cell adhesion, in a process called acantholysis, probably due to desmosomal damage. In PV, acantholysis (which is not observed in mucous membrane pemphigoid) is localized in the basal cell layer and in the cells directly above it, forming a suprabasal intraepithelial blister [209, 210] (Fig. 5.21). Acantholytic cells show a more spherical shape than normal ones (Tzanck cells) and can be detected with a simple cytological examination (Tzanck cytodiagnostic test) [209].

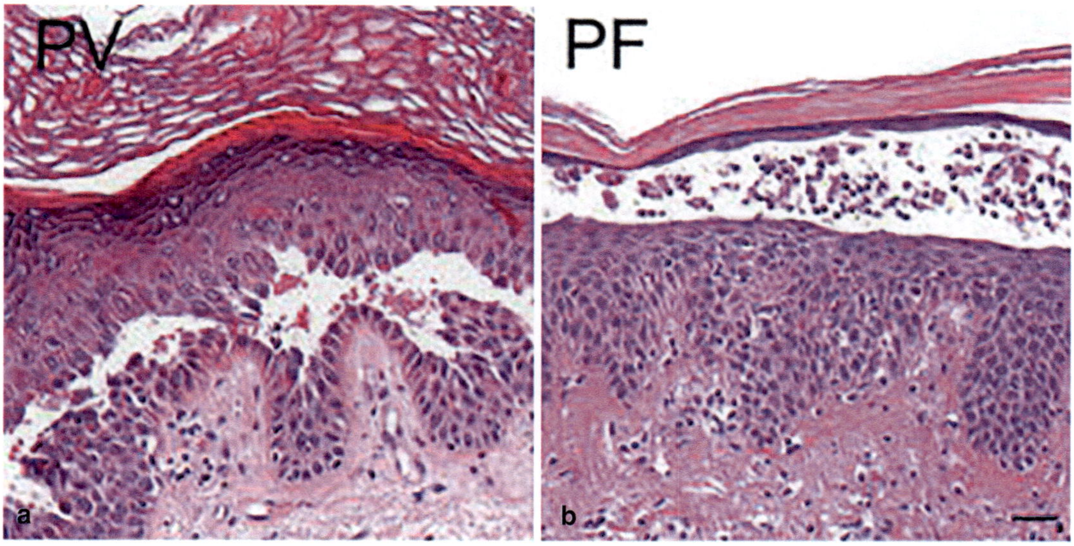

Fig. 5.21 Typical histology of epidermal lesions from pemphigus patients. Hematoxylin eosin-stained paraffin sections from PV (**a**) and PF (**b**) patients showed suprabasal epidermal cleavage in the PV and superficial granular blistering in PF. *Scale bar* is 50 μm. From [213] with permission

This examination consists of scraping the base of the lesion with the sharp edge of the scalpel [232]. In the oral mucosa, it is possible to use a blunt spatula or a brush because they cause less bleeding [233]. The detected material is transferred to a slide, stained, and examined under an optical microscope [232]. Basal keratinocytes often lose cell-to-cell adhesion (but not the basement membrane-to-cell relationship) and assume a cuboidal or rectangular shape, forming a so-called row of tombstones [210]. The stroma may show the presence of a non-specific inflammatory infiltrate by several cells of the immune system, including neutrophils and eosinophils [209].

In addition to the histological examination, which must demonstrate the phenomenon of acantholysis with the relative epithelial separation at the level of the spinous layer, for the PV diagnosis, it is necessary to perform the DIF [209] which allows to detect intercellular deposits especially of IgG and C3, but also of IgM and IgA on the periwound epidermis, with a characteristic lattice morphology, offering 100% sensitivity [209–211]. It is also important to perform the IIF on serum, almost always positive in the case of PV, which allows to highlight, in 80% of patients with PV, the title of circulating IgG autoantibodies directed against the cell surfaces of keratinocytes [209, 210] (Fig. 5.22). IIF is of great usefulness not only for diagnosis but also for therapeutic monitoring [209]. The ELISA test which uses recombinant Dsg1 and Dsg3 to measure anti-Dsg1 and anti-Dsg3 antibodies in serum may also be useful; and, when the diagnosis remains uncertain, immunoprecipitation and immunoblotting techniques may be employed [211].

As for the treatment, given the wide variety of clinical presentation, more or less severe, the therapy must be individualized on the basis of the clinical aspect and immunological data (antibody titer detected with IIF) but also on the possible presence of comorbidities that indicate a contraindication to systemic corticosteroid treatment for a long period of time. These patients should therefore be treated in specialized centers and monitored over time to detect any adverse effects due to chronic immunosuppressive therapy [209]. In patients with extensive oral lesions or skin involvement, standard therapy consists of the combined administration of corticosteroids and systemic immunosuppressants to achieve symptom remission. Once this goal is achieved, a maintenance regimen is started, using the lowest

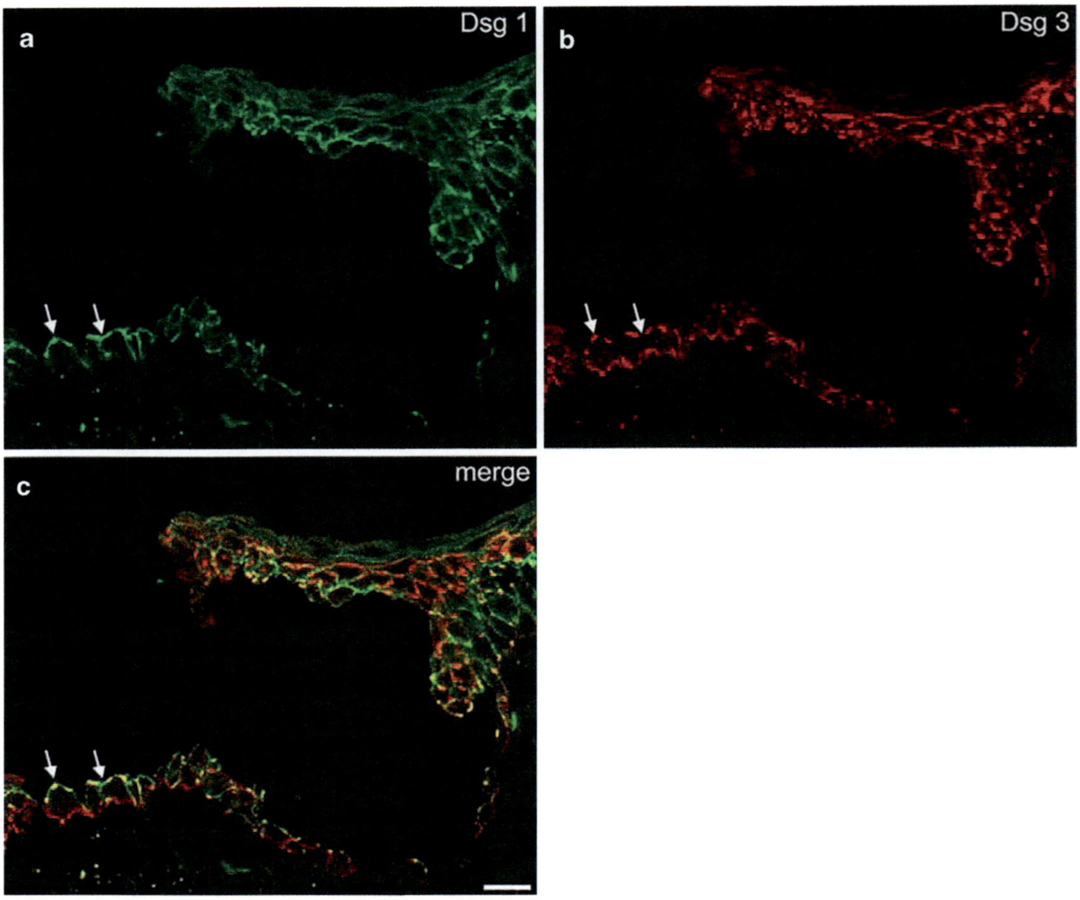

Fig. 5.22 Immunostaining of Dsg1 and Dsg3 in PV lesional epidermis. Epidermis from a patient with mucocutaneous PV was stained for Dsg1 (**a**) and Dsg3 (**b**). A merge of both panels is shown in (**c**). Both Dsg1 and Dsg3 are expressed in the basal layer underneath the blister as well as in keratinocytes in the blister roof. However, Dsg3 staining appears to be fragmented throughout the epidermis, whereas Dsg1 staining is more continuous. Note that in the level of the cleavage plane, the apical membrane of basal cells shows strong immunostaining for Dsg1 and Dsg3 (*arrows*). Therefore, based on the desmoglein compensation hypothesis, the expression patterns of Dsg1 and Dsg3 cannot explain why the cleavage plane is located suprabasally in PV but not in other epidermal layers. *Scale bar* is 20 μm. From [213] with permission

possible dose capable of controlling the disease in order to minimize the side effects of these drugs [211]. The treatment of choice is systemic immunosuppression with corticosteroids (prednisone 1–2 mg/kg/day) [209], which begins to show its effectiveness, along with other systemic corticosteroids, quite quickly (within a few days) [210]. A second immunosuppressive drug such as azathioprine (1–2 mg/kg/day), cyclophosphamide (1–3 mg/kg/day), and mycophenolate mofetil (2–3 g/day), which are able to reduce the production of antibodies, can be used to reduce the dosage of corticosteroids and increase its therapeutic efficacy [209, 234–236]. These drugs do not target autoantibody-producing cells [210] and they are not effective on their own [209].

Oral lesions are more challenging than skin lesions because their response to treatment is much slower [224]. Oral mucosal lesions in patients with low circulating antibody titer can be controlled (at least temporarily) with corticosteroid-based topical mouthwashes or creams, e.g., 0.1% triamcinolone acetonide in orabase, 0.05% fluocinolone acetonide, 0.05% clobetasol propionate (conveyed with hydroxyethyl cellulose gel), and 0.05% halobetasol [209, 210], but local agents are rarely effective in monotherapy [209]. In refractory lesions, intralesional injections of triamcinolone acetonide (20 μg/L) or paramethasone can be given every 7–15 days, but treatment should be stopped if symptoms do not improve after three injections [210]. At completion to treatment with local or systemic corticosteroids, further measures can be taken to improve the comfort of patients: occasional administration of analgesics, maintenance of strict oral hygiene associated with the use of antiseptic mouthwashes (chlorhexidine), periodontal treatment, diet free from irritants, control of prosthetic restorations and tooth margins (to prevent local trauma to mucous membranes), and application of antifungal therapy in patients on long-term corticosteroid treatment [214, 220, 224, 237]. Factors that can exacerbate the onset of injuries include sun exposure, X-rays, stress, and trauma. Since oral trauma can trigger or worsen PV, Bystryn et al. recommend prophylactic administration of prednisone 20 mg/day in addition to the patient's normal needs for 5–7 days prior to any dental procedures associated with mucosal trauma [224]. Advances in research have expanded the therapeutic arsenal which now includes several treatments: high doses of intravenous immunoglobulin, plasmapheresis, immunospecific immunoadsorption, PUVA, anti-TNF-α, cholinergic antagonists, and anti-CD20 monoclonal antibodies (e.g., rituximab) [221, 223, 238]. Among these, plasmapheresis and immunoadsorption can be highly effective tools in rapidly reducing abnormal serum levels of pathogenic antibodies, but they remain adjuvant treatment strategies that must be combined with systemic immunosuppression to prevent rebound of newly synthesized antibodies [239, 240]. Administration of anti-CD20 antibodies (rituximab) leads to a depletion of peripheral $CD20^+$ B lymphocytes for a duration of at least 1.5 years, after which reconstitution of the repertoire of B lymphocytes derived from the stem cell pool is observed [241, 242]. Rituximab is used primarily as a second-line treatment, although studies for its use as a first-line therapy are ongoing [210]. Sometimes it is administered in combination with intravenous immunoglobulins or immunoadsorption. Rituximab induces clinical remission in 50% or more of patients, but relapses frequently occur, requiring additional courses of use [240, 243, 244].

Finally, close cooperation between dentists and dermatologists is required to properly treat this disease [212].

As seen, therefore, the differential diagnosis between PV and OLP is important in the case of oral erosive lesions. Clinically, the distinction is sometimes not easy, but histologically the two pathologies present some differences. The results of the DIF and IIF are also different between PV and OLP.

5.5.7 Bullous Pemphigoid (BP)

The term "pemphigoid" indicates a family of relatively common chronic bullous disorders that manifest themselves with the appearance of subepidermal vesicles and erosions on the erythematous surface [212, 245]. Within this family are bullous pemphigoid (BP) and its variants (urticarial, vesicular, dyshidrosiform, seborrheic, vegetans, localized, and prurigo nodularis-like BP), gestational pemphigoid (or herpes), mucous membrane pemphigoid (in the past called "cicatricial"), ocular pemphigoid, acquired epidermolysis bullosa, herpetiform dermatitis, linear IgA bullous dermatosis, and lichen planus pemphigoides [209, 210, 246].

Bullous pemphigoid (BP) is a chronic autoimmune vesiculo-bullous disorder of the skin and mucous membranes characterized by the loss of adhesion of basal keratinocytes to the basement membrane, due to the production of autoantibodies directed against hemidesmosomes (which mediate adhesion to the membrane baseline) [210, 212] (Fig. 5.23). BP shows a lower morbidity and mortality rate than PV [243] and tends to occur mainly in patients over the age of 60 (the average age of onset is 76 years) and usually has a duration of 5 years [231]. The pathophysiological mechanisms of BP are summarized in Fig. 5.24.

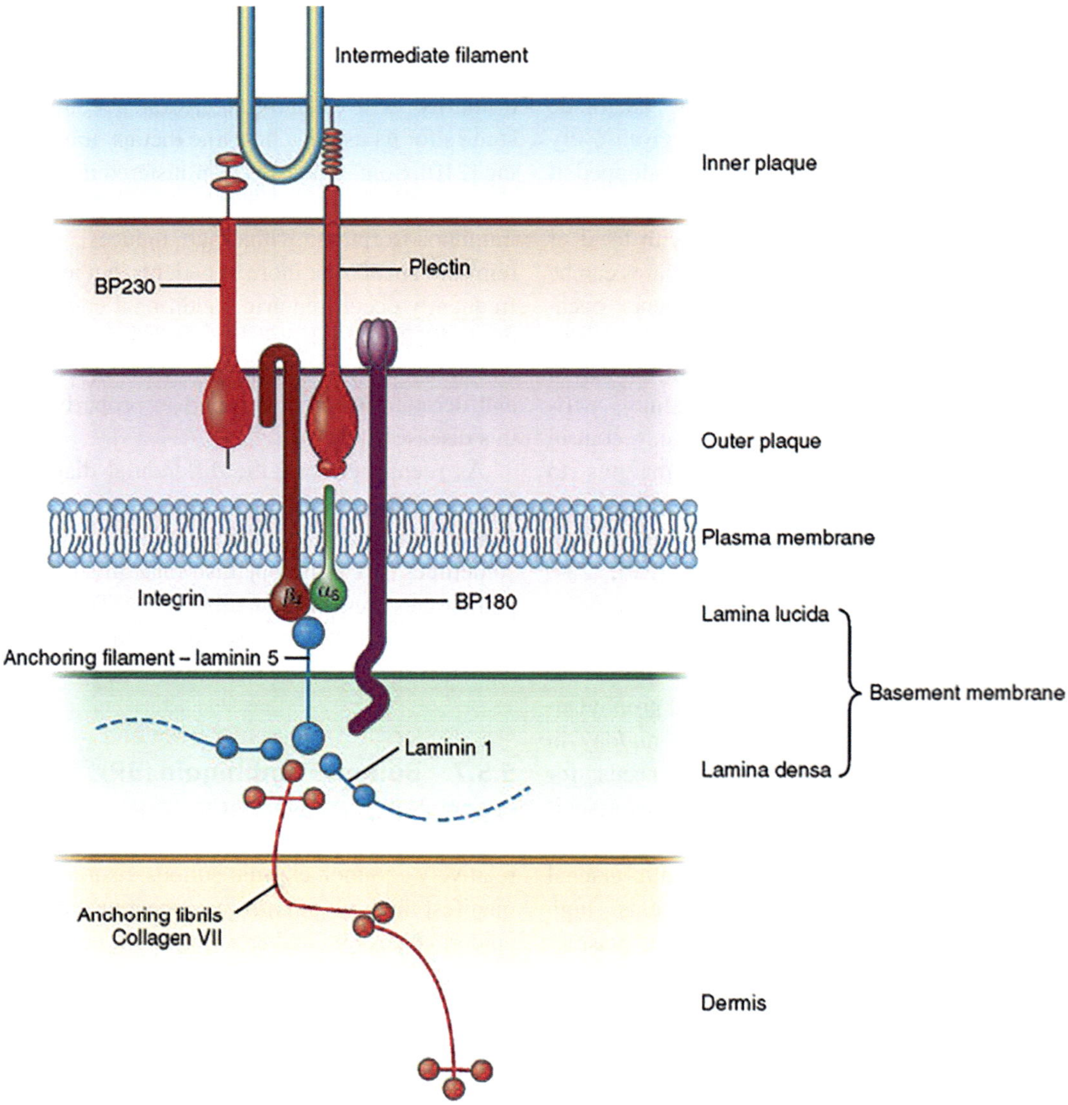

Fig. 5.23 Molecular components of the hemidesmosome. From [247] with permission

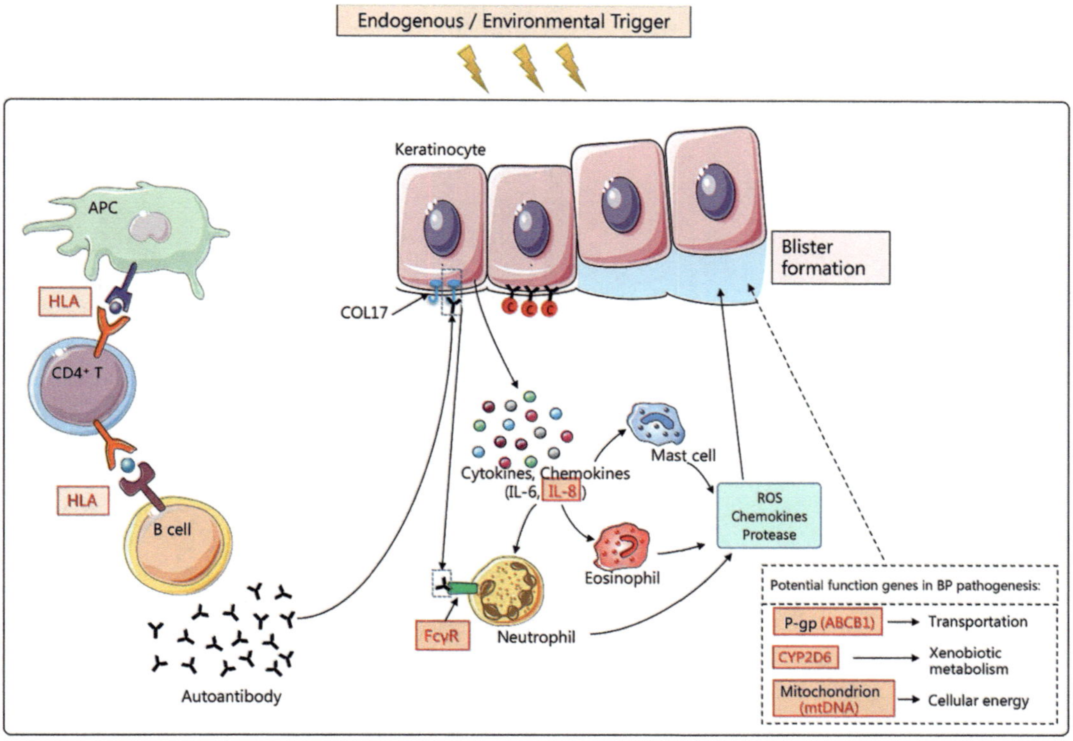

Fig. 5.24 Major pathways and cell types involved in BP, with BP-susceptibility genes shown in the pathway in which they are presumed to function. The interaction between BP autoantibodies, including IgG and IgE, and their target antigens, BP180 and BP230, leads to pathogenic events in complement-dependent and complement-independent pathways. The release of proteases by neutrophils results in tissue damage, which is enhanced by IL-8 from mast cells. On the other hand, the degranulation of mast cells is implicated in the activation of eosinophils. Therefore mast cells stimulate the activity of neutrophils, establishing a vicious circle, and in turn can also exacerbate the activity of eosinophils, favoring the appearance of urticarial lesions. Sensitized mast cells can express on the surface IgE capable of recognizing BP180EC and BP230, stimulating further degranulation of mast cells, and causing, due to the recognition of BP230, damage to the basal cells. Many of these pathways have been demonstrated in mouse models. Although neutrophils are critical for the formation of subepidermal blisters in mice, in humans the infiltrate is usually rich in eosinophils, with very few neutrophils. APC, antigen-presenting cell. C, complement. COL17, BP180. From [248]

Clinically we distinguish:

- *Skin lesions*: BP is characterized by the formation of tense blisters which occur on normal or erythematous skin and which are not as fragile as those observed in PV [249, 250] (Fig. 5.25). In this case Nikolsky's sign is generally negative, and the disease is often associated with skin itching that can precede the formation of blisters by months [210].
- *Oral lesions*: Some authors report that oral lesions in BP are relatively common (40%), although it is generally believed that they occur only in a minority of patients [210] and, unlike PV, they usually appear after cutaneous lesions [217]. Generally, oral BP lesions are smaller, slower growing, and less painful than oral lesions associated with PV [251, 252]. Oral blisters break rapidly, thus forming erosions that mainly involve the buccal mucous membranes, palate, gums, tongue, and lower lip [212]. The gingiva can also be affected in 16% of BP patients and present with erosion and/or desquamation [217]. Therefore oral lesions may appear as erosions, white-coated erosions, erythematous patches, and/or vesicles [253].

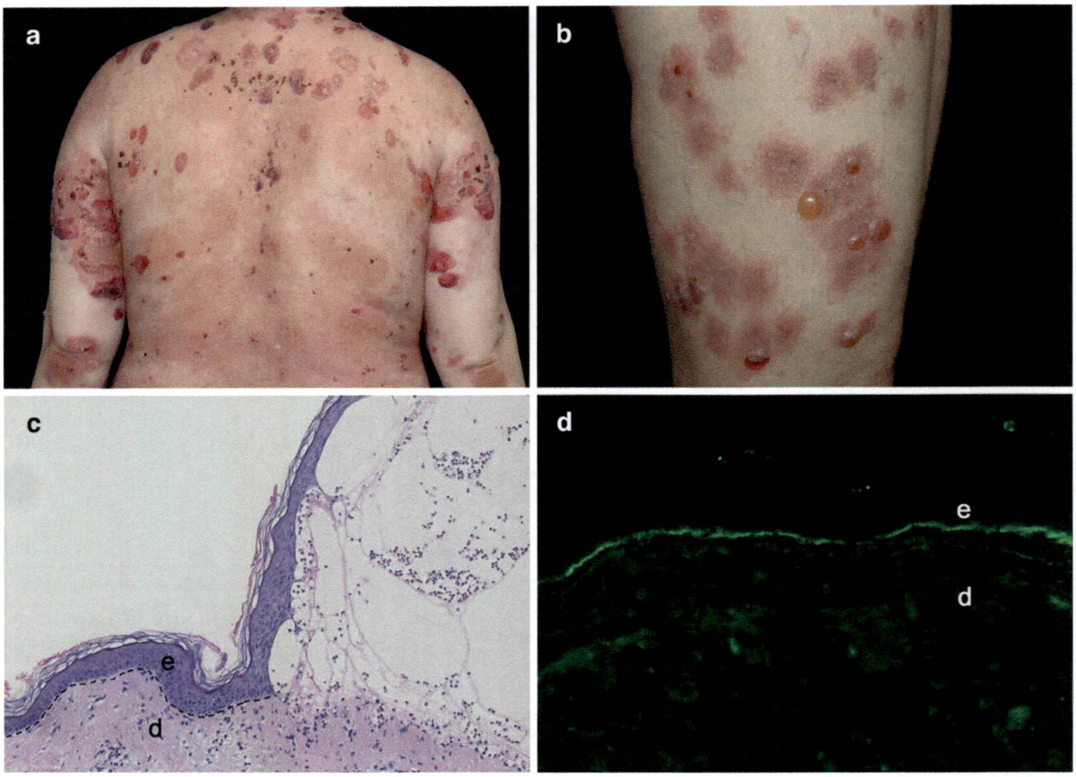

Fig. 5.25 Clinical and immunopathological characteristics of bullous pemphigoid. Tense blisters and erosions on the back, both arms (**a**), and right leg (**b**) of patients with BP. (**c**) Histopathology of a lesional skin specimen shows subepidermal splitting with inflammatory infiltrate of eosinophils and neutrophils. The intact dermal-epidermal junction in C is indicated by a dotted line. (**d**) Direct immunofluorescence microscopy of lesional specimen reveals linear deposits of IgG at the dermal-epidermal junction. e, epidermis. d, dermis. From [248] with permission

- *Other lesions*: Very rarely it is possible to report the appearance of pharyngolaryngeal lesions in patients with BP [253].

From a histopathological point of view, the hallmark of BP is the presence of subepidermal vesicles [249, 250] (Fig. 5.25). An inflammatory cell infiltrate is almost always present in the superficial dermis containing eosinophils (often seen in the vesicle cavity and intact basement membrane area, where they can degranulate before vesicle formation) [210].

DIF of the periwound skin shows linear deposits of C3 complement (Fig. 5.25) and, in most cases, of IgG. In fact, if DIF is negative for C3, the diagnosis of BP is questioned [210]. Immunohistochemical staining of formalin-fixed biopsies for complement proteins C3 (C3d) and C4d can be used to support a diagnosis of BP when only paraffin-embedded tissue and not fresh frozen is available [254, 255]. In most cases, the IIF shows circulating IgG that bind to the basement membrane [210].

Performing histological analysis and immunological tests will allow for an easy differential diagnosis between bullous OLP and BP in case of clinical doubt.

Current therapeutic strategies for BP include systemic immunosuppression by corticosteroids or immunomodulatory drugs sparing corticosteroid therapy: these approaches, however, allow for a non-specific reduction in autoantibody production [210]. Treatment with rituximab has been shown to be effective in cases resistant to non-specific therapy. In fact, this drug reduces the anti-BP180 and anti-BP230 IgG antibody titer within 1 month indicating that the autoantibodies are probably derived from short-lived plasma cells. However, IgE anti-BP180 antibodies decreased to a lesser extent than IgG anti-BP180 during treatment and follow-up, potentially making it more difficult to treat patients with predominantly IgE BP (e.g., the urticarial variant) [256]. Treatment with omalizumab (a monoclonal antibody that prevents IgE from binding to its own receptors) may be effective in patients who have high levels of anti-BP180 IgE, eosinophilia, and show urticarial skin lesions and resistance to standard therapeutic regimens [257].

The management of patients with pemphigus and pemphigoid associated with oral lesions is largely based on a multidisciplinary approach involving dermatologists, oral pathologists, internists, endocrinologists, otolaryngologists, and ophthalmologists, necessary to improve the prognosis of these diseases [212].

5.5.8 Lichen Planus Pemphigoides (LPP)

If, through diagnostic tests, the differential diagnosis between OLP and PV/BP can prove to be easy in clinically doubtful cases, it becomes more complex in other disorders such as lichen planus pemphigoides (LPP). LPP, a member of the pemphigoid family, is a rare mucocutaneous bullous disease (incidence about 1:1000000 patients) that shows clinical and histopathological features of both LP and pemphigoid (BP or MMP) [250, 258, 259]. In most cases, the lesions are found only on the skin, but occasionally (24% of cases), there is involvement of the oral mucosa [258, 260, 261]. The disease can occur in both adults and children [262]. Contrary to MMP (which usually occurs later, between the sixth and eighth decade of life), LPP appears to have a similar demographics to OLP, with a slight female predominance (in a ratio of 5:4 compared to men) and with onset about the fifth decade of life (average age of onset: 46 years) [96, 258, 259]. LPP always arises in LP (i.e., it is preceded by lichenoid lesions), and the time from the development of LP lesions to that of LPP vesiculo-bullous lesions can be from concomitant to subsequent up to 17 years [263], with an average duration of 8.3 months [258]. LPP has been associated with a wide range of conditions including malignant tumors (lymphoma, hemangiopericytoma, and colon adenocarcinoma), viral infections (HBV [contrary to OLP which is associated to HCV infection], varicella zoster), HBV vaccine, and some therapeutic approaches including statins (simvastatin), ACE inhibitors (ramipril, captopril), anti-H1 antihistamine (cinnarizine), loop diuretics (furosemide), NSAIDs (paracetamol and ibuprofen), Chinese herbal medicine, narrowband UVB, PUVA phototherapy, and immunotherapeutic agents such as anti-programmed death-1 (PD-1) antibodies (nivolumab) [258, 259, 262, 264–274].

LPP nature and pathogenesis is a debated argument. Actually it is considered a variant of BP; also bullous OLP is a variant of classic OLP. LPP is characterized by the release of autoantibodies anti-BP180 (or type XVII collagen) [275, 276]. The main target is the immunodominant non-collagenous region 16A (NC16A) of the BP180 ectodomain, similar to BP [250]. However, LPP patients' serum is characterized by autoantibodies preferentially reacting against the C-terminal rather than the N-terminal epitopes of the NC16A domain of BP180 [276]. Interestingly, even in milder BP forms, autoantibodies against the C-terminal portion of BP180 have been detected. Therefore, some scholars have considered LPP as a milder variant of BP [277]. Conversely, it has been showed that autoantibodies detected in LPP serum reacted against a different epitope within the C-terminal NC16A domain of BP180 antigen (MCW-4) compared to BP serum autoantibodies (MCW-0–MCW-3). Therefore, other scholars believe that LPP is a pathological entity distinct from BP [276]. Furthermore, LPP is also characterized by autoantibodies also targeting BP230, Dsg1, and two unidentified antigens of 130 and 200 kDa, respectively [275, 278–280]. The heterogeneity of autoantibodies detected in LPP patients could also explain the heterogeneity of clinical manifestations. Indeed it is possible to hypothesize that anti-NC16A domain of BP180 and anti-BP230 autoantibodies could promote a BP-like pattern, whereas anti-C-terminal portion of BP180 autoantibodies could promote a mucosal-dominant MMP-like pattern [281]. These findings suggest that in OLP an exposing of different antigens by the apoptotic basal oral keratinocytes to the autoreactive T lymphocytes could be present [278]. This results in the formation of pathogenic autoantibodies that lead to the formation of subepithelial blisters. Therefore, the development of vesiculo-bullous lesions may be due to the *epitope spreading phenomenon* resulting from apoptotic damage at the basement membrane. This is not uncommon in autoimmune diseases [250, 259, 277]. The epitope spreading phenomenon was first described in the early 1990s to define the capacity of the autoreactive B and T lymphocytes to carry out the immune response from a single determinant of endogenous epitopes to many other subdominant epitopes on the same or other proteins during the release of self-antigens during a chronic inflammatory process. The establishment of this phenomenon determines a vicious circle as the recruitment of autoreactive lymphocytes will favor the further release of "hidden" autoantigens with the possibility of triggering an autoimmune response directed against various auto-epitopes [282–284]. Two kinds of epitope spreading phenomenon exist: intramolecular (involving the same protein) and intermolecular (involving the same tissue or protein complex) [283]. The epitope spreading phenomenon has been described in different autoimmune mucocutaneous blistering diseases such as PV or pemphigus foliaceus via both intramolecular and intermolecular epitope spreading phenomena within the desmoglein ectodomain [285, 286]. This phenomenon can also occur between one immunological disorder and another, such as psoriasis and LP related to BP, Stevens-Johnson syndrome with cicatricial pemphigoid, or ulcerative colitis with linear IgA disease [284]. It is believed that at least three different factors could be involved in the initiation and perpetuation of this phenomenon: the nature of the "hidden" self-antigen which becomes "visible" and able to trigger an autoimmune response, the pattern of cytokines, and the type of APC involved in the perpetuation of the autoimmune inflammation [287]. In this regard, Mignogna et al. reported two cases of patients initially diagnosed with OLP that developed (in 3–11 years) a MMP and hypothesized that LPP might be a simple epitope spreading phenomenon from OLP to BP/MMP where lichenoid lesions precede vesiculo-bullous lesions or vice versa [264]. More specifically, the basement membrane zone (BMZ) break induced by MC degranulation could represent the crucial moment in which "hidden" epitopes of BMZ proteins may be exposed, such as BP180, α6β4 integrin, and laminin-322, that may trigger an autoimmune humoral response (Fig. 5.26). It seems that this process may take several years (from 3 to 11 years) due to a progressive loss of autoimmune control mechanisms, such as (1) the alteration of Treg suppressor lymphocytes and their subpopulation (Tr1) (as demonstrated in PV); (2) the "epitope theft" phenomenon by reducing the efficiency of lower-affinity naïve $CD8^+$ T lymphocytes priming and/or preventing the activation of lower-affinity specific $CD8^+$ effector T lymphocytes; or (3) a slow and delayed spreading from ordered to disordered epitopes. This process of progressive loss of control of autoimmune response induces an exposition of self-epitopes that were before invisible to B and T lymphocytes [264].

LPP should not be confused with bullous OLP. In bullous OLP the blisters' formation is the result of an extensive mucosal inflammatory infiltrate determining significantly vacuolar alterations in oral basal keratinocytes and dermal-epidermal separations. However, autoantibodies directed against components of the BMZ are absent in bullous OLP [258]. But some studies reported the presence of serum anti-BP180 antibodies in LP and vulvar LP patients targeting the NC16A domain [288, 289]. Serum and skin analyses revealed that in OLP a predominant Th1/Th17 profile was directed against Dsg3 and BP180, whereas a significantly incremented Th2 response was showed in PV and BP [290].

LPP patients show lichenoid skin papules and plaques with blisters spread on healthy and

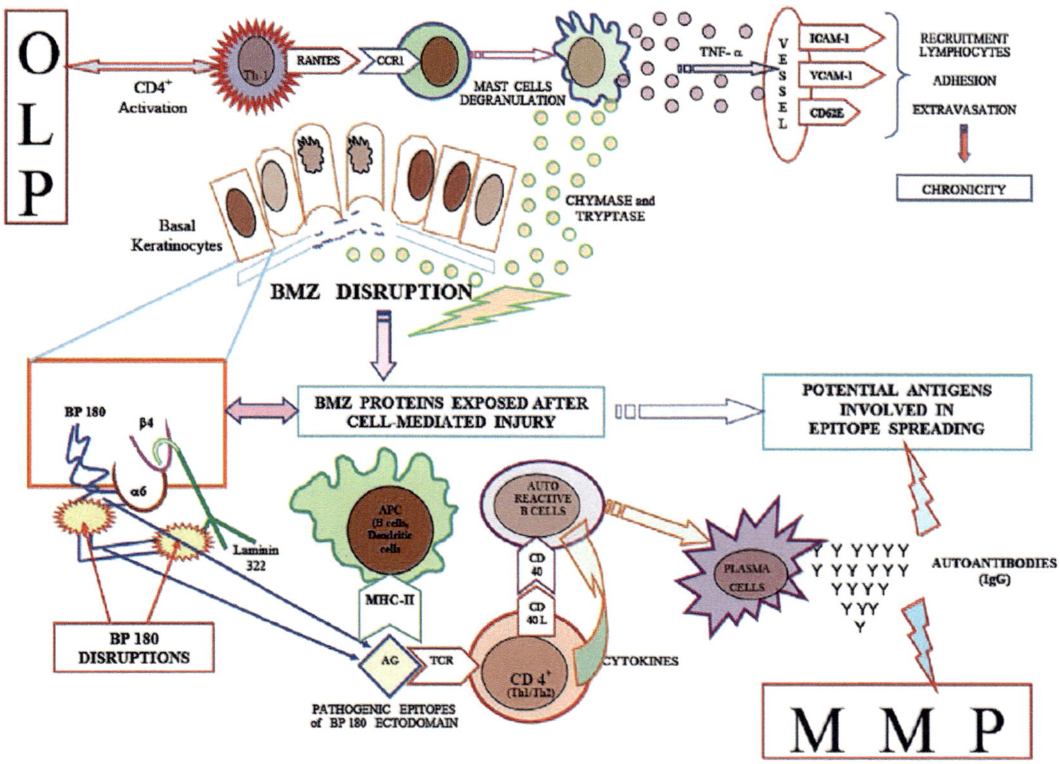

Fig. 5.26 LPP pathogenic hypothesis showing a schematic model of the probable phenomenon of "epitope spreading" from oral lichen planus (OLP) to mucous membrane pemphigoid (MMP) (Mignogna et al.). *MHC-II* major histocompatibility complex class II; *AG* antigen; *TCR* T-cell receptor; *Th1/2* T helpers 1 and 2; *TNF-α* tumor necrosis factor-α; *APC* antigen-presenting cells; *CD4* lymphocytes cluster of differentation 4; *RANTES* regulated upon activation, normal T cell expressed and secreted; *CCR1* chemokine (CC motif) receptor 1; *ICAM-1* intercellular adhesion molecule 1; *VCAM-1* vascular cell adhesion molecule-1; *CD62E* lymphocytes cluster of differentation 62E; *BMZ* basement membrane zone; BP180, bullous pemphigoid Ag 180; *b4* integrin b4; *a6* integrin a6; *CD40* lymphocytes cluster of differentation 40; *IgG* immunoglobulin G. From [264] with permission

affected skin. The skin lesions are usually localized on the extremities and sometimes the nails may be also involved (longitudinal ridging like LP) [259]. Cases of oral LPP have been occasionally reported without any involvement of the skin or other mucous membranes [258, 260]. Clinically LPP is characterized by the formation of tense vesiculo-bullous lesions, before, during, or after papular eruptions of cutaneous LP; blisters can appear both on normal and LP-affected skin [260, 262]. LPP oral lesions are typical of OLP (multifocal whitish reticular papules, plaque lesions, ulcer-erosive or desquamative gingivitis) with or without vesiculo-bullous lesions: these clinical features are indistinguishable from OLP [258]. LPP can affect various oral sites such as the palate, buccal mucosa, lip, gums, and rarely tongue [96, 258] (Figs. 5.27 and 5.28). Rarely LPP may extend to the pharynx and esophagus. Although LPP has clinical mucocutaneous manifestations very similar to bullous OLP, the prognosis is better than LP and BP with a recurrence rate in about 20% of cases [259].

The diagnosis of LPP is made in the presence of clinical, histopathological, and immunological features that suggest the concomitance of both the LP and the PB [260, 262, 275]. Histopathologically, LPP shows the characteristics of LP, MMP, or both [32] (Fig. 5.28d), namely, the presence of orthokeratosis, hypergranulosis, irregular acanthosis, hydropic degeneration of the basal keratinocytes with formation

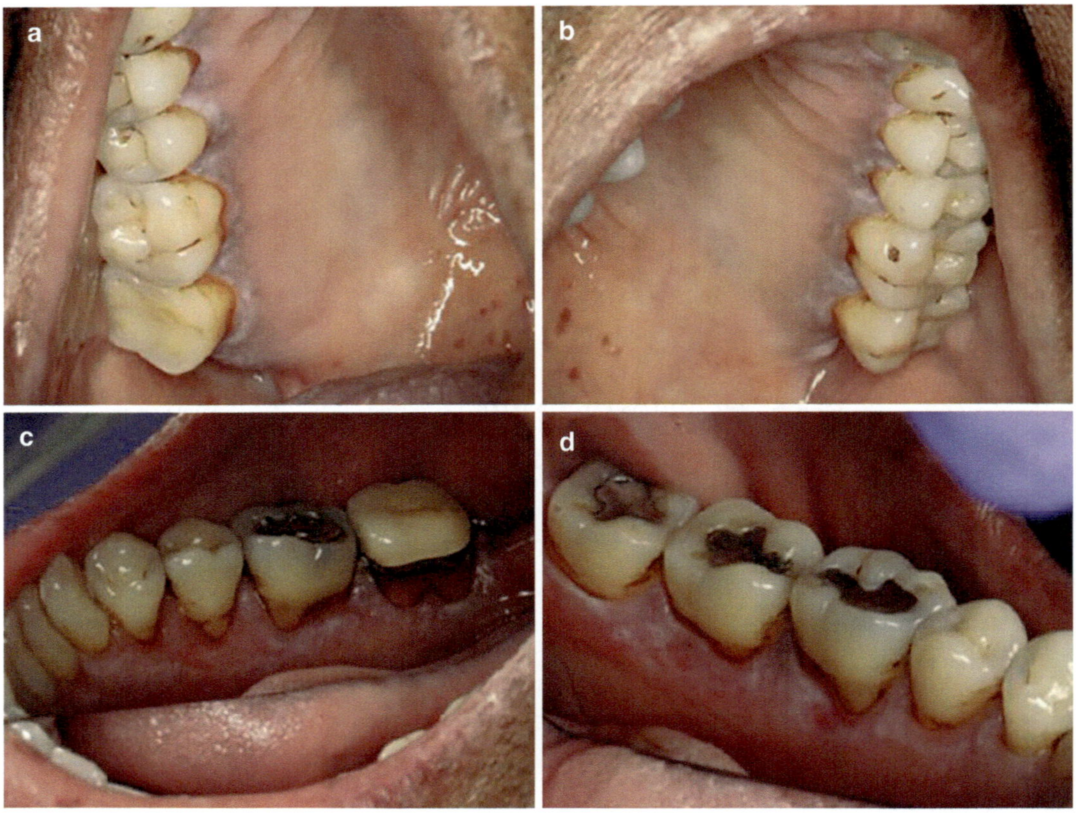

Fig. 5.27 Initial presentation. Wickham's striae with post-inflammatory hypermelanosis on the right (**a**) and left (**b**) sides of the palatal gingiva. Wickham's striae and mild and irregular erythema of the right (**c**) and left (**d**) lingual mandibular gingiva. From [263] with permission

of cytoid bodies, and subepidermal blister (at the level of lamina lucida). The inflammatory skin infiltrate is inconstant (basically with eosinophils and neutrophils rather than lymphocytes) and can be rich or poor in cells, of the lichenoid or perivascular type, and eosinophilic spongiosis can also be an additional feature [260, 280, 291].

To distinguish LPP from bullous OLP, it is imperative to demonstrate the presence of autoantibodies binding to the dermal-epidermal junction [259]. In this regard DIF is essential for diagnosis [32]. DIF is usually negative in bullous OLP, but sometimes globular IgM deposition in the Civatte bodies and linear/shaggy fibrinogen deposits in the dermal-epidermal junction may be observed [259]. In contrast, DIF shows a linear deposition of Ig (very often IgG) and/or C3 along the basement membrane at the level of the subepidermal blister in LPP, i.e., the same results observed in MMP [32, 96] (Fig. 5.29). IIF-SSS also shows in 50% of LPP patients the presence of circulating IgG antibodies to the basement membrane that are deposited on the epidermal side of the separated skin with 1.0 mol/L of NaCl [96]. The autoantigens found in LPP are BP180 and BP230 [258]. With immunoblotting, sera from LPP patients react against BP180 (the same target in BP), and in particular the autoantibodies bind to the C-terminal portion of NC16A, a noncollagenic region of BP180 recognized by the vast majority of patients with BP and MMP [276, 292]. In this context, the commercially available ELISA based on NC16A may contribute to the diagnosis [96]. This ELISA procedure includes antigen coating; blocking of non-specific binding sites; incubation of the serum-coated antigen of

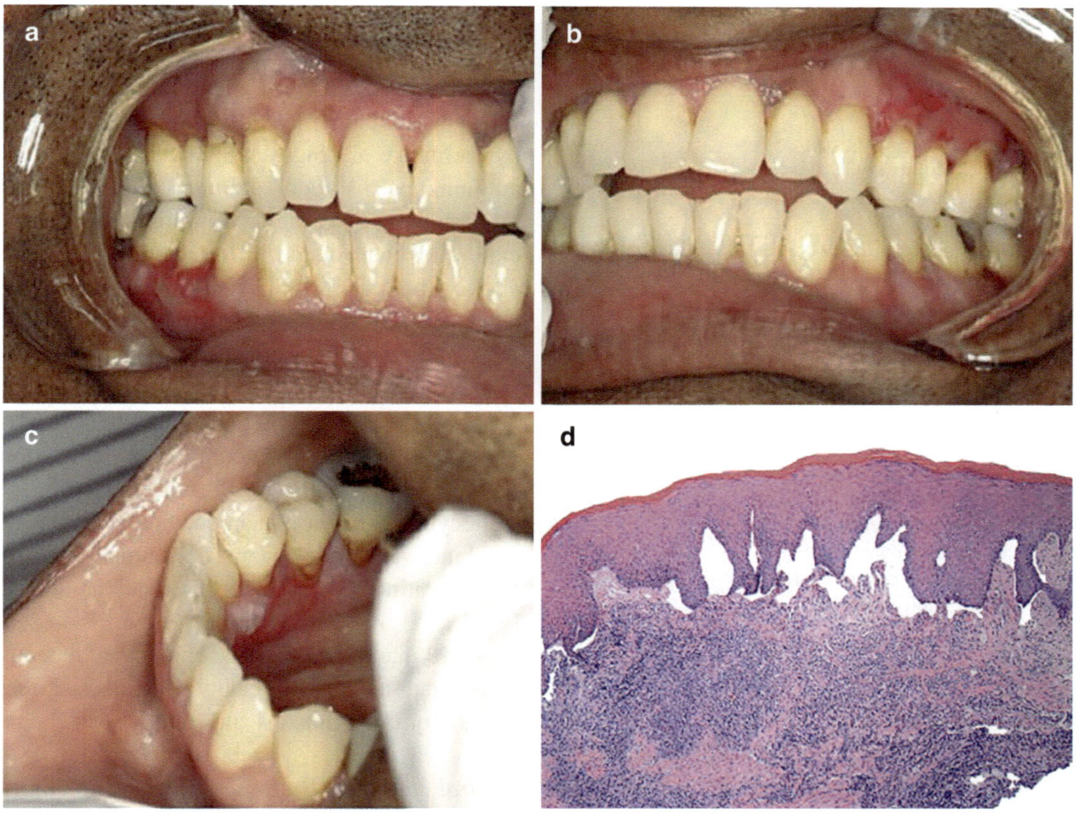

Fig. 5.28 Same case as Fig. 5.39 after 12 months. Ulcerations and erythema of the right mandibular buccal gingiva (**a**), left maxillary buccal gingiva (**b**), and right mandibular lingual gingiva ulcer (**c**). (**d**) Hyperkeratosis, acanthosis, subepithelial fissuring with preservation of the basal layer, and irregular lymphocyte band at the interface (H&E, original magnification x 100). From [263] with permission

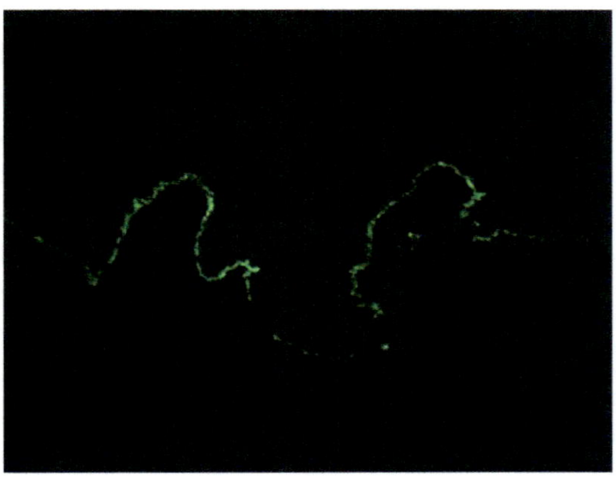

Fig. 5.29 Direct immunofluorescence study showed linear deposition of immunoglobulin G along the basement membrane zone (H&E, original magnification ×100). From [263] with permission

normal healthy individual (NHI) and LPP; washing to remove unbound autoantibodies; incubation with antihuman IgG antibody conjugated with Hrp (horseradish peroxidase); and addition of peroxidase substrate and stop which produces colored products [67].

Several therapeutic protocols of the LPP have been proposed in the literature (Table 5.5). Dapsone as monotherapy or combined with corticosteroid showed excellent results, especially in children. Topical corticosteroids were usually effective in the treatment of the oral lesions. However, the majority of cases were resolved successfully with systemic corticosteroids (from 10–15 mg/day to 1 mg/kg/day) or dapsone as monotherapy or combined [259].

Since LPP is a disorder that manifests in LP, it is not surprising that a patient is initially diagnosed with OLP (based on clinical, histopathological, and DIF findings), but subsequently the disease evolves into LPP, and this diagnosis is later established through the repetition of a

Table 5.5 Treatment options in LPP

LPP therapy
Topical
Corticosteroids Tacrolimus
Systemic monotherapy
Acitretin Azathioprine Cyclosporine Corticosteroids[a] Dapsone[a] Doxycycline Intravenous immunoglobulin Methotrexate Mycophenolate mofetil Ustekinumab
Systemic combination therapy
Corticosteroids + acitretin Corticosteroids + cyclosporine Corticosteroids + dapsone[a] Corticosteroids + methotrexate Tetracycline + nicotinamide

[a]This therapy was one of the most utilized and effective treatments based on literature

biopsy examination during the follow-up period for therapeutic purposes [263, 264]. The LPP is an example that demonstrates how the LP diagnostic process cannot end after an initial biopsy with confirmed LP diagnosis [32].

5.5.9 Mucous Membrane Pemphigoid (MMP)

Mucous membrane pemphigoid (MMP), formerly known as cicatricial pemphigus/pemphigoid, is a mucocutaneous autoimmune disorder belonging to the pemphigoid family and characterized by the formation of subepithelial blisters and vesicles [32, 209] The lesions mainly involve the oral and ocular mucosa (but occasionally also other systems) [209].

The epidemiology of MMP is not clear, as some data indicate a seven times lower prevalence compared to BP, while retrospective immunofluorescence studies suggest a three times higher frequency of pemphigus [209]. MMP predominantly affects women and can occur in any age group, rarely in children and more frequently between the fifth and eighth decade of life [32, 209].

MMP is probably an autoimmune disease of idiopathic etiology. It is occasionally stimulated by the intake of drugs and associated with other autoimmune disorders and neoplasms. There is no specific geographic distribution, but an association has been found with the HLA-DQB1*0301 allele. About 50% of patients show circulating autoantibodies to major BP antigens (BP180 and BP230) and anti-laminin 5, all present at the hemidesmosomal junction. As regards the pathogenesis, it is believed that the action of autoantibodies mediated by complement activation probably involves the recall and stimulation of leukocytes with consequent enzymatic release of cytokines and subsequent detachment of the basal keratinocytes from the basement membrane [209].

MMP mainly affects the conjunctival mucous membranes and the oral cavity but can also affect the skin or other mucous sites [209].

- *Oral lesions*: Bullous lesions (sometimes filled with blood) are almost always present in any site of the oral cavity (buccal mucosa, palate, alveolar ridge, tongue, and lower lip) but mainly in the gingiva beyond the 60% of cases of oral MMP. In fact, MMP is one of the main causes of desquamative gingivitis and in these cases it can clinically mimic EOLP [32, 209] (Fig. 5.30). Nikolsky's sign is commonly positive in MMP, but this is also found in bullous OLP [32]. Due to the frequent intraoral trauma, it is difficult to observe intact vesiculobullous lesions in MMP, but erosions covered by yellowish fibrin pseudomembranes are found which, on healing, give rise to scarring lesions, including stenosing [32, 65, 209]. Post-inflammatory atrophy can mimic the atrophic form of OLP [293]. Unlike erythema multiforme (EM) and PV, lesions to the lips are infrequent [209].
- *Ocular lesions*: These lesions (often neglected by odontostomatologists) can culminate in blindness. In the initial stages, there is usually a chronic conjunctivitis associated with symptoms of burning, irritation, and excessive lac-

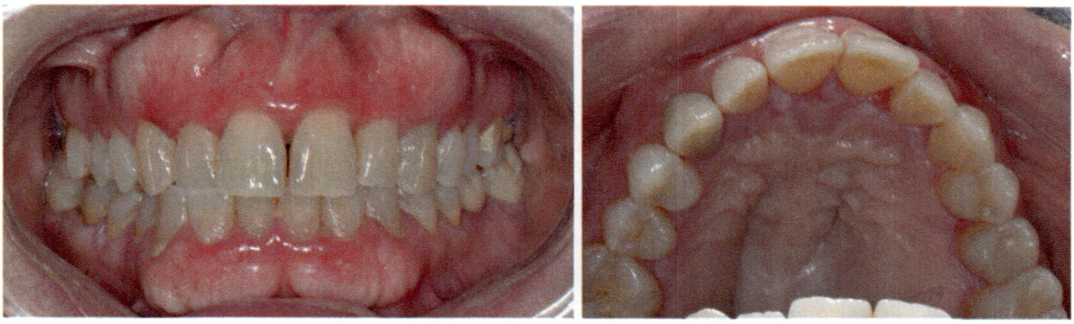

Fig. 5.30 MMP presenting as desquamative gingivitis, miming atrophic OLP. The vesicles often rupture giving rise to areas of erosion

rimation; the conjunctival narrowing is followed by a reduction in the fornix depth and finally the formation of a fibrous synechia which tends to fuse the bulbar sclera with the eyelid conjunctiva (symblepharon); fibrosis may then produce the progressive inversion of the eyelid margins (entropion) which brings the cilia against the corneal surface (trichiasis), thus causing a reduction in visual acuity [209].

- *Other less common lesions*: They may be present in other parts of the body covered by stratified squamous epithelium, such as the larynx or esophagus (where it can reach stenosis), the nasal cavities, the vulva, the penis, or the anal mucosa. Skin blisters are rarely observed [209].

From a histopathological point of view, MMP shows a subepithelial fissure similar to EOLP with separation of the epithelium from the lamina propria (Fig. 5.31) and resulting in the formation of a subepithelial blister [32, 209]. The pathologist should suspect a MMP when observing an epithelium clearly detached from the underlying lamina propria or the absence of connective tissue [32]. Contrary to OLP, basal keratinocytes in MMP do not show hydropic degeneration with the formation of cytoid bodies [156, 159]. MMP shows a mixed inflammatory infiltrate consisting of plasma cell lymphocytes and scattered eosinophils, and, unlike BP, tends to contain fewer eosinophils, but unfortunately this aspect is not constant [32, 209].

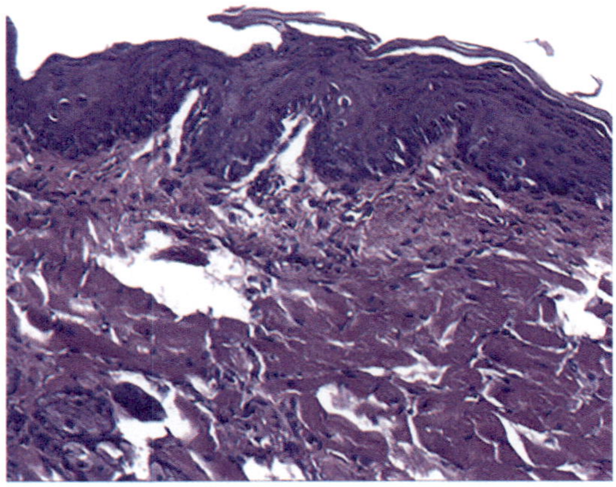

Fig. 5.31 Histopathological features of MMP, showing the typical subepithelial cleavage. Unlike OLP, the basal cells are intact and the superficial lamina propria contains a low to moderate inflammatory infiltrate consisting of lymphocytes and plasma cells. From [294] with permission

DIF represents the test of certainty in MMP and should highlight (in 80–100% of patients) linear deposits of IgG and C3 (more rarely also of IgM and IgA) along the basement membrane [293], allowing the distinction between MMP and OLP [32] (Fig. 5.32). IIF is usually negative for the detection of circulating antibodies in MMP, however the salt split skin technique (IIF-SSS) allows to increase its sensitivity, and it is possible to detect circulating antibodies located on the roof or on the floor of the separation, based on the specific distribution of MMP autoantigens in the basement membrane [250, 295, 296]. Furthermore, serological tests (immunoblotting and ELISA) can help in immunological subtyp-

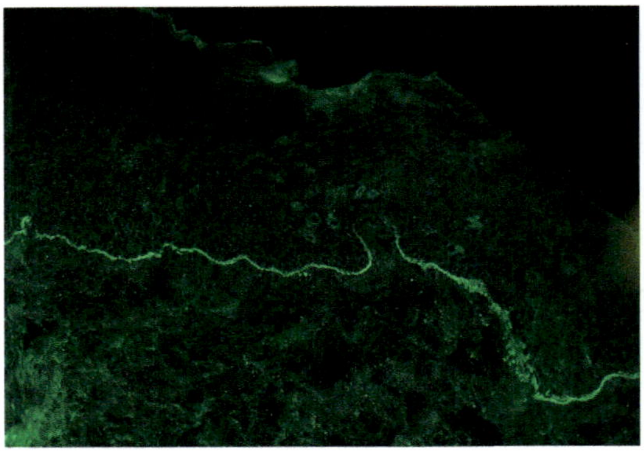

Fig. 5.32 DIF microcopy of a perilesional oral biopsy from a patient with mucous membrane pemphigoid shows linear deposits of IgG at the basement membrane zone. From [294] with permission

ing in the diagnosis of MMP [296]. As mentioned above, one of the main target antigens in MMP is a hemidesmosomal transmembrane molecule known as BP180 [67] (BP230 is an intracytoplasmic component of the hemidesmosome). It is interesting to note that, by immunoblotting of cultured keratinocyte cell extract, low levels of circulating anti-BP180 IgG were detected in up to 17% of patients with OLP (while almost all were negative if less sensitive techniques were used), and this is considered an example of the phenomenon of epitope spreading [297]. The epitope represents the component of an antigen that binds the specific antibody. The epitope spreading is a phenomenon that, in autoimmunity, consists in the development of immune responses to multiple epitopes during the progression of an autoimmune disease originally caused by the breakdown of tolerance mechanisms toward a single epitope. This phenomenon probably occurs following further disruptions of the tolerance mechanisms and the release of additional tissue antigens as a consequence of the inflammatory process stimulated by the initial response. In particular, in the phenomenon of epitope spreading, the immune response spreads from an epitope of an antigenic molecule to another epitope of the same antigenic molecule (which does not present with this a cross-reactivity), or alternatively to an epitope of different peptides which are part of a larger complex. The epitopes involved are frequently those against which the immune response has not developed a tolerance, since they are not normally presented by the MHC molecules in sufficient concentrations. These so-called "cryptic" epitopes are normally expressed in insufficient concentrations or are "hidden" during the differentiation and development of lymphocytes. However, during an infection or an inflammatory response, there may be damage to the tissue or cell that causes the release or expression of the cryptic or hidden epitopes of the autoantigens, and these become targets for the immune response. Since these epitopes were hidden, the immune system had not developed tolerance toward them. Therefore, the spread of the epitope seems to be responsible for maintaining the initiated immune response, through a continuous recruitment of specific autoreactive T lymphocytes for normal "cryptic" auto-peptides [298].

The correct diagnosis of MMP is fundamental to establish the correct therapeutic regimen, which is highly variable among the various pathologies. Several clinical entities can present in a similar way to MMP; therefore the diagnosis must be based on the history, clinical and histological examination, and DIF. It is important to make a differential diagnosis from other oral ulcer-erosive lesions, especially PV and hemorrhagic bullous angina, while in the case of desquamative gingivitis, it is necessary to differentiate MMP from OLP [209]. The clinical appearance of desquamative gingivitis in OLP and PMM and the microscopic presentation of EOLP and PMM often overlap, and a definitive diagnosis of MMP requires the DIF [32, 65]. Sometimes, to differentiate OLP from MMP, additional immunological tests such as IIF-SSS, immunoblotting/immunoprecipitation, and ELISAs are required [152]. However, such techniques are not universally available and are not commonly used in dentistry [67]. Consequently, the misdiagnosis of MMP and OLP is unfortunately common in dentistry [153].

MMP is not a single entity, therefore the clinical course is highly variable between patients, from mild to devastating forms, and for this reason individual patient treatment is required. Most of the therapeutic experience was made on

BP. Generally, oral MMP seems to have a relatively benign course compared to the forms that affect, in addition to the oral cavity, also other districts, therefore simple oral localizations should be treated initially with topical drugs, while in patients with multiple and persistent lesions not responding to the local therapy, aggressive systemic therapy should be used (where the same considerations made for PV to side effects are valid; see Sect. 5.5.6) [209].

- The treatment of first choice is topical corticosteroids, especially for oral lesions, among which the activity of clobetasol propionate 0.05% conveyed in hydroxyethyl cellulose gel stands out; for exclusively gingival lesions, the drug should be used with special drug-holder trays packaged on patient impressions. In case of *Candida* superinfection, this can be remedied with a miconazole gel therapy and chlorhexidine rinses [209].
- If oral lesions persist, worsen, or involve other districts, it is advisable to start therapy with systemic corticosteroids (prednisone or prednisolone): given that most reactions to corticosteroid therapy occur after 2–3 weeks, medium-high dosages (1–2 mg/kg/day) for short periods are generally preferred. Systemic therapy can be combined with topical therapy for further clinical benefits. At the systemic level, other immunosuppressive drugs such as azathioprine, cyclophosphamide, dapsone, sulfonamides, and tetracyclines can be used, mostly in combination with systemic steroids (alone they would not be equally effective) but with the exception of cyclophosphamide which appears to be effective also in monotherapy in patients with ocular lesions [209].

5.5.10 Lichen Planus-Like Variant of Paraneoplastic Pemphigus (PNP)

In 1990 Anhalt et al. [299] described for the first time a particular autoimmune syndrome which was given the name of paraneoplastic pemphigus (PNP). It is an autoimmune bullous disease of the epithelia associated with neoplasms, especially lymphoproliferative diseases: non-Hodgkin's lymphoma (38.6%), chronic lymphocytic leukemia (18.4%), Castleman's disease (18.4%), thymoma (5.5%), Waldenstrom's macroglobulinemia (1.2%), Hodgkin's lymphoma (0.6%), and monoclonal gammopathy (0.6%) [96, 300, 301]. Other possible associations of PNP can be given by squamous carcinomas of epithelial cells (8.6%) [302] and by mesenchymal lines sarcomas (6.2%) [303]. Eighty-four percent of cases of paraneoplastic pemphigus are associated with the presence of a neoplasm or hematological disorders. In the literature there are rare cases of association of PNP with gastric cancer [304] or with the intake of some drugs including fludarabine [305] and bendamustine [306], which are two antineoplastic molecules.

The mortality rate is very high (up to 90%) and early diagnosis is not easy; therefore PNP, although rare, is considered the most severe form of pemphigus [307]. It occurs more frequently in patients between the ages of 45 and 70 but can also affect children and adolescents [308]. In this subset of patients, PNP is often associated with Castleman's disease and malignant hematological disorders. On the other hand, no significant differences in incidence were observed between males and females [300].

Although the term PNP is widely accepted and used, this disorder actually consists of a spectrum of at least five different clinical and immunopathological mucocutaneous variants: pemphigus-like, pemphigoid-like, EM-like (EM, erythema multiforme), GvHD-like, and LP-like. Therefore, the most appropriate and comprehensive term of "paraneoplastic autoimmune multiorgan syndrome" (PAMS) has been suggested [309].

LP-like PNP is often associated with Castleman's disease, a rare lymphoproliferative disease [310], a non-clonal tumor of lymphatic origin, also known as giant lymph node hyperplasia or benign giant cell lymphoma [67]. Castleman's disease most commonly develops in the lymphatic areas of the retroperitoneal spaces or the chest, and evidence shows that the tumor may be present for very long periods before PNP develops [96]. The hyaline-vascular form is the most common histological variant of Castleman's disease associated with PNP [67].

The pathogenesis of PNP is not yet fully understood, but the key role of both humoral and cell-mediated immunity has been demonstrated [299, 300]. Cell-mediated immunity is characterized by the involvement of $CD8^+$ T lymphocytes [311]. IgG is mainly involved in humoral immunity, although in some cases a role of IgA has been reported [312, 313]. The autoreactive B and T lymphocytes therefore cause the detachment of keratinocytes from each other with consequent formation of vesiculo-bullous lesions. The most common targets of T lymphocytes and autoantibodies are different antigens belonging to the plakins family which are part of the intracellular plaque of desmosomes and/or hemidesmosomes [96]. These include envoplakin (210 kDa), periplakin (190 kDa), desmoplakin I and II (250 and 210 kDa), plectin (500 kDa), and BP230 (230 kDa) [314, 315]. The components of desmosomes such as desmogleins 1 (Dsg1) and 3 (Dsg3) are also involved [316]. Other more recently recognized antigens are placophilin 3 and desmocollins 1 and 3 [317, 318], and finally another antigen highly recognized in the serum of PNP patients is alpha-2-macroglobulin-like-1, a protease inhibitor recognized by autoantibodies circulating cells present in 69% of affected patients [319, 320]. Furthermore, there appears to be an association with HLA-Cw*14 and DRB1*03, respectively, in Chinese and French patients [321, 322], but this association has not yet been confirmed in other populations [96]. Two hypotheses have been formulated that may explain the association between PNP and neoplasia:

1. The onset of a tumor induces an immune response that targets the epithelial antigens expressed by the tumor or tumor antigens cross-reactive with epithelial antigens, resulting in an autoimmune response to the skin and mucous membranes.
2. According to the other hypothesis, which could explain the association with lymphatic tumors or sarcomas of dendritic cells, there could be a direct role of the immune cells involved in the autoreactive response.

Anamnesis is important to detect a recent or suspected history of cancer in patients with oral and/or skin lichenoid lesions. In these cases, a possible diagnosis of PNP must be considered [96].

Clinically, PNP has extremely polymorphic characteristics (Fig. 5.33) and the lesions are detectable on the skin and various mucous membranes. Usually the onset of the disease is characterized by the formation of widespread and very painful bullous and ulcer-erosive lesions in the oral mucosa; stomatitis is frequent [323]. Other mucous membranes such as the nasopharyngeal, esophageal, and anogenital mucosa can also be affected: often well-demarcated erosion with hyperkeratosis and reddish-violet erythema of the genital mucosa can be detected, and many can be distributed between the hard palate and pharynx [300]. In 70% of patients, there is also ocular involvement: cases of painful ocular irritation, worsening of vision, and mucosal secretion have been reported as symptoms, while clinical signs may include conjunctival erosions, thickening of the eyelid margin, corneal erosions, and pseudomembranous conjunctivitis [324, 325]. Skin lesions can be distributed on all surfaces of the body, especially on the trunk, head, neck, and proximal extremities [326], and are very variable in appearance; therefore this form of pemphigus is not always easily distinguishable from other

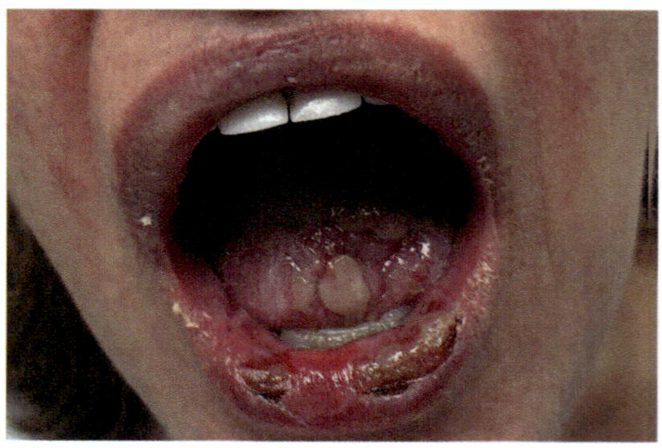

Fig. 5.33 Painful ulcerations of the tongue related to PNP manifesting in a patient treated with pembrolizumab for urothelial carcinoma. From [331] with permission

mucus diseases, such as PV, EM, PB, and LP. Patients may present with red and inflamed patches, scaly plaques, fluid-filled blisters, or intensely itchy ulcerative lesions [309, 327, 328]. Furthermore, PNP also affects the epithelium of the respiratory tract in up to 93% of cases [329], causing dyspnea, obstructive pulmonary disease, and obliterative bronchiolitis (with consequent respiratory failure), causing death in these patients [96, 330].

Histopathology may show acantholysis with necrotic keratinocytes and vacuolation of the basal layer with underlying inflammatory infiltrate; however these findings are not of much help [96, 332]. DIF may show linear deposits of IgG and C3 (more rarely IgA and IgM) in the junction between keratinocytes and sometimes in the dermoepidermal junction, but it can also be negative [332]. IIF analysis of sera from PNP patients shows the presence of anti-epidermals (typical of PV) and basement membrane (typical of BP) autoantibodies. Therefore routine immunological tests such as DIF and IIF can be negative or controversial, showing the characteristics of multiple pathological entities [96]. To discriminate between PV and PNP, it is possible to employ IIF with special substrates, such as rat bladder epithelium, which does not contain Dsg1 and Dsg3 (recognized in the serum of PV patients) but only plakins, such as desmoplachins, envoplachins, and periplakin (recognized in patients with PNP): this greatly increases the sensitivity (75–86%) and specificity (83–98%) of the test and also helps to differentiate PNP from patients with seropositive pemphigus autoantibodies that react against plachins [333, 334]. Other advanced diagnostic assays may also be conducted in specialized centers. For example, there are numerous ELISA tests on the market capable of detecting reactivity against certain antigens in PNP: BP180, BP230, Dsg1, Dsg3 (MBL, Nagoya, Japan), and envoplakin (EUROIMMUN, Lübeck, Germany) [67]. In particular, an ELISA based on the N-terminal domain of envoplachin is able to detect serum reactivity in 80.6% of patients with PNP [335, 336]. Immunoblotting may exhibit a family-directed plakin profile including envoplakin, periplakin, bullous pemphigoid antigen 1 (BPAG1), and plectin [96]. However, the gold standard for diagnosing PNP is still the immunoprecipitation (IP) of keratinocyte extracts. Historically, the first technique used for the identification of autoantibodies in PNP was immunoprecipitation using radiolabeled keratinocyte extracts [299]. The sensitivity of this technique exceeds that of immunoblotting, rat bladder IIF, and envoplachin-based ELISA [96] and also allows to identify anti-α-2-macroglobulin-like-1 reactivity undetectable from immunoblotting of sera from PNP patients [319]. However, due to the use of radioactive material, this technique is not widely available [96]. Recently, nonradioactive immunoprecipitation has been introduced which appears to show similar diagnostic performance [337].

PNP is one of the forms of pemphigus most resistant to medical treatment [328] and is generally refractory to standard treatments [96]. In case of PNP suspicion, as suggested by Frew et al. [338], the following are important: the stabilization of vital parameters to reduce the high mortality rate, evaluation of any underlying tumors (if not already known), accurate diagnosis, tumor removal or specific anti-tumor therapy; drug treatment with immunosuppressants and immunomodulators; and plasmapheresis. High-dose corticosteroids, effective for skin lesions, but not always for mucosal lesions, are indicated as first-line treatment [339, 340]. The association between prednisolone and other drugs such as azathioprine, cyclosporine, mycophenolate mofetil, cyclophosphamide, intravenous Ig, and plasmapheresis has been shown to have a good efficacy and safety profile [341, 342]. In patients with PNP caused by B lymphoma, treatment with rituximab (anti-CD20) has been shown to be effective both as monotherapy and in combination with corticosteroids and immunosuppressants [338, 343]. Supportive treatments may also be important, such as early antimicrobial therapy due to the risk of sepsis resulting from loss of skin integrity and immunosuppression [328] and analgesic therapy to reduce the pain caused by extensive erosions.

PNP has often a poor prognosis, with a high mortality rate, usually related to systemic complications including sepsis, gastrointestinal bleeding, and bronchiolitis obliterans [328, 344]. It has also been reported that PNP and the underlying neoplasm do not necessarily have a parallel evolution; in fact the lesions can progress even after removing the neoplasm or when the latter is under control [300]. But cases of PNP with Castleman's disease have also been reported in which tumor removal led to marked clinical improvement [345, 346].

5.5.11 Chronic Ulcerative Stomatitis (CUS)

Chronic ulcerative stomatitis (CUS) is a rare mucocutaneous disease that can mimic both EOLP and MMP [65]. It was first described in 1990 by Jaremko et al. [347] and is characterized by the formation of chronic oral ulcerations that may occasionally involve the skin [348–356].

The incidence of CUS is unknown and, to date, less than 100 cases have been reported in the English literature since its first description in 1990 [65, 357, 358]. Similar to OLP, CUS has a female predilection and arises in the fifth and sixth decade of life [32, 65].

The clinical appearance of the oral lesions of CUS is practically indistinguishable from that of EOLP and MMP [32, 65, 96]. Similar to EOLP, white striae may be detected peripherally to the erosive lesions. CUS can involve any oral anatomical site, most commonly the gums, tongue, and buccal mucosa and less commonly the palate, lower lip, and lingual gingiva [32]. Gingival involvement appears as desquamative gingivitis, with erosion and ulceration indistinguishable from OLP and MMP [162, 351, 352] (Fig. 5.34).

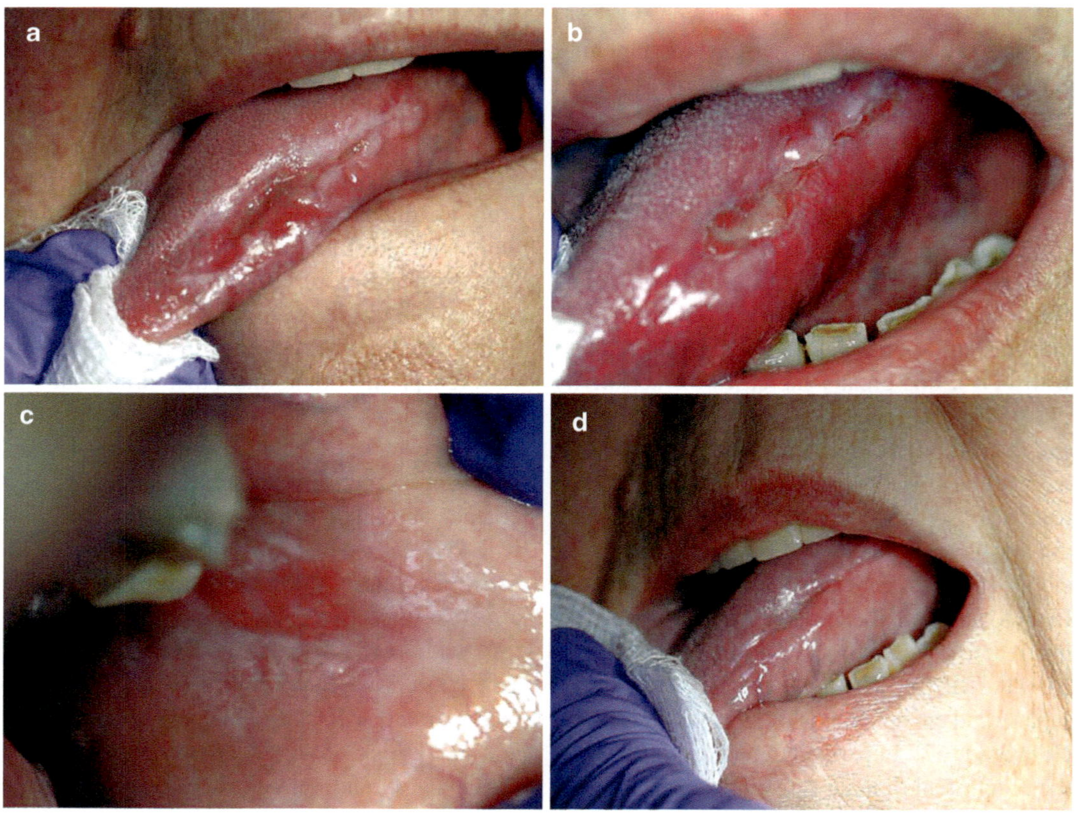

Fig. 5.34 (**a**) Oral examination of the tongue that revealed faint leukoplakia of the left lateral tongue with a 2.5 × 0.6 cm linear crateriform ulcer involving the left anterolateral aspect and the adjacent ventral and lateral areas. (**b**) Enlarged image of the same area. (**c**) Left buccal mucosa exhibiting an erythematous and eroded rectangular lesion measuring approximately 1.5 × 1.0 cm and surrounded by white striations. (**d**) Tongue exhibiting near-complete resolution of the ulcerations at 6 months' follow-up after initiation of hydroxychloroquine pharmacotherapy. From [351] with permission

The histopathological features of CUS (Fig. 5.35) are non-specific and vary according to the biopsy site [32, 96]. Often, features are indistinguishable from those found in OLP: atrophic epithelium with sawtooth epithelial ridges, liquefactive degeneration of basal keratinocytes, cytoid bodies, epithelial atrophy, and a dense inflammatory band infiltrate predominantly lymphocyte [67, 351, 357]. However, ulcerative lesions may present non-specific features with mixed inflammatory cell infiltrate [32].

The diagnosis of CUS requires immunofluorescence [359]. DIF may allow a distinction between OLP and CUS [65].

DIF of the periwound tissue reveals the presence of IgG in the nuclei of the basal keratinocytes and of the lower third of the epithelium, according to a speckled and/or granular pattern [352, 355, 357]. This characteristic result on DIF is known as the stratified epithelium-specific antinuclear antibody (SES-ANA) pattern (or model) [355] (Fig. 5.36). In addition, other autoimmune diseases, such as SLE, systemic sclerosis, CREST syndrome (calcinosis, Raynaud's phenomenon, esophageal involvement, sclerodactyly, and telangiectasia), and mixed connective tissue disease (MCTD), may also demonstrate a similar ANA pattern in the epithelium; however, these autoantibody deposits, unlike CUS, are typically found in the spinous cell layer [32, 352]. However, the tangential orientation of the tissue sections can make the interpretation of IgG localization problematic. Sometimes a linear band of fibrinogen with a "shaggy" appearance can be identified in the basement membrane, but this result of DIF is not specific for CUS; in fact it is also found in OLP [32, 65]. IIF, in patients with CUS, also allows the identification of circulating antibodies that exhibit the SES-ANA pattern using the monkey or guinea pig esophagus as a substrate [348, 355]. Circulating IgG in SLE, CREST syndrome, and MCTD patients [348, 360, 361] are usually detected using human HEp-2 neoplastic

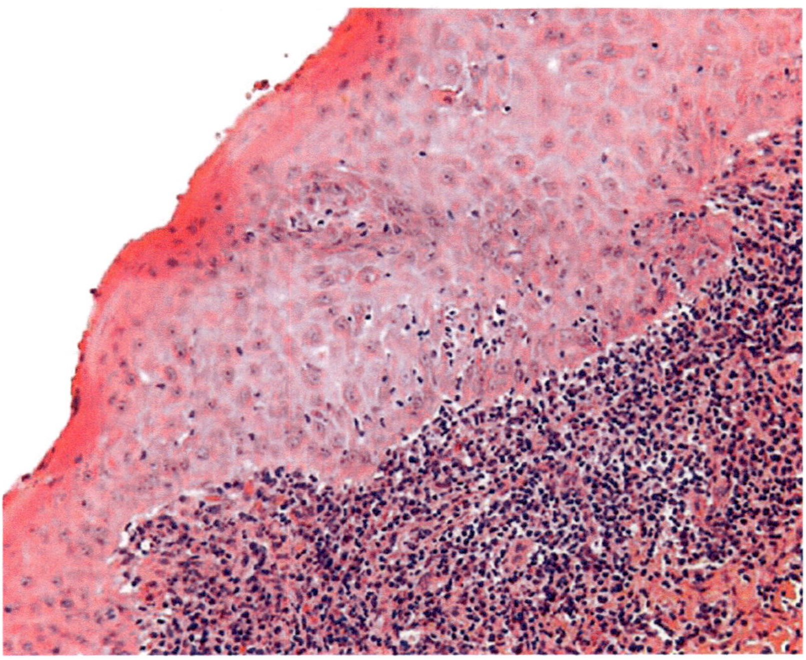

Fig. 5.35 Routine HE-stained section of oral mucosal lesion revealing histopathologic similarity to lichen planus exhibiting partly atrophic epithelium with sawtooth rete ridge formation and a subepithelial eosinophilic coagulum. Interface stomatitis (leukocytic exocytosis) and a dense band-like inflammatory infiltrate composed mainly of lymphocytes and a few plasma cells in the superficial lamina propria and in the epithelium-connective tissue interface are also noted (magnification ×20). From [351] with permission

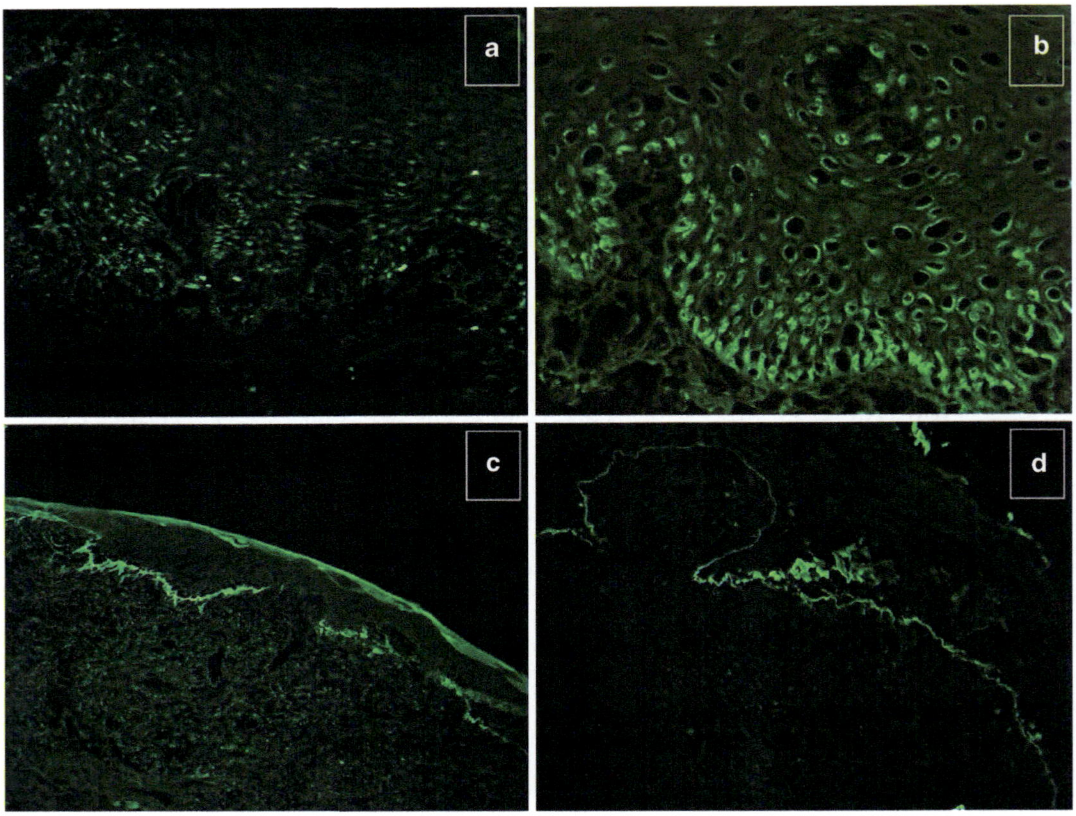

Fig. 5.36 Images of direct immunofluorescence (DIF) antibody staining from biopsy taken from case 4. (**a**) DIF of lesional and perilesional tissue revealing a speckled finely granular SES-ANA pattern of IgG deposition in the nuclei of keratinocytes (magnification ×10). (**b**) Higher-power view (magnification ×20). (**c**) DIF with basement membrane zone staining for fibrinogen (magnification ×10). (**d**) Higher-power view of DIF staining for fibrinogen (magnification ×20). From [351] with permission

cells or rodent kidney cells as substrates, but are not suitable for IIF of suspected CUS cases. SLE, systemic sclerosis, and MCTD may also be positive for ANA on esophageal substrates, but the pattern is different because antibodies should be distributed across the surface epithelial layers [352].

Immunoblot studies have led to the recognition of a keratinocyte protein of 70 kDa in some cases of CUS [362–364]. Further research has led to the identification of a nuclear protein normally present in the basal and parabasal cells of the stratified squamous epithelium called ΔNp63α, which is believed to be the presumed specific antigen of CUS [365]. ΔNp63α belongs to the family of nuclear transcription factors, including p63, p73, and the tumor suppressor gene p53, with which it shares a considerably homologous sequence [366]. It is still debated whether ΔNp63α is specific for CUS, since, according to what some authors have reported, patients with OLP may have circulating autoantibodies against this protein [364].

Two noncommercial ELISA systems have been developed for the detection of anti-ΔNp63α antibodies [260]. In the first, the N-terminal part of the protein (considered the immunogenic portion) is used to coat the ELISA plates [352]. Instead the other group of researchers used the whole protein [367].

The therapeutic management of CUS is different from that of OLP and similar [32]. In fact, according to some authors, in case of resistance to treatment with glucocorticoids, a possible case of CUS should be considered [356]. In the treatment of CUS, corticosteroids and dapsone were found to be less effective than hydroxychloroquine, which induced clinical remission and a reduction in autoantibody titer [351, 352].

Due to the limited number of reported cases, understanding of the etiopathogenesis, natural history, and optimal management of CUS is limited [32].

5.5.12 Erythema Multiforme (EM)

The term erythema multiforme (EM) indicates a particular syndrome that includes very different clinical pictures including a variant characterized by simple oral lesions (oral EM); another self-limited, mild, exanthematic, cutaneous variant with minimal oral involvement (EM minor (EMm)); and an aggressive, progressive, fulminant, severe variant with extensive mucocutaneous epithelial necrosis (EM major [EMM] or Stevens-Johnson syndrome [SJS] and toxic epidermal necrolysis [TEN]) [209, 368]. All these conditions are considered to be sequelae of a cytotoxic immune reaction against keratinocytes expressing non-self-antigens [369]. EM therefore consists of an acute, immune-mediated, uncommon mucocutaneous condition that is usually caused by HSV infection and the use of certain drugs. About 70% of patients with EM may have oral involvement, and sometimes this may be the only site affected [67]. However, this fact has often been overlooked in most published classifications, especially by dermatologists [370]. Rarely EM may be persistent and associated with some viruses, including HCV [371]; therefore oral EM has sometimes been diagnosed and published as fixed drug eruption [372], unspecified oral ulceration [373], or atypical erosive OLP [374].

EM usually affects apparently healthy young adults and males are more involved than females [67]. The peak age of the disease is between 20 and 40 years, although 20% of cases can occur in children over 3 years or adolescents [209, 375–377]. The estimated incidence varies from 1.1 cases/106 inhabitants per year in Germany to 3.7 cases/106 inhabitants per year in the USA, up to 5–10 cases/106 inhabitants per year in Sweden. Relapses occur in 37% of cases, often with a severe clinical increase in attacks [209].

From an etiological point of view, although many factors seem to be involved in the pathogenesis of EM (Table 5.6), the two main causes seem to be the use of some systemic drugs (in particular antibacterials, antimycobacterials, NSAIDs, analgesics, hormones, diuretics, antiepileptics) and the organic reaction to particular infectious agents (mainly herpes simplex virus [HSV] and *Mycoplasma pneumoniae*), but

Table 5.6 Well-documented etiological factors of EM

Main known etiological agents of EM	
Infectious agents	Fenoprofen
A. *Virus*	Ibuprofen
Herpes simplex[a]	Isoxicam *
Epstein-Barr	Ketoprofen
Orf virus	Phenylbutazone [a]
Vaccine virus	Feprazone [a]
B. *Bacteria*	Naproxen
Yersinia	Piroxicam [a]
C. Mycobacteria	Sulindac
Tuberculosis	Tenoxicam
D. *wMycoplasma pneumoniae**	E. *Antiepileptics*
	Carbamazepine *
E. *Mycetes*	Phenytoin
Histoplasma capsulatum	Phenobarbital [a]
Systemic drugs	F. *Hormones*
A Antibacterials	Glucagon
Tetracyclines	Estrogen
Penicillins [a]	Glucocorticoids
Cephalosporins	G. *Diuretics*
Fluoroquinolones (ciprofloxacin)	Furosemide
	H. *Antidiabetics*
Sulfonamides and trimethoprim	Chlorpropamide
	I. *Cytostatics*
Lincosamides (clindamycin)	Alkylating substances (cyclophosphamide)
Amphenicol (chloramphenicol)	Antimetabolites (methotrexate)
B. *Antimycobacterials*	J. *Others*
Isoniazid	Allopurinol [a]
Ethambutol	Phenolphthalein
Rifampicin	Arsenical
C. *Antiprotozoals*	Ethanol
Aminoquinoline (quinine)	Imiquimod
D. *NSAIDs and analgesics*	**Physical agents**
	Radiotherapy
Acetylsalicylic acid	
Benoxaprofen [a]	
Codeine	
Diclofenac	

[a]Most frequently related causative agents

recently other causative agents have also been found [209, 378–380]. However, sometimes the triggering cause remains unknown, especially if the lesions occur only orally [209].

EM appears to be associated with some HLAs, mainly with HLA-B15 (B62), HLA-B35, HLA-A33, HLADR53, and HLA-DQB1*0301 [67], and the latter has been strongly related to EM associated with HSV infection [381]. Given the possibility of even fatal skin reactions (including SJS and TEN) linked to some HLA alleles, the EMA (European Medicines Agency) and its Member State agencies have recommended testing for the HLA gene before starting a specific drug treatment [67]. Specifically, three drugs were identified that cause significant drug hypersensitivity reactions in patients with the following HLA alleles: abacavir and HLA-B*57:01, carbamazepine and HLA-B*15:02/A*31:01, and finally allopurinol and HLA-B*58:01 [382].

Regarding the pathogenesis EM appears to be the result of a cell-mediated immune reaction to a precipitating agent (e.g., HSV-DNA fragments). This agent is expressed as an antigen in the keratinocyte membrane and is recognized by $CD4^+$ Th1 lymphocytes (specific, e.g., for HSV) that release IFN-γ, a potent inflammatory mediator that leads to an overproduction of pro-inflammatory cytokines and chemokines from different cell types, inducing a further recruitment of autoreactive T cells and the consequent tissue damage. It also seems that the mechanisms of tissue damage in EM induced by drugs or viruses are different from each other and different from those of SJS and TEN [375].

From a clinical point of view, oral, skin, and ocular lesions may appear. Skin lesions present typically with a "target pattern" and are symmetrical and consist of erythematous macules or papules [67]. Ocular changes, when present, are similar to those of PMM (dry eye, symblepharon), and SJS can lead to sicca syndrome or Sjögren's syndrome [375, 376, 383]. Oral lesions may be isolated or precede lesions in the other stratified squamous epithelia. They usually early appear on the lips that become swollen and chapped, bleeding, and encrusted, and typically bilateral and diffuse oral ulcerations appear, generally and more pronounced in the anterior areas of the oral cavity. Mucosal lesions may sometimes be accompanied by flu-like symptoms, fever, sore throat, headache, arthralgia, myalgia, pneumonia, nephritis, or myocarditis, and these occur more frequently in EMM, SJS, and TEN [67].

The course of the pathology, in general, is mostly acute, self-limiting, and recurrent, particularly during the change of seasons [209]. As already mentioned, four clinical variants are distinguished:

1. *Oral EM*. It usually affects adults. Acute oral lesions generally tend to resolve in 1 to 3 weeks but can sometimes persist and worsen. Usually these are widespread erythematous and ulcer-erosive lesions. The lips may have crusty lesions, but no skin lesions or systemic symptoms are present [209] (Fig. 5.37).

2. *EM minor (EMm)*. It affects adolescents and young adults and this form seems to be particularly associated with HSV. Oral lesions are absent, or, at most, appear in the form of simple erosions. On the other hand, skin lesions are always present (typically with a

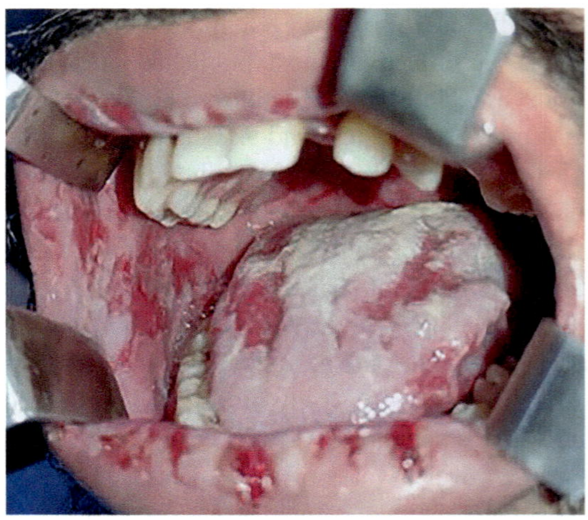

Fig. 5.37 Oral EM following intravenous ceftriaxone. From [384] with permission

"target" appearance) and have a duration of 1–4 weeks. These particular lesions are characterized by an erythematous central ring (with or without bullous lesions), an intermediate edematous area, and an erythematous outer ring and symmetrically involve the extensor surface of the limbs, the back and palm of the hands, and the soles of the feet. In this form, systemic symptoms may occur [209].
3. *EM major (EMM)* or *Stevens-Johnson syndrome (SJS)*. It can affect any age group and the lesions have an average duration of 1–6 weeks. The mucous lesions (oral, genital, and anal) have an ulcer-erosive aspect and involve at least two different districts. Skin lesions are always present, but they are not always with a "target pattern" but may have an atypical appearance. Skin lesions generally involve less than 30% of the entire body surface. Systemic symptoms occur in 10–30% of cases [209].
4. *TEN (toxic epidermal necrolysis or Lyell's syndrome)*. It affects adults and the lesions last for 1–3 weeks. In 85–90% of cases, there are mucous lesions which, even in this case, affect at least two different districts. Skin lesions involve more than 40% of the total body surface. Nikolsky's sign is positive, i.e., the skin and mucous membranes tend to detach from the underlying stroma due to a modest trauma in apparently healthy areas. Systemic symptoms are also present [209].

EM diagnosis is primarily based on clinical presentation and a careful history which generally includes acute onset of oral and/or skin lesions, possibly preceded by HSV infection or recent drug use [67, 209]. There are no specific diagnostic tests for EM, so diagnosis is usually made by excluding other causes [67]. It is essential to keep in mind that EM episodes are usually acute, self-limiting, and recurrent, often preceded by flu-like systemic symptoms (fever, headache, rhinorrhea). In addition, it is necessary to distinguish oral EM from that with more generalized manifestations that also involve other districts [209]. Cases with only oral and more persistent manifestations are more difficult to diagnose. In fact, the absence of skin lesions represents a diagnostic challenge for the clinician due to a wide spectrum of differential diagnostic conditions such as primary herpetic gingivostomatitis (EM hardly affects the keratinized gingiva), recurrent aphthous stomatitis, EOLP, MMP, PV, and fixed drug eruption [209, 372].

There is no specific histopathological feature for EM. During the first clinical manifestations, the superficial dermal vessels dilate, and therefore a perivascular infiltrate of lymphocytes and macrophages appears that arrives toward the epithelial-connective tissue interface [209]. Intra- and intercellular edema is often observed on the epithelium, early spongiosis, with necrosis of satellite cells (single necrotic eosinophilic keratinocytes surrounded by lymphocytes) and some intra- and subepithelial vesicles [67, 209]. Severe stromal edema is frequently observed in the papillary areas, and vacuolar degeneration of the basement membrane accompanied by intense lymphocytic infiltration may also be found [67, 209]. On the oral sample, a pronounced presence of intraepithelial neutrophils and an irregular elongation of the epithelial crests should also be noted [209]. However, the histological aspect may be variable and the immunostaining is not specific for EM [67].

Immunopathological studies may also not be specific for the diagnosis of EM although, especially in early lesions, with DIF it is observed that the dermis vessels present intraparietal deposits of IgM, C3, and fibrin. Furthermore, DIF may be useful to exclude other bullous diseases such as PV and MMP [209]. DIF and IIF and, in some cases, the Tzanck smear test and the tampon for HSV-PCR can facilitate the distinction between EM and other types of diseases including OLP [67].

Foedinger et al. [385] in patients with severe forms of EM, characterized by suprabasal acantholysis in lesional skin and mucous membranes, found anti-DSP-I and anti-DSP-II autoantibodies (DSP, desmoplachins) using various biochemical tests, including immunoblotting of epidermal section lysates and immunoprecipitation of cultured radiolabeled human keratinocyte protein extracts.

The same authors also developed an ELISA for the detection of peptide-specific anti-DSP autoantibodies based on a synthetic peptide containing the respective amino acid sequence [386]. It has also been hypothesized that DSP^{+} patients represent a subgroup of pemphigus patients with an unusual phenotype of EM patients, and the rare reactivity against DSP-I and DSP-II detected in sera from EM patients represents only one epiphenomenon that carries out a secondary role in the pathogenesis of the disease [387, 388].

It is essential, in the treatment of EM, to differentiate the various clinical forms, bearing in mind that an initial oral involvement can turn into a major form, even very severe in a short time.

- *Oral EM*. Any triggering drug must be identified and stopped. In the case of lesions easily manageable with topical treatment, it is possible to use clobetasol ointment 0.05% in adhesive hydroxyethylcellulose gel two times/day under antifungal coverage (chlorhexidine + miconazole) until the lesions are reduced by at least 50% and then once/day until the resolution is obtained. Patients should be instructed to dry the area before applying the topical agent which should not be rubbed and should be asked to refrain from talking, drinking, and/or eating for 1 h. In the case of oral lesions that are widespread or not easily manageable with topical treatment, prednisone 50 mg/day for 3 days is recommended, followed by 25 mg/day for 3 days and then three tablets every other day.
- *EMm*. If related to HSV, acyclovir is given (1–2 g/day) until the lesions are reduced by at least 50%, after that the dosage is gradually decreased. If unrelated to HSV, oral lesions should be treated like oral EM lesions, while skin lesions can be treated with medium-strength topical steroids (e.g., triamcinolone acetonide) and an antihistamine (e.g., hydroxyzine 50 mg/day) to reduce itching.
- *EMM* or *SJS*. If drug related, it is necessary to suspend it and administer prednisone 50 mg/day for 3 days, 25 mg/day for 3 days, and then three tablets every other day, or prednisone 50 mg/day until a reduction of at least 50% of the lesions and after that the dosage is gradually decreased. If due to *Mycoplasma pneumoniae* infection, use erythromycin 0.5–1 g/day.
- *TEN*: Hospitalization in centers for burns and water reintegration, parenteral nutrition, and antimicrobial and local therapy are mandatory [209].

5.5.13 Discoid Lupus Erythematosus (DLE)

The term lupus erythematosus (LE) indicates a connective tissue disorder comprising at least three main subgroups: systemic LE (SLE), subacute cutaneous LE, and discoid LE (DLE). All subgroups but most commonly SLE and DLE can give rise to oral lichenoid lesions, which may appear similar if not identical to those of OLP [96].

DLE represents the most common form of chronic cutaneous LE and can be distinguished into a localized and a generalized form [67]. The diffuse form is more frequently associated with laboratory abnormalities [389]. DLE has been associated with HLA region genes and non-MHC loci (HLA-B7, -B8, -Cw7, -DR2, -Dr3, -DQw1, ITGAM, CTLA4, TYK2, IRF5), but the evidence is weaker than LES [390–392].

DLE can only involve the skin, especially that exposed to the sun (face, ears, scalp), but it can also affect some mucous membranes (usually only the oral and anogenital) [393–400]. But up to 28% of patients with DLE are susceptible to developing SLE [401]. Patients with DLE rarely meet four or more of the criteria used to classify SLE [402].

Around 15–20% of DLE cases have oral involvement [67] and the clinical presentation can mimic OLP (Fig. 5.38), especially the atrophic or erosive forms [32]. Generally the affected sites are the buccal mucosa, vermilion, gingiva, and palate [67]. Typical oral lesions appear as central atrophic areas or superficial erosions characterized by white lines at the margins that are much less clearly defined than in OLP [96]. The lesions are often unilateral and can be localized on the hard and soft palate and on the outer

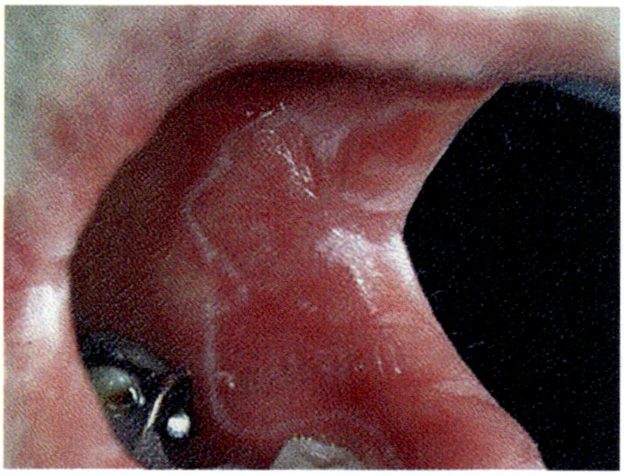

Fig. 5.38 Discoid lupus lesions on the right buccal mucosa. From [405] with permission

side of the lips, these usually spared in the OLP; this type of injury could also be the unique manifestation of the disease [96]. However, while OLP manifests in most cases only oral lesions, patients with LE present much more frequently concomitant skin lesions with clinical indication of photosensitivity [32]. Furthermore, unlike the OLP, DLE lesions are more often distributed asymmetrically in the oral cavity [67]. Lip lesions may tend to spread from vermilion to the surrounding lip skin, obscuring the vermilion boundaries, but this is not a constant feature [403]. Rarely, long-standing oral DLE lesions can evolve into OSCC [404].

Histopathology can sometimes help but is often equivocal or not specific enough, particularly in distinguishing DLE from OLP. There is usually a regular or focal thickening of the basement membrane. A deeper, perivascular inflammatory infiltrate is sometimes detectable. Vessel walls may be prominent with endothelial swelling. Variable edema and mucin deposits may be present [67]. The presence of mixed clinical and histopathological features of LE and LP has been defined as lupus erythematosus/lichen overlap syndrome (LE/LP) [406].

DIF may show a possible granular deposition of Ig and/or complement in the basement membrane (positive lupus band test or lupus band test), but this finding, although characteristic, is not pathognomonic of SLE or DLE; in oral lesions, among other things, the DIF is usually negative [67]. The lupus band test is neither sensitive nor specific and has mostly been replaced by advances in serological testing [407]. DIF is positive in about 70% of patients with LED, while the IIF is usually negative in oral lesions [32, 67]. Therefore, although immunofluorescence studies can be useful to distinguish LE from LP [408], they do not always allow a differential diagnosis between the two disorders [406].

Serological abnormalities are particularly rare in localized forms, unlike diffuse ones [67]. The predominant autoantibody in patients with DLE remains unknown, and only low-titer anti-Ro (60 kDa) antibodies have been found in many of these patients [409]. A study using autoantigen arrays hypothesizes nonpathogenic roles for specific IgM autoantibodies found in DLE [410].

5.5.14 Systemic Lupus Erythematosus (SLE)

SLE is a systemic autoimmune disease attacking various organs and systems, with an indefinite etiology and complex pathogenesis [67].

A meta-analysis identified an association with HLA-DR2 and -DR3 in European populations [411], while a genome-wide association study found a greater association with the MSH5 gene, belonging to the class III region [412]. Other associations were found with IRF5, ITGAM, STAT4/STAT1, FcGR2A, and PTPN22 [67]. Given the large number of recognized loci linked to the susceptibility of SLE, it is believed that the genetic risk of this pathology derives from the variation of many genes, each with modest effects [413]. Therefore, their clinical utility is unlikely to matter at present [67].

From a pathogenetic point of view, SLE is characterized, in the presence of appropriate antigens, by the formation of soluble immune complexes composed mainly of IgG and IgM [413]. The model is that of a type III hypersensitivity reaction triggered by an endogenous antigen which can be generalized or organ-specific [414] (Table 5.7). Due to the affinity of the antibody and the size of the immune complexes, the kid-

Table 5.7 Hypersensitivity reactions

Type	Antibodies involved	Mechanism	Clinical examples
Type I hypersensitivity	IgE	IgE binds to basophils and mast cells, releasing histamine, trypsin, and arachidonic acid. The manifestations are local and systemic	Conjunctivitis, asthma, anaphylaxis
Type II hypersensitivity	IgG, IgM	Antibodies bind to cell surfaces, triggering the immune response through complement activation	Transfusion reaction, Hashimoto's thyroiditis
Type III hypersensitivity	Soluble IgG and IgM aggregates	Antibody complexes are deposited in various tissues such as skin, kidneys, or joints, triggering the immune response by activating complement	Serum sickness, Arthus reaction, SLE
Type IV hypersensitivity	Cell-mediated immunity (delayed hypersensitivity)	Cytotoxic T cells ($CD8^+$) and T helper cells ($CD4^+$) recognize the antigen in a major histocompatibility complex, resulting in further macrophage-mediated proliferation of T helper lymphocytes	Contact dermatitis, contact arteritis, graft rejection, OLCL, OLDR

neys, lungs, and joints are the most frequently affected areas in subjects with SLE; tissue damage is caused by platelets and neutrophils [415]. The lesions contain mainly neutrophils and deposits of immune complexes and complements, namely, C3a, C4a, and C5a [414]. Macrophages infiltrating later stages are involved in the healing process [415]. Genetic factors and specific genetic loci are important in the pathogenesis of SLE [413]. In susceptible people, environmental triggers, including exposure to sunlight (photosensitivity), drugs (pharmacogenetics), and infections (particularly with Epstein-Barr virus), are thought to precipitate the development of SLE [416].

SLE manifests itself as a mixture of symptoms affecting different districts, with skin, musculoskeletal, and hematological involvement. However, some patients may present predominantly hematological, renal, or neuropsychiatric manifestations [417].

Skin manifestations of SLE are present in 85% of affected patients. The most typical skin lesion of LE consists in the appearance of an erythema on the malar eminences and on the bridge of the nose (the so-called butterfly erythema) [67].

Oral lesions appear in 40% of SLE cases [66, 418] and, rarely, may be the presenting sign. Oral manifestations of SLE may be similar to those of DLE: atrophic-erosive oral lichenoid lesions and reticular hyperkeratotic striae [96]. Oral lesions are predominantly distributed on the hard palate, buccal mucosa, and gingiva and generally present as a central area of ulceration or atrophy, with erythema surrounded by white radiating streaks (Fig. 5.39a). Lesions of the palate can be purely erythematous and irregular in distribution [32]. LE lesions can also involve the lip and are not usually distributed in a symmetrical manner, an element that could help make a differential diagnosis with OLP [65]. It is also possible to observe non-specific oral ulcerations, which constitute one of the criteria of the European League Against Rheumatism and the American College of Rheumatology for the diagnosis of SLE [419, 420] (Table 5.8 and Fig. 5.40). In particular, according to the American College of Rheumatologists, the diagnosis of SLE requires the satisfaction of at least 4 of the 11 criteria, in series or simultaneously, during any observation period [417]. Diagnosis of SLE also presents a challenge, as the typical signs and symptoms may take a long time to settle [67]. In any case, the presence of systemic inflammatory manifestations can help distinguish this pathology from OLP. Notably, most patients with oral manifestations of LE have also concomitant skin lesions and other features of LE such as photosensitivity [394].

The histopathological and immunofluorescence characteristics are similar to those of DLE (Sect. 5.5.13). The histopathology of the oral LE is highly variable; it is influenced by the anatomi-

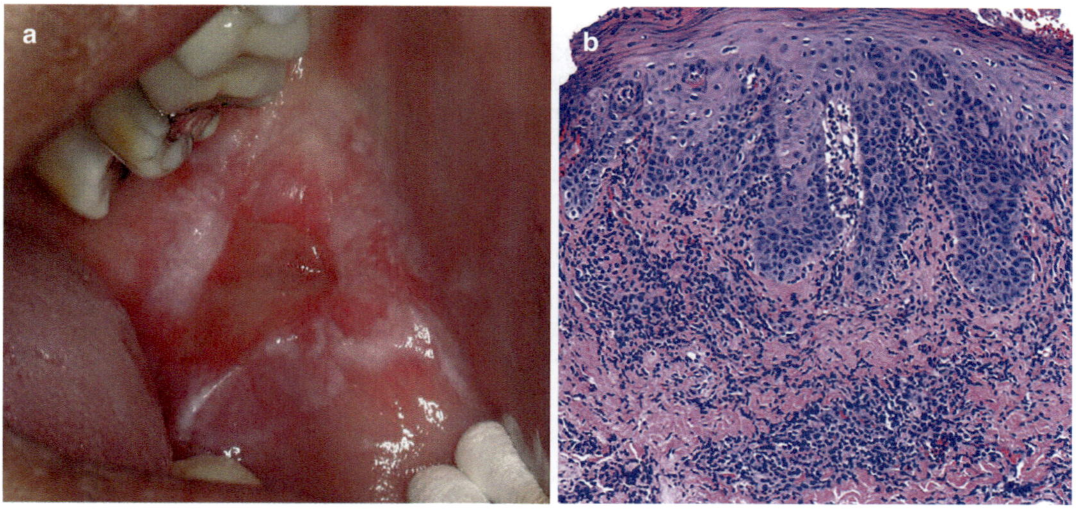

Fig. 5.39 (**a**) Intraoral presentation of LES of the buccal mucosa which presents as a central area of erosion surrounded by white radiating striae similar to EOLP. (**b**) Biopsy of an oral lesion of LE showing acanthotic epithelium with disordered infiltrate of inflammatory cells in the lamina propria (H&E x250). Unlike OLP, inflammation of LE extends into deeper connective tissue and perivascular inflammation is observed. From [32] with permission

cal site and the age of the lesion and often overlaps with that of OLP, OLDR, and OLCL [32]. In fact, the epithelium may present atrophy or pseudoepitheliomatous hyperplasia with keratin plug and a thickened basement membrane that shows reactivity with PAS (periodic acid-Schiff) reactive staining [67, 421, 422]. The lamina propria is often edematous, and the inflammatory cell infiltrate in the superficial lamina propria can range from paucicellular to lymphocyte-rich, but the infiltrate can also be mixed (Fig. 5.39b). Sometimes cytoid bodies, mucositis of the interface, and melanin incontinence adjacent to the epithelium can be observed [32, 65]. Superficial and deep perivascular inflammatory infiltrates are often present, a feature also present in OLDR and OLCL [32].

DIF in both SLE and DLE shows granular or "shaggy" deposits of IgG, IgM, and/or C3 in the basement membrane [67, 162, 421], typical of type III hypersensitivity reactions [415]. These results are useful in differentiating LE from OLP and immunoglobulin deposits are practically found in all cases of SLE [32].

The diagnosis of SLE must be confirmed by the pattern of autoantibodies, in particular ANA (antinuclear antibodies), a serological sign in SLE [65, 67]. The traditional view has been questioned that autoantibodies directed against the double-stranded DNA (dsDNA) are the main pathogenic effectors of LE [424] and the detection of other autoantibodies in SLE is common (besides ANA and dsDNA), such as anti-Sm (anti-Smith), anti-RNP (anti-ribonucleoproteins), anti-Ro/SSA, anti-La/SSB, aPL (antiphospholipids), and aCL (anticardiolipin) [67]. Some SLE autoantibodies are pathogenic, others are protective, and some appear neutral and/or have roles that may not be directly related to pathogenesis or protection [424].

The technologies and diagnostic platforms available to detect ANA and related autoantibodies have grown dramatically in recent decades, from the LE cell test dated in the 1950s to the IIF in the 1960s; immunodiffusion; ELISA; dot blot; linear immunoassays and more recently multiplexed immunoassays (i.e., capable of detecting multiple autoantibodies simultaneously) such as addressable laser bead immunoassays (ALBIA), planar antigen arrays, nanobarcoding, chemiluminescence, and lateral flow assays; and other point-of-care testing (POCT) systems and other promising new technologies that continue to emerge [67, 424]. These new technologies have shown the existence of heterogeneity among SLE patients and also the practicality of being able to

Table 5.8 LE oral manifestations

Classification	Type of lesion	Localization	Key characteristics	Clinical significance
LE-specific oral ulcers	Palatal erythematous ulcer	Masticatory mucosa (especially hard palate)	Painless, single/multiple erythematous ulcer(s)	Sign of acute disease, sometimes the first manifestation of SLE without skin lesions. In case of a large patch also extending to the soft palate, consider early onset of oral DLE
	Oral DLE	Lining mucosa (especially buccal mucosa and soft palate). Sometimes also masticatory mucosa (without radiating streaks), vermilion, and tongue	Atrophic plaque with white radiant keratotic striae and painful telangiectasia	The radiant white striae can sometimes recall Wickham's striae of OLP; necessary histological analysis to distinguish
	Honeycomb plaque	Lining and masticatory mucosa. In the soft palate, minor hyperkeratosis	Chronic well-circumscribed erythematous plaque with white lacy hyperkeratosis	Very rare incidence in SLE. Possible morphological variant or late stage of oral DLE
	Verrucous LE	Lining mucosa	Raised, intense keratotic plaque	Rare variant reported in LES
LE-non-specific oral ulcers	Aphthous ulcer	Lining mucosa	Painful white/yellowish ulcer with erythematous halo. Often multiple or clustered lesions. Aphthae classified into minor (<1 cm, no scar), major (>1 cm, often having scar), herpetiform (>10, small ulcers), severe (minor ulcers lasting >1 month)	More common in juvenile LS and in the acute phase of the disease. They are usually minor aphthous ulcers (<10)
	Lupus cheilitis	Lining mucosa (especially lower lip)	Lips with small or widespread erythema/edema or painful and crusty ulcer(s)	Area exposed to light, therefore associated with photosensitivity in juvenile LES. Extensive erosions of both lips manifest in active juvenile LES
	Bullous LES	Buccal mucosa, face, neck, trunk	Multiple and tense bullous lesions in the skin	Presence of autoantibodies against collagen VII at the subepidermal level. In the oral mucosa, it is associated with both juvenile and adult SLE

divide them on the basis of autoantibody dosages. This growing body of data and diverse responsiveness profiles could lead to patient-appropriate medical decisions and therapies in the future [67].

The management of SLE is based on the prevention, resolution of inflammation, the maintenance of remission states, and the alleviation of symptoms [416, 425].

Prevention consists of UV protection in order to avoid flare-ups of skin lesions [426]. Avoidance of sun exposure is also recommended in patients with lupus cheilitis and oral DLE on the lips, since UV rays are an aggravating factor [427, 428]. Routine wet dressing can relieve pain and it is necessary to keep chapped lips moist using petrolatum ointment or lipstick (with UV protection) [423].

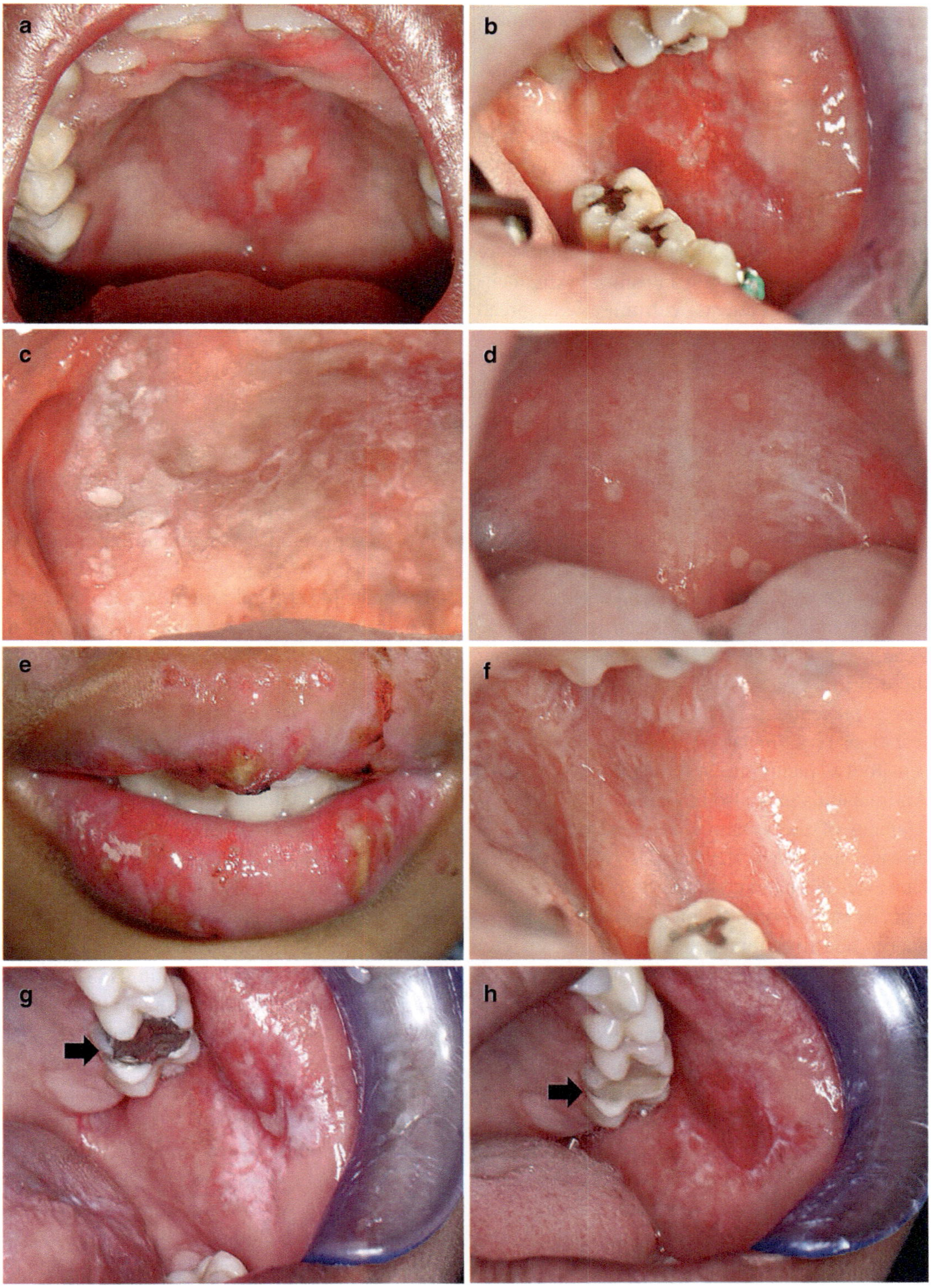

Fig. 5.40 Oral ulcers in patients with juvenile SLE and their differential diagnoses. (**a–c**) *LE-specific oral ulcers*: (**a**) a hard palatal erythematous ulcer; (**b**) painful oral DLE with well-demarcated radiating white striae on the left buccal mucosa; (**c**) verrucous LE on the alveolar ridge. (**d–e**) *LE-non-specific oral ulcers*: (**d**) multiple aphthous ulcers with erythematous halo on the soft palate; (**e**) erosive lupus cheilitis extended to both upper and lower lips. (**f–h**) *Differential diagnoses*: (**f**) OLP with typical white reticular striae (Wickham's striae) on the left buccal mucosa and retromolar trigone; (**g**) OLCL associated with an extensive amalgam filling of the left maxillary first molar (arrow); (**h**) clinical improvement 2 weeks after replacement with a nonmetallic restoration. From [423] with permission

From a pharmacological point of view, there are many molecules that can be used in the management of SLE. Generally NSAIDs (including selective COX-2 inhibitors) and antimalarials are effective for musculoskeletal disorders and mild serositis [429, 430], but NSAIDs only provide symptomatic relief of pain and are of little benefit in more severe forms. High- and medium-potency corticosteroids and calcineurin inhibitors are used as topical therapies for localized skin manifestations [431]. Patients with more widespread skin lesions can benefit from taking antimalarials such as hydroxychloroquine [426]. Systemic corticosteroids remain the cornerstone of therapy in SLE and are particularly useful for the control of disease flare-up [432]. Systemic corticosteroids, such as prednisone, are in fact indicated in patients with significant involvement of various organs, in particular the kidneys and the central nervous system, and with systemic vascular diseases [416, 429]. Hydroxychloroquine associated with systemic corticosteroids can be a first-line treatment in patients requiring systemic therapy; these drugs can be used on their own in mild cases of juvenile SLE with mucocutaneous manifestations (e.g., malar rash, discoid rash, photosensitivity, including oral ulcers) [433, 434]. Antimalarials may also be important in the management of the systemic manifestations of the disease and have fewer side effects [432]. However, the patient should be monitored periodically with a complete blood count, eye examination, and liver function tests, as drug toxicity may occur in children [423]. However, as the signs and symptoms resolve, the dosage of the corticosteroid should be progressively decreased [426]. However, some patients may require a maintenance dose to remain in remission [429]. However, chronic corticosteroid intake involves several side effects: impaired immunity, atherosclerosis, hypertension, hypercholesterolemia, hyperglycemia, cushingoid aspect, acne, cataract, avascular necrosis of the hip, severe osteoporosis, drug-induced adrenal insufficiency, opportunistic infections, and steroids-induced diabetes [426, 432]. Epidemiological studies have shown that it is important to try not to exceed prednisone doses of 10 mg per day or less to minimize the risk of cardiovascular complications. Other molecules sirolimus, methotrexate, and intravenous immunoglobulin (IVIg) have also been used in SLE, but data to support efficacy are scarce [432]. Other immunosuppressive agents such as cyclophosphamide, methotrexate, and azathioprine are reserved for severe organic diseases such as advanced lupus nephritis [429, 435]. In particular, pulsed cyclophosphamide for induction of remission followed by quarterly infusions for maintenance has been the cornerstone of modern therapy for severe SLE, particularly for lupus nephritis [432]. Despite its high level of efficacy, cyclophosphamide is toxic, with a high frequency of complications such as hemorrhagic cystitis, bladder cancer, and ovarian failure. Recently, maintenance with other less toxic agents such as mycophenolate mofetil (MMF) and azathioprine has been shown to have an efficacy equivalent to that of quarterly cyclophosphamide with fewer side effects [432]. Oral retinoids (such as acitretin and isotretinoin), analogues of vitamin A, thanks to their keratolytic and anti-inflammatory effects, are very useful in forms of refractory cutaneous LE, especially in very crusty forms, such as hyperkeratotic DLE and subacute LE [436]. However, retinoids require careful monitoring due to serious side effects, including teratogenicity (patients of childbearing age must adhere to two forms of contraception), hypercholesterolemia, hypertriglyceridemia, hypertransaminemia, depression, and diffuse interstitial skeletal hyperostosis [437]. Patients should also be advised that eyes and dry skin can be treated symptomatically with lubricating and moisturizing agents. Several biological drugs are also being studied in the treatment of SLE. For example, rituximab (anti-CD20), which acts on B lymphocytes, has been shown to be of benefit in refractory bullous SLE and acute cutaneous lupus, while its role in subacute LE and DLE is less clear [436]. An important breakthrough was the approval of belimumab (anti-BAFF, B-cell activating factor, which plays a role in B-cell differentiation and proliferation) in the treatment of SLE: this was the first new drug specifically approved for the SLE in 50 years [432]. Patients who respond best to this drug are those with skin and musculoskeletal manifestations [436]. Currently, other biologics are in clinical trials for SLE, including antibodies against other BAFF-related targets [432]. Other biological anti-interferon drugs are also being tested: sifalimumab (anti-IFN-α, which however does not act on the other IFN-I, leaving them free to bind to the IFNAR) and anifrolumab (anti-IFNAR, which appears to be effective in moderate-severe forms of SLE) [436]. One study showed the ineffectiveness of an anti-IFN-γ drug in the treatment of DLE [438]. Pharmacological protocols in the treatment of SLE are summarized in Table 5.9.

As for oral lesions, one of the most commonly used drugs is topical corticosteroids (e.g., 0.1% oral triamcinolone paste), capable of improving the course and reducing the severity of oral ulcers; the duration of their use depends on the severity of the lesions [423]. In case of refractory to treatment, more potent corticosteroids (e.g., betamethasone or clobetasol in the oral preparation) or systemic drugs may be needed [439]. However, some oral ulcers are very difficult to treat even when a high-potency topical corticosteroid is applied, particularly erythematous palatal ulcers and oral DLE lesions [440]. Intralesional corticosteroid injection is rarely used, especially in children (in the case of juvenile SLE), due to pain [423]. In case of worrying side effects from corticosteroids, calcineurin inhibitors (such as tacrolimus 0.03% or 0.1%) are indicated [441, 442]. Systemic corticosteroids are frequently prescribed for the treatment of juvenile SLE because most patients develop multiple organ involvement and these drugs greatly improve clinical signs and symptoms, including oral ulcerations [421, 428].

Dental management of the patient with lupus must take into account the complex pathological manifestations of the disease, including oral aspects and complications of immunosuppressive treatment [432]. Good oral hygiene and prevention of secondary bacterial infection of oral ulcers with chlorhexidine-based oral rinses are advised [439, 443]. An infection should be suspected when oral ulcers become painful or bleed. If infection is suspected, local antibiotics and antifungal agents (e.g., nystatin) should be considered [423]. Dentists must apply all preventive treatments to prevent infectious complications, as patients with SLE are predisposed to the develop-

Table 5.9 Recommended treatment scale for SLE patients

Severity	Clinical-pharmacological protocols
Mild	– Photoprotective methods – Topical steroids/immunomodulators – Intralesional steroids (2.5–10 mg/ml)
Moderate/refractory[a]	– Prednisone (up to 0.5 mg/kg per day) for rapid reduction of symptoms – Hydroxychloroquine (200 mg qd-bid) (based on weight) – Quinacrine (100 mg qd) – Chloroquine (125–250 mg qd) (based on weight)
Moderate/severe/refractory[b]	– Prednisone (up to 1 mg/kg per day) – Mycophenolate mofetil (1000–1500 mg bid) – Methotrexate (7.5–25 mg qwk) – Azathioprine (2–3 mg/kg per day) – Cyclophosphamide (500–750 mg/m^2 per month) – Thalidomide (25–100 mg qhs), lenalidomide (2.5–10 mg qhs) – Retinoids, e.g., acitretin (10–50 mg qd), isotretinoin (0.5–1 mg/kg per day) – Dapsone (25–100 mg bid) – Intravenous immunoglobulins (2 g/kg per month)

bid two times per day; *qd* every day; *qhs* every night at bedtime; *qwk* every week.

[a]Photoprotection and topical creams ± intralesional steroids are often continued in patients with cutaneous lupus erythematosus with moderate and/or refractory disease.

[b]Antimalarials (hydroxychloroquine or chloroquine ± quinacrine), photoprotection, and topical creams ± intralesional steroids are often continued in patients with cutaneous lupus erythematosus with moderate/severe/refractory disease. From [436] with permission

ment of severe head and neck infections. Often these infections are silent and difficult to detect due to the scarcity of pain and swelling, but nevertheless they can progress rapidly due to disease or therapy-induced immunosuppression [426]. To complicate matters further, SLE patients may have overlapping antiphospholipid antibody syndrome that predisposes them to thromboembolic events, such as arterial and venous thrombosis, pulmonary embolism, stroke, and myocardial infarction [435]. It is therefore important to document whether these patients are managed with anticoagulant therapy, aspirin or warfarin, and recent laboratory tests (platelet count, prothrombin time, and international normalized ratio (INR)) are indicated prior to dental surgery. It is always necessary to consider the possible intraoperative need for additional local measures to maintain hemostasis. Some patients with SLE may also experience further complications, such as Libman-Sacks endocarditis: it is a form of nonbacterial endocarditis with valve damage associated with SLE that requires prophylaxis of subacute bacterial endocarditis [426]. Furthermore, lupus nephritis is a serious complication of SLE affecting 30% of patients [435, 444]. Impaired renal function will affect the choice and dosage of medications prescribed by dentists (Table 5.10).

In addition, patients suffering from chronic kidney failure are often on dialysis. In these cases, oral surgery should be scheduled 1 day after dialysis treatment to ensure the elimination of administered drugs and their by-products.

Dentists must carefully monitor the appearance of orofacial pain to assess their nature: odontogenic, Temporomandibular joint (TMJ), or myofascial type. In fact, patients may present with temporomandibular disorders (TMD) caused by arthralgia and/or arthritis. They should also consider the possibility of a reduction in the level of oral hygiene due to pain triggered by oral ulcers. They may also be affected by a Sjögren-like syndrome (keratoconjunctivitis sicca, xerostomia, and generalized hypohidrosis) which can favor the appearance of carious lesions [426]. A multidisciplinary approach and the comparison between different medical figures will allow the best possible management of these complex patients.

Table 5.10 Medicines commonly prescribed by dentists with predominantly renal elimination

Commonly prescribed dental drugs and SLE patient management
Drugs with predominantly renal elimination
NSAIDs
Acetylsalicylic acid
Penicillins
Cephalosporins
Tetracyclines
Antifungals
Suggestions
Consider increasing the dose intervals and decreasing the dosage
Consider contacting the doctor if kidney function is not known
Be aware of the possibility of drug interactions because this group of patients may be taking many different drugs
Suggested alternatives
Paracetamol
Narcotics
Clindamycin

Prognosis is often good when the disease course is intermediate in severity and only a few organs are involved [445]. The disease can also be fatal in the case of renal pathologies with hypertension and rapid evolution toward renal failure leading to patient death [446–448].

5.5.15 Leukoplakia and Erythroplakia (LK, ELK, EK, PVL)

Leukoplakia is a white lesion of the oral mucosa that cannot be traced, clinically or histologically, to any known pathology. Erythroplakia, on the other hand, is an intense red lesion that cannot be traced, clinically or histologically, to any known pathology. Mixed lesions with the appearance of non-homogeneous leukoplakias with areas of fire red typically erythroplastic are called erythroleukoplakias, which have biological and clinical features such as those of erythroplakia [209]. All of these constitute potentially malignant lesions (including OLP), a term indicating the morphological alterations of the oral mucosa at the level of which the onset of a carcinoma is statistically more frequent than the surrounding healthy tissue [449].

Leukoplakia has a prevalence of between 0.2% and 5%, with a predilection for male sex and an age of onset usually greater than 40 years, while erythroplakia is a rarer lesion. Leukoplakia most frequently affects the retrocommissural, the alveolar, and the labial mucosa, while the tongue, oral floor, soft palate, and palatine pillars are less affected (although in these sites and in the lower lip, these lesions show histological features of dysplasia or with a tendency to degeneration). The lingual dorsum is a rare site of onset of leukoplakia, usually in association with luetic infection. Erythroplakia, unlike leukoplakia, is mainly localized in the oral floor, in the lingual edges, in the retromolar trigone, and in the soft palate (i.e., those areas covered by a thin mucosa); however its onset is possible in any location [209].

Clinically, there are several forms of leukoplakia (LK):

- *Homogeneous leukoplakia*: It is characterized by a uniform and flat white plaque with well-defined margins [450] (Fig. 5.41).
- *Non-homogeneous leukoplakia*: It presents with white areas fragmented into islands of different sizes, prominences, and intensities, sometimes with a verrucous/nodular appearance and mixed with areas of red color or erosions. Therefore, these forms of leukoplakia can present erythroplastic/erythroleukoplasic areas and more commonly show histological pictures of dysplasia [209].
- *Proliferative verrucous leukoplakia* (PVL): This is considered by the WHO to be a particularly aggressive form of non-homogeneous leukoplakia. It is more common in women (ratio of M:F = 1:4); usually the lesions appear in people over 50 years of age; less than 45% of cases were associated with the habit of tobacco use [209, 451]. It may begin with the presence of hyperkeratotic lesions clinically and histologically attributable to a homogeneous leukoplakia without dysplasia. However, during the follow-up, the lesions become multifocal, with a tendency to a verrucous appearance, rapid spread, and clinical-histological alteration assuming the characteristics of non-homogeneity and dysplasia (Fig. 5.42). The main sites involved are the keratinized gingiva (including the fibromucosa of the edentulous alveolar ridges) and the hard palate, while less frequently the lesions are localized in the alveolar and buccal mucosa and tongue [209]. The rate of malignant transformation is much higher than in other forms of leukoplakia (70–100%) [451]. PVL must be carefully distinguished from localized leukoplakia (Table 5.11) and by OLP; therefore it has been further explored subsequently.

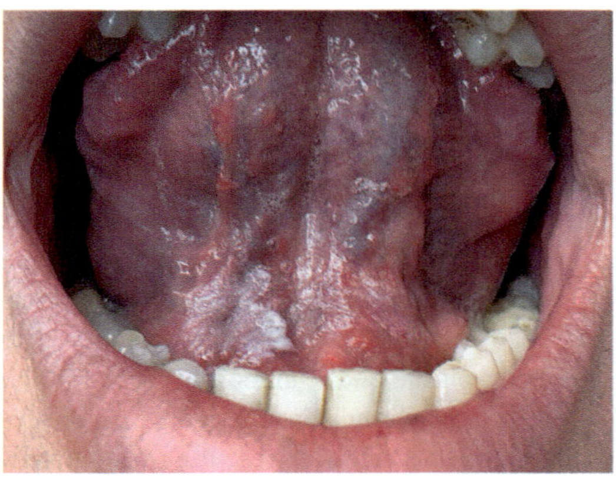

Fig. 5.41 Homogeneous leukoplakia of the oral floor presenting as a plaque with a surface of just over 1 cm^2 in a man who has been a smoker (about 20 cigarettes a day) for 15 years

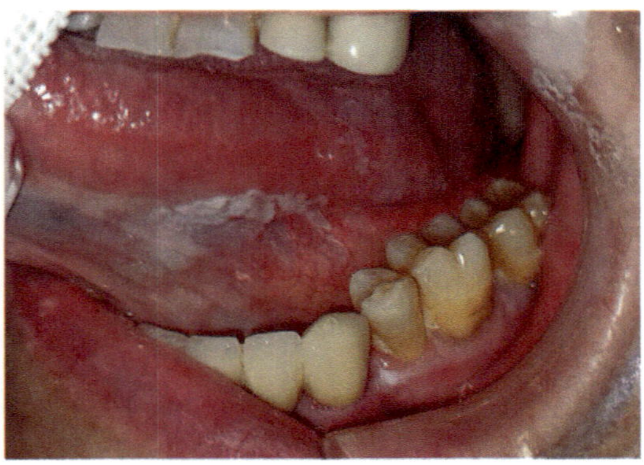

Fig. 5.42 Proliferative verrucous leukoplakia of the tongue and gingiva presenting as multiple irregular plaques in a nonsmoker woman. Note the erythroplastic areas in the posterior part of the tongue

Table 5.11 From [451] with permission

Main differences between localized and proliferative leukoplakia	
Localized leukoplakia	Proliferative leukoplakia
Mainly men	Mainly women
Strong association with cigarette smoking	Weak association with cigarette smoking
Single site	Multifocal
~40% are dysplasia or carcinoma at the time of the first biopsy examination	<10% shows dysplasia or carcinoma at the time of the first biopsy, mainly atypical verrucous hyperplasia or keratosis of unknown significance
Overall malignant transformation: 3–15%	Overall malignant transformation: 70–100%
Malignant transformation by year: 1–3%	Malignant transformation by year: 10%
Easy to eliminate or remove because it is localized	Difficult to treat because it is multifocal

- *Candidal leukoplakia/chronic hyperplastic candidosis*: Hyperplastic oral candidiasis can give rise to particular oral manifestations, including candidal leukoplakia which clinically appears more frequently as a non-homogeneous leukoplakia (small white nodules on erythematous mucosa, sometimes with areas of erosion). The diagnostic suspicion occurs in the presence of PAS-positive hyphae when a biopsy of leukoplakia with a typical histopathological picture is performed: presence of pseudoepitheliomatous hyperplasia, psoriasiform, acanthosis-parakeratosis, epithelial microabscesses, strong inflammatory infiltrate in the connective tissue, or possibility of various degrees of dysplasia. It is not known whether chronic candidiasis represents superinfection or the cause of the lesion itself. Tobacco smoke and prostheses may be important etiological factors of candidal leukoplakia, and the presence of the fungus makes the possibility of malignant short-term degeneration more likely. Therefore, early diagnosis and adequate local and/or systemic treatment (antifungals) are essential, and usually the therapy allows both the degree of dysplasia and the clinical appearance to regress, which becomes more homogeneous. The lesions will in any case be followed up and if medical therapy is not sufficient, surgical excision will have to be resorted to [209]. A recent WHO consensus concluded that the use of antifungal treatment should be part of the diagnostic process—even if many cases improve with antifungal treatment, they do not disappear completely. However, since the definition of leukoplakia excludes specific causes and the Working Group noted that candidal leukoplakia was now a deprecated term [28].
- *Erythroleukoplakia* (*ELK*) may be confused with OLP due to its white and red components; however the former does not possess the typical white reticular changes and is usually a one-sided lesion associated with well-demarcated plaques [451].
- *Erythroplakia* (*EK*) usually appears as a fiery red macula of very variable size (even a few millimeters), with clear or slightly blurred margins. Sometimes it can appear as a slightly raised plaque and small whitish areas may be observed in the vicinity (Fig. 5.43). This severe precancerous disease must be distinguished from the common areas of inflammation subjected to trauma or poor oral hygiene, as well as from lichen and various forms of stomatitis; an important element of differential diagnosis is a positive toluidine blue test. False positives (inflammatory lesions) are possible, while hyperkeratotic lesions with areas of underlying degeneration are falsely negative: hyperkeratotic lesions are therefore not among the indications of the vital dye [209].

Leukoplakia and erythroplakia are exclusively clinical terms; therefore they do not correspond to precise histological entities: in leukoplakia these can range from simple hyperkeratosis to severe dysplasia and carcinoma in situ [209, 451], while erythroplakia is a more severe precancerous disease always presenting with moderate or severe dysplasia [209]. A suspected leukoplakia on clinical examination could turn out to be histologically a frictional keratosis or OLP, for example [451]; therefore biopsy is still

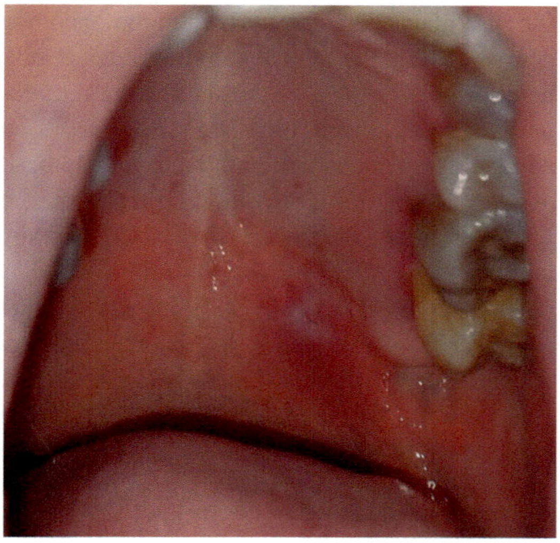

Fig. 5.43 Erythroplakia of the soft palate in a nonsmoker woman

Table 5.12 LSCP classification of leukoplakia

LSCP classification of leukoplakia
L = size of the lesion
Lx = not specified
L0 = absence of lesions
L1 = maximum diameter < 2 cm
L2 = maximum diameter 2–4 cm
L3 = maximum diameter > 4 cm
S = site of the lesion
Sx = not specified
S1 = any location except oral floor and tongue
S2 = oral floor and/or tongue
C = clinical aspect
Cx = not specified
C1 = homogeneous
C2 = not homogeneous
P = histopathological features
Px = not specified
P1 = absence of dysplasia
P2 = mild dysplasia
P3 = moderate dysplasia
P4 = severe dysplasia

Table 5.13 LSCP staging of leukoplakia

LSCP staging of leukoplakia				
Stage	L	S	C	P
Stage 1	Any L	S1	C1	P1 or P2
Stage 2	Any L	S1	C2	P1 or P2
		S2	C1	P1 or P2
Stage 3	Any L	S2	C2	P1 or P2
Stage 4	Any L	Any S	Any C	P3 or P4

indicated (as well as for the identification of dysplastic areas).

The diagnosis of true leukoplakia is based on a combination of patient history, clinical considerations, and histopathology and is typically an exclusion diagnosis [452].

During an international workshop held in 1994, an interesting classification of leukoplasic lesions based on clinical and histological characteristics [453] has been proposed (Tables 5.12 and 5.13). Staging is based on clinical parameters of size (L), site (S), and clinical appearance (C) and on histopathological characteristics (P) (presence and severity of dysplasia): LSCP (lesion-site-clinic-pathology). From Table 5.10 (relating to staging), it can be seen that the extent of the lesion is an irrelevant parameter, while the presence of moderate-severe dysplasia is of fundamental importance in the prognosis of the lesions [209].

The evolution of leukoplasic lesions is unpredictable: about a third of cases show regression and improvement of the lesions, others remain stationary for long periods of time, and still others progress assuming the characteristics of non-homogeneous leukoplakias; the transition from one form to another seems to be progressive but reversible at any stage. The probability of cancerization in the short to medium term is evaluated on the basis of three parameters: the clinical aspect (homogeneous or non-homogeneous), the histological aspect (absence or presence of dysplasia), and the site of onset (in the tongue; oral floor degeneration is more frequent) [209]. Homogeneous leukoplakias have a lower risk of malignant transformation (0.6%–5%) than non-homogeneous ones (20%–25%) [450]. PVL is the most aggressive form of leukoplakia, with a malignant transformation rate of 70 to 100% if followed up over the long term [451]. Many non-dysplastic keratotic lesions (hyperkeratosis without dysplasia or keratosis of uncertain significance (KUS)) can also degenerate in a malignant sense (11–30%). Dysplasias also have a high rate of malignant transformation (5–36%) [450].

The evolution of erythroplakia is particularly frightening; in fact this can arise in association with other pathologies in whose clinical aspect it goes unnoticed (other potentially malignant disorders, OLP, and in the context of oral carcinomas themselves). Erythroplakia typically undergoes volumetric variations and color intensity (due to changes in the inflammatory component of the lesion). In Western countries, erythroplakia has the characteristics of a severe precancerous disease with probably obligatory transformation. It is not clear whether in some cases it can be reversible [209].

Malignant transformation of leukoplakia is driven by multiple genetic or epigenetic alterations [451]. Leukoplakia may share some of the same genetic mutations seen in oral cancer and lead to similar chromosomal instability, such as loss of DNA aneuploidy, loss of heterozygosity (LOH), and telomerase dysfunction, which have been linked with the initiation of the neoplastic process and malignant transformation [454–456]. DNA hypermethylation in specific loci (e.g., CDH1, CDKN2A, and MGMT) in dysplastic lesions and tumors was also detected, as well as impaired expression of mi-RNAs (e.g., miR-345, miR-21, and miR-18b), which are associated with the onset and progression of oral potentially malignant lesions [457–459]. In particular, aberrant expression of p53, p16INK4a [460–462], and gene mutations on 3p, 9p, and 17 (particularly TP53) may be associated with an increased risk of cancer [463]. Current evidence suggests that development from preinvasive dysplastic lesion to invasive cancer, based on patterns established at other sites (e.g., cervical cancer and melanoma), involves the gradual accumulation of genetic changes until invasion develops [464]. The three steps leading to cancer include a breakthrough phase, an expansion phase, and an invasive phase [464]. During the breakthrough phase, a cell develops a driver gene mutation (i.e., one that favors the development of a carcinoma) and begins to divide abnormally. Lesion tissue (presumably as in leukoplakia) becomes clinically visible after several years. In the expansion phase, an additional driver genetic mutation occurs which gives rise to neoplastic growth. During the invasive phase, the tumor invades surrounding tissues [451]. More recently, preclinical data have suggested that immuno modulation may play a critical role in oral carcinogenesis [465]. With recent advances in immuno-oncology demonstrating the efficacy of immune checkpoint inhibitors, such as those targeting the programmed cell death protein-1 (PD-1) axis in advanced squamous cell carcinoma of the head and neck [466, 467], there is significant interest in understanding the impact of anti-PD-1 therapy in early OSCCs and cancer prevention [450]. A recent study by Yagyuu et al. [468] showed that nearly 50% of high-grade leukoplakia samples were positive for PD-1 ligand (PD-L1). Furthermore, PD-L1 positivity and $CD8^+$ T-cell counts were significantly associated with the degree of dysplasia of these samples ($p < 0.001$). These results suggested that anti-tumor immunity may be suppressed through upregulation of PD-L1 in leukoplasic lesions, which could promote oral carcinogenesis.

Management and treatment of leukoplakia remain challenging especially for large lesions and PVL. Often, patients present with noncontiguous multifocal lesions (PVL) with a histopathologic diagnosis of "hyperkeratosis without dysplasia," but 70–100% will develop cancer over time [450]. The first fundamental therapy (to be implemented also in other oral potentially malignant diseases) consists in the patient's motivation, in the abolition of risk factors (smoking and alcohol), and in dental treatment that may be necessary to eliminate or reduce chronic trauma [209].

Current strategies for oral leukoplakia include surgery, a "look and see" approach, and medical therapies [469–471]. Surgical removal is not always the first choice of treatment for oral potentially malignant lesions. In the case of homogeneous leukoplakia, without dysplasia and localized in sites not considered to be at high risk of malignant transformation (stage 1 of the LSCP classification), it is advisable to follow the course of the lesion over time and subsequently decide whether to proceed with surgical removal in case of evolution of the lesion. On the contrary, in the case of erythroplakia or non-homogeneous leukoplakias or homogeneous leukoplakias localized in risk sites (tongue or oral floor) or with dysplasia (stages 2, 3, and 4 of the LSCP classification), immediate surgical removal is indicated, given the greater risk of neoplastic degeneration. The extension of the lesion to be removed, especially in the presence of a red component, must be highlighted by the toluidine blue, and the margins of the exceresis must extend on the surface by 5 mm beyond the edges of the lesion, while for the depth it is advisable to reach the muscular plane or the periosteum. In the case of large-area lesions, grafts can be used or, alternatively, it can be removed in several stages [209]. Villa and Woo [451] instead suggest a removal of the lesion with margins that must extend from 2 to 3 mm beyond the lesion.

The latest-generation lasers prove to be more versatile and manageable than traditional surgery, especially if they are used by vaporization; in fact they have several advantages: marked hemostasis, limited vaporization of the soft tissues, remarkable precision, the possibility of not suturing the wound, and reduction of postoperative discomfort and healing procedure; however, their superiority in achieving the primary goal of precancerous therapy has not been demonstrated. With the scalpel and with the laser in the cutting function (not vaporization), it is possible to obtain the operative piece for histological evaluation, and this is a very important advantage because it allows to better define the removed lesion and to detect any microscopic foci of microinvasive carcinoma [209]. A recent systematic review on the use of CO_2 laser for the management of leukoplakia demonstrated that the laser technique was reliable and reproducible with low morbidity [472]; however, relapse rates and malignant transformation rates ranged from 0 to 15%.

Vohra et al. [473] systematically reviewed photodynamic therapy (PDT) studies for the management of leukoplakia, erythroplakia, and their variants. When leukoplakia was considered, the results showed a complete (27–90%), partial (5–48%), or absent (4–25%) response to PDT, and the relapse rate ranged from 10 to 25%.

It must be specified that some cases of dysplasia (in particular mild dysplasia) have regressed over time, however it has been shown that several cases of mild dysplasia in reality could represent reactive epithelial atypia from trauma, and therefore regression and relapse could be expected [470].

In the case of severe dysplasia and carcinoma in situ, in these cases the exeresis must have wider safety margins, as the preoperative diagnosis, based on an incisional biopsy, cannot exclude with certainty the presence of a microinvasive carcinoma in some lesion areas. The margin of the exeresis must therefore be more extended both on the surface and in depth; in case of supraosseous lesions, it may sometimes be advisable to perform a corticotomy [209].

In cases of proliferative verrucous leukoplakia (PVL), the removed lesions tend to recur frequently; therefore the therapy in this case consists in a close clinical and histological surveillance with surgical removal of only the areas of dysplasia or carcinoma that may have arisen [209]. Villa and Woo [451] proposed a decision tree for the management of oral leukoplakia (Fig. 5.44).

Actinic keratosis (sun-induced dysplasia) of lip vermilion can be successfully treated with topical 5-fluorouracil (5-FU) twice daily for 2–4 weeks (2% or 5% cream) or with a 5% imiquimod-based topical cream two to three times a week for up to 4 months [474, 475] (Fig. 5.45). The results are more consistent with 5-FU [451].

In general, the relapse after conventional surgical excision varies from 0% to 35%, from 0% to 15% when the CO_2 laser was used, and from 10% to 25% in patients undergoing photodynamic therapy [450]. Following repeated post-treatment relapses, several topical agents for oral cancer chemoprevention have been tested in recent decades [476].

During the 1990s, several studies were conducted to evaluate the efficacy of vitamin A and its analogues, both natural (β-carotene) and synthetic (retinoids), on oral precancerous lesions; although the results obtained are encouraging in terms of research, they have not been such as to suggest its application in clinical practice. In fact, the daily use of these products is not free from significant side effects (dermatitis, conjunctivitis, liver damage, etc.) [209]. In addition to topical retinoids, various other agents such as bleomy-

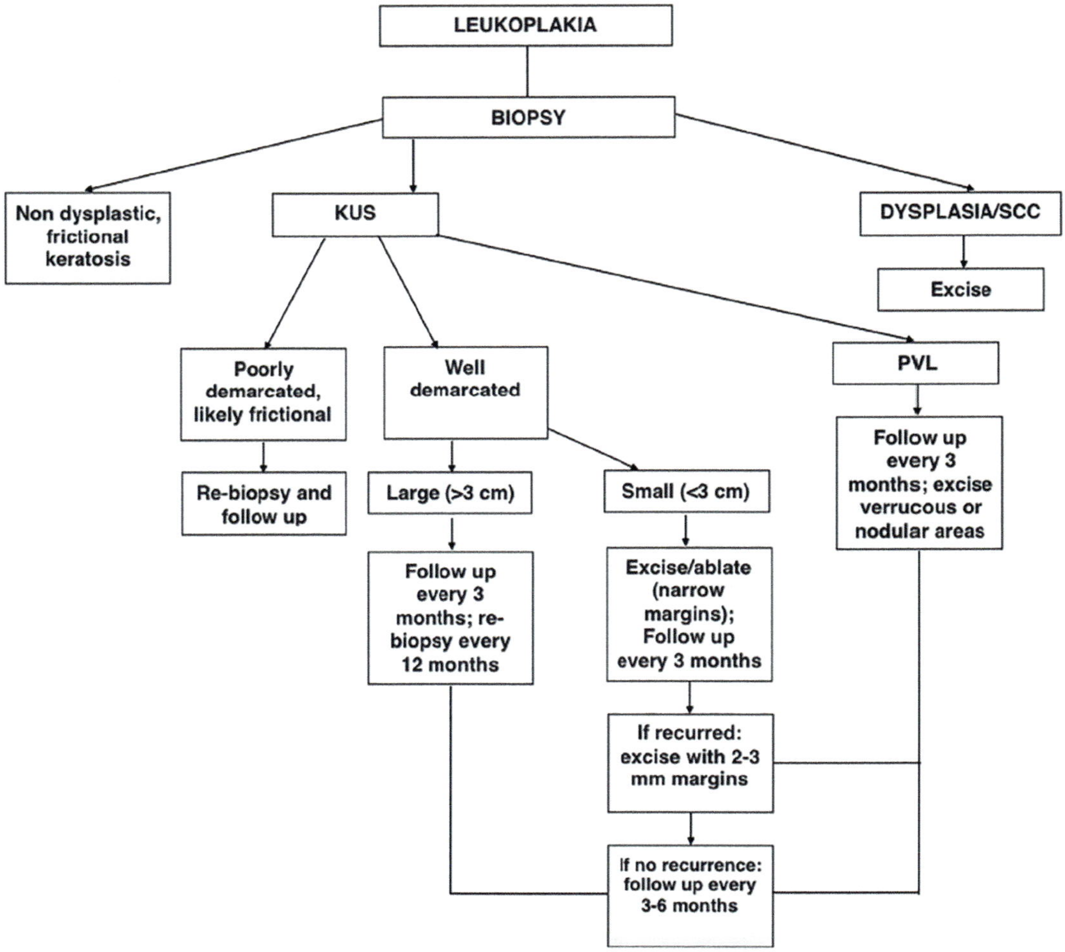

Fig. 5.44 Diagnosis and management of leukoplakia. From [451] with permission

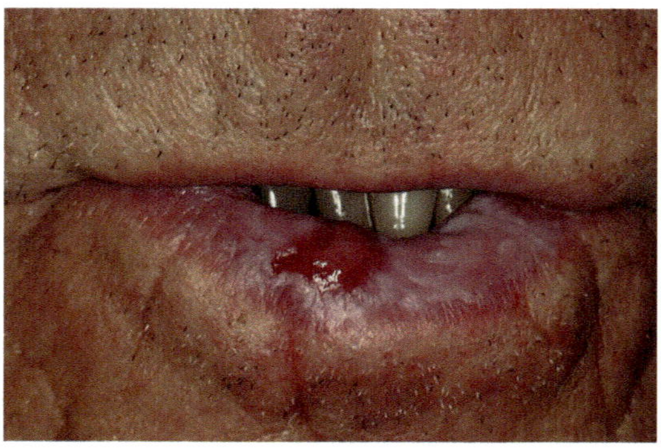

Fig. 5.45 Actinic keratosis of the lower lip. From [451] with permission

cin, adenovirus (gene therapy), cyclooxygenase inhibitors, and phytochemical-enriched agents have been tested [476]. A recent systematic review of the literature [476] showed that the mean complete response rate to topical retinoid therapy was 32%, for 1% bleomycin it was 40.2%, and for 0.5% bleomycin it was 25%. However, all of these agents have again been associated with disease recurrence.

A recent Cochrane review [469] evaluated the evidence in the literature on interventions for the treatment of leukoplakia and the prevention of neoplastic transformation. First of all, the experts noted that surgical interventions, including laser therapy and cryotherapy, have never been studied by means of a RCT (randomized controlled trial) that included a treatment-free or placebo group. Regarding medical therapy, the studies included in the review concern vitamin A and retinoids (four studies); beta-carotene or carotenoids (three studies); NSAIDs such as ketorolac and celecoxib (two studies); herbal extracts (four studies) including tea components, Chinese herbal blend, and freeze-dried black raspberry gel; bleomycin (one study); glycopeptide antibiotic with antitumor action; Bowman-Birk inhibitor (one study); and a serine protease inhibitor with anticarcinogenic properties. Some individual studies have suggested that some proposed treatments, namely, systemic vitamin A, beta-carotene, and lycopene, are effective in achieving clinical resolution of lesions more than placebo. Likewise, individual studies have found that systemic retinoic acid and lycopene may provide some benefits in terms of improving histological characteristics. Some studies have also reported a high relapse rate. There is currently no evidence, according to experts, of an effective treatment to prevent the development of oral cancer. Treatments such as vitamin A and beta-carotene can be effective in healing oral lesions, but relapses and adverse effects are common. In general, the authors of the Cochrane review rated the overall quality of the evidence as low or very low, so the results are uncertain and more research is needed.

In all cases, periodic checkups (every 3–6 months) throughout life are of fundamental importance; in fact, in many of these patients, treated or not, relapses or new lesions occur in a short or long time [209, 451]. Frail older patients may undergo long-term follow-up, while it may be more appropriate to remove lesions in younger patients. White lesions with a histopathologic diagnosis of "hyperkeratosis without dysplasia" or KUS should be reevaluated clinically to rule out frictional keratosis and evaluate the feasibility of complete removal. It must be specified that the recent consensus of the WHO Working Group [28] did not recommend the use of the term "keratosis of unknown significance." In fact this term would indicate a histological entity of hyperkeratosis with minimal to no epithelial dysplasia or cellular atypia, a condition compatible with oral leukoplakia (which is idiopathic by definition). The Working Group observed that there is no rationale to apply this term in the clinical context since over 50% of leukoplakia will be in this histologic category.

Focal lesions with poorly defined margins are likely frictional and may require annual follow-up with a possible biopsy examination only if the lesion progresses, if nodular or verrucous or red areas develop, or if there is evidence of induration. However, if there is no clinical evidence of clear pathogenesis and the lesion has clearly demarcated margins, it should be followed up closely, periodically, re-examined by biopsy, or excised/ablated depending on the clinical context. White multifocal lesions with a diagnosis of "hyperkeratosis without dysplasia" should be followed up every 3 months, with excision of verrucous or nodular areas [451].

5.5.16 Proliferative Verrucous Leukoplakia (PVL)

PVL goes into differential diagnosis with OLP and therefore requires further attention. PVL is an unusual, extremely aggressive form of leukoplakia that can mimic OLP clinically and microscopically [65, 156, 159, 477, 478]. Some aspects of PVL have been discussed above (see above).

The etiology of PVL is unknown and does not appear to be associated with the usual risk factors for oral cancer including tobacco and alcohol use, and no association with HPV or other viruses has been found [65].

The diagnosis of PVL is often made retrospectively, as this precancerous condition can be difficult to diagnose, particularly in its earlier stages; lesions typically grow slowly over a few years or decades [32]. PVL shows several common features with OLP such as multifocal presentation and propensity for the gum, palate, tongue, and buccal mucosa [477–479] (Fig. 5.42). On the other hand, the lingual belly and the oral floor are not commonly affected by PVL [32]. Lesions vary in appearance and may appear in the form of hyperkeratotic plaques, erythematous atrophic regions, and ulcerations [479]. More precisely, the clinical features of PVL vary from a white and flat lesions, to focal keratosis that becomes more widespread over time: the lesions can progress to a verrucous surface and have erythema and eventually can progress to verrucous or other squamous cell carcinoma forms of OSCC [65, 479].

From a histopathological point of view, PVL typically shows hyperkeratosis that may be associated with mucositis of the interface, similar to OLP, especially in the earlier stages where dysplastic alteration may not be present [32, 65]. As the disease progresses, the epithelium may change toward a verrucous epithelial architecture, called "atypical verrucous hyperplasia," which distinguishes PVL from OLP [32] (Fig. 5.46). PVL lesions often present with verruciform epithelial hyperkeratosis, more often orthokeratosis rather than parakeratosis [65], and often exhibit basal cell expansion, nuclear crowding, and varying degrees of cell atypia

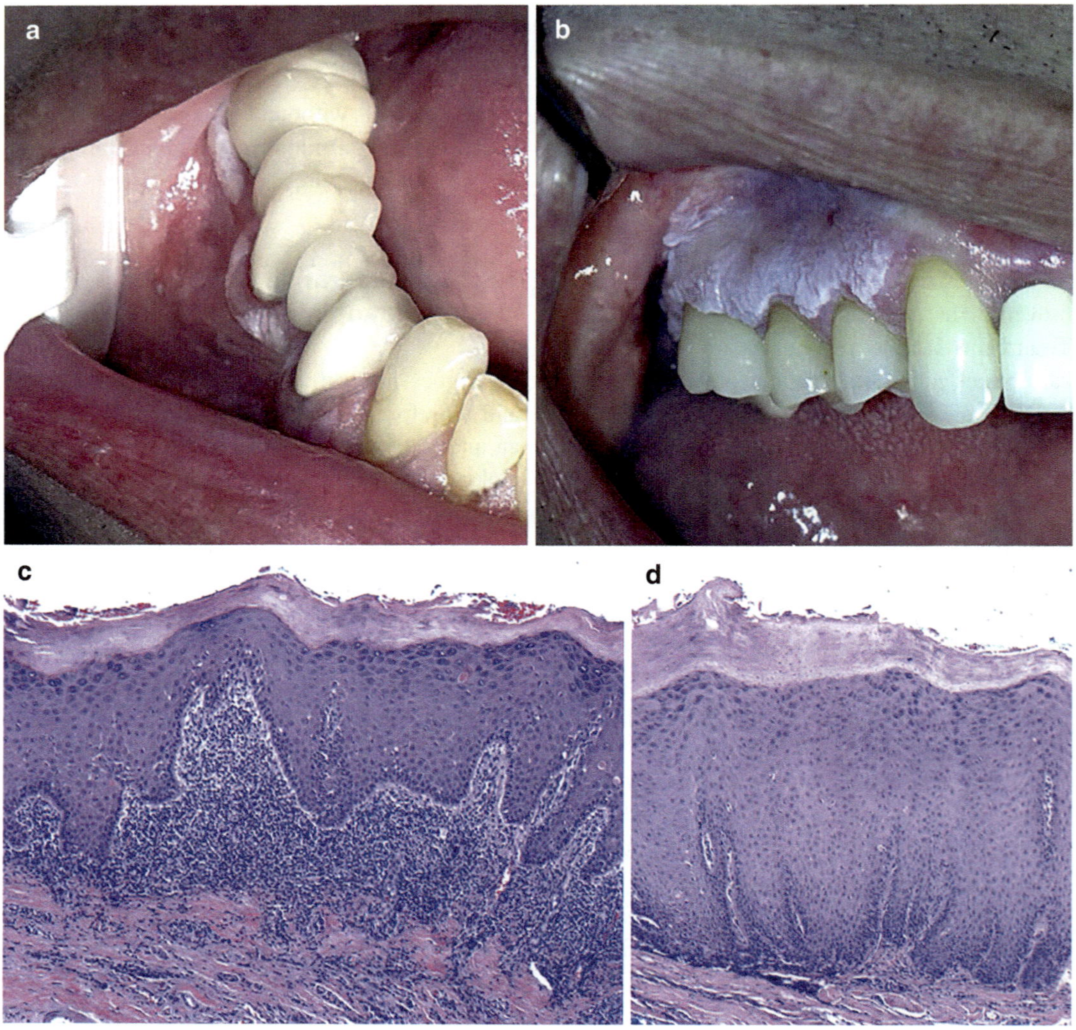

Fig. 5.46 Clinical and histopathological features of PVL in a 58-year-old nonsmoker. White, thickened plaques with irregular and rough surface changes are reported on the gingiva of the mandible (**a**) and maxilla (**b**). Other sites were also involved. (**c**) Biopsy of (**a**) showed hyperorthokeratosis, a prominent granular cell layer, and verrucous epithelial architecture associated with mucositis of the interface. The absence of basal cell degeneration (H&E ×250) is noted. (**d**) Biopsy of (**b**) revealed several histopathological features, including a verrucous epithelial architecture with thickened and acanthotic ridges (H&E ×250). Note the lack of inflammation compared to the image in (**c**). Based on the clinical and histological findings, the patient was given an operative diagnosis of PVL. From [32] with permission

[32]. Progressive lesions may present with dysplasia [65].

It has been observed that verrucous hyperplasia/hyperkeratosis can show, through DIF, a deposition of fibrinogen at the level of the basement membrane in about 42% of cases and a deposition of fibrinogen and C3 in about 3% of cases [159]. Therefore, DIF cannot be used to distinguish OLP from PVL and the differentiation between these two disorders is based on histopathological characteristics. The overlapping clinical and histopathological features between OLP and PVL remain a major challenge in diagnosing OLP, especially in the early phase of PVL, when the verrucous architectural change and/or the degree of cellular atypia are often mild [32].

5.5.16.1 Lichenoid Dysplasia (LD)

The term "*lichenoid dysplasia*" was coined in 1985 by Krutchkoff and Eisenberg [83] to describe lesions that clinically and histologically resemble OLP but also show epithelial dysplasia: in particular, the term refers to those lichenoid lesions that have two or more histological features of epithelial dysplasia. Eisenberg [480] later suggested that this term should be avoided, as it creates confusion, and dysplastic OLP is better assigned to the category "other dysplastic conditions." The debate on the possibility of OLP to determine dysplasia and/or on the consideration of evaluating lichenoid dysplasia a clinical entity other than OLP has been very long, and to date the WHO discourages the use of the term "oral lichenoid dysplasia" to describe an entity among OLP or lichenoid disorders which show dysplastic changes. Unlike what was established by the various classification criteria proposed in the past in which the presence of dysplasia excluded the diagnosis of OLP, the WHO established that if dysplasia is present, the diagnosis should be "*oral epithelial dysplasia with lichenoid features*" (i.e., if the latter features are indeed evident) or "*OLP with dysplasia*" [28].

Oral epithelial dysplasia is sometimes associated with a chronic inflammatory band infiltrate in the superficial lamina propria which, if observed with low-power microscopy, can offer substantial histopathological mimicry of OLP: this condition had been sometimes defined as "lichenoid dysplasia" [65]. In this regard, Fitzpatrick et al. revealed about 29% of oral dysplasia/OSCC may show histopathological lichenoid features [82].

Detectable classic features of oral epithelial dysplasia include irregular epithelial stratification, loss of basal cell polarity, drop-shaped epithelial ridges, increased number of mitoses and figures, premature keratinization, and hyperchromasia [65]. However, the discrimination of mild epithelial dysplasia with chronic OLP interface mucositis with reactive cellular atypia can be challenging, requiring a subjective evaluation [32]. However, objective criteria such as a predominant versus mixed lymphocyte infiltrate can sometimes be useful in distinguishing true OLP from epithelial dysplasia with lichenoid features [65] (the latter should be considered as a maturative disorder of the epithelium, while OLP is an immune-inflammatory disorder). The evaluation of factors such as the maturation pattern and cytological distortion of keratinocytes is complicated by the impact of chronic interface mucositis on the basal cell layer, on the maturational sequence of the lower layer of spiny cells, and on degenerative changes of keratinocytes, with potential mimicry of cytological atypy. Since the microscopic changes supporting the diagnosis of mild epithelial dysplasia are largely confined to the lower basal and spinous cell regions, the implications of an inflammatory process affecting the microscopic appearance of this area are evident [32]. In this situation, the inflammatory cell infiltrate—typically mixed in epithelial dysplasia with lower proportions of lymphocytes in favor of plasma cells and other cell types—tends to counteract the predominance of lymphocytic infiltrates present in OLP [83, 156, 159]. This distinction, although useful, cannot be considered as a surrogate for the assessment of epithelial maturational status. Where the clinical presentation is an isolated lesion, oral dysplasia should be strongly suspected. On the other hand, in the case of a multifocal lesion, the differential diagnosis becomes more problematic, particularly in patients with a history of tobacco use and in patients in whom the clinical appearance of mucosal lesions does not reach a definitive lichenoid model [32]. Cheng et al. suggest to pathologists, in cases deemed likely to represent OLP with significant reactive cellular atypia, to include in the histological report a comment that recognizes a level of pathological uncertainty regarding the significance of the observed maturational alterations. In such situations, a diagnosis of OLP must be considered provisional, and the patient must be guaranteed continuous follow-up [32].

In addition to the possibility of a cellular atypia reactive to the chronic inflammatory insult of OLP that could mimic epithelial dysplasia (with different prognostic significance and with different therapeutic implications), the question arises as to whether OLP is capable (due to chronic inflammation) to lead over time to dysplastic alterations of the epithelium, up to carcinoma. The possibility of OLP to evolve into squamous carcinoma has already been discussed in Sect. 4.5. As for dysplasia, the question still remains open. There are two possibilities:

1. In many cases, the dysplastic lichenoid lesion may represent de novo dysplasia and the lesion may have no relation to OLP. This is supported by the fact that it is common to observe oral epithelial dysplasia with varying degrees of submucosal lymphocytic infiltrate. Such clinically white lesions are more likely a form of leukoplakia than OLP, especially when they present as single plaque-like lesions.
2. On the other hand, in some cases there may actually be a relationship between OLP and dysplasia, and the dysplastic lesions of the lichenoid may actually represent OLPs that have undergone dysplastic changes. Once again it could be hypothesized that these dysplastic lichenoid lesions may have originally been OLPs which, under the influence of oral carcinogens or chronic inflammation, have undergone dysplastic changes.

However, the only compelling way to show that OLP develops in dysplastic lichenoid lesions would be, as has been suggested by Zhang et al. in 2000, to undertake prospective studies and demonstrate that clinically and histologically confirmed cases of OLP become dysplastic [481]. Until recently, the presence of dysplasia excluded the diagnosis of OLP; therefore "lichenoid dysplasia" was thought to be a distinct disease entity. However, it is also likely that "lichenoid dysplasia" may be an early stage in the path of malignant transformation from "true" OLP to OSCC, i.e., a form of OLP lesion capable of becoming dysplastic [29], and this is suggested by a series of clinical observations (post-2000) by Mignogna et al. [482–484] who performed a large retrospective study on a sample of 45 patients with histologically confirmed OLP without dysplasia at the time of initial diagnosis: 20 patients subsequently encountered a single transformation event, and 25 had multiple transformation events including multifocal dysplasia and/or malignancy. These results suggest that not only OLP itself constitutes a risk factor for malignant transformation, but that there may also be a field cancerization in OLP [484]. To date, therefore, the WHO discourages the use of the term "lichenoid dysplasia" and recognizes the possibility that OLP may be associated with the presence of dysplasia; therefore the recommendation is to use the terms "*oral epithelial dysplasia with lichenoid features*" and "*OLP with dysplasia*" [28].

It can be difficult to distinguish OLP and oral epithelial dysplasia with an underlying lichenoid immune reaction histopathologically. It cannot be stressed enough that OLP diagnosis requires the correlation and comparison of clinical and histopathological features. If a lichenoid immune reaction is present and OLP is not suggested clinically, the histopathologist should search carefully for other features of epithelial dysplasia. Sequential biopsy may be required for definitive diagnosis. Therefore, it is recommended that the term "lichenoid dysplasia" should not be used, and pathologists should diagnose all oral epithelial dysplastic lesions with lichenoid immune reactions as dysplasia, unless clinicopathological correlation produces compelling reasons to consider that OLP is present. This recommendation is based on the fact that many early biopsies in PVL show lichenoid features with minimal dysplasia which have been frequently misdiagnosed as oral lichen planus [485].

5.5.16.2 Other Oral Lichenoid Lesions

Various other disorders have been reported in the literature characterized by lichenoid reactions. For example Eisenberg [480] discussed other lichenoid entities, such as non-specific lichenoid stomatitis and atypical lichenoid stomatitis.

- *Non-specific lichenoid stomatitis* (*NLS*). The histopathological characteristics of OLP have already been described. As already mentioned, these are not always emblematic of OLP: for example, it is not unusual to detect superficial parakeratosis, Civatte bodies, and fibrous deposits at the epithelial-connective tissue interface. These findings are also present in other disorders already treated in the previous paragraphs. These conditions of interface mucositis that have more ambiguous clinical-histological characteristics have been called "non-specific lichenoid stomatitis" (NLS). Currently this term has fallen into disuse. The recent WHO workshop agreed to the van der Meij and van der Waal (2003) consideration establishing that lichenoid disorders which do not present the clinical and/or histopathological characteristics considered typical (but compatible) with OLP are considered as *oral lichenoid lesions* (*OLLs*). OLLs include [28]:
  - Atypical OLP and unilateral lichenoid lesions [89, 97, 98]
  - OLCHR (lichenoid lesions in close contact relationship to a dental restoration, often amalgam) [95, 99]
  - OLDR [95]
  - Oral lesions following intake of food or some substances, such as cinnamon (cinnamon stomatitis)
  - OLL-GvHD
- *Atypical lichenoid stomatitis* (*ALS*). This term refers to cases in which non-specific cellular peculiarities or disorders of maturation are observed which could represent local inflammatory influence or possibly subtle characteristics of incipient dysplasia [486]. OLP usually presents a profile of normal cytomorphology, maturation, and epithelial architecture. In some cases, in the presence of oral lichenoid reactions with maturation disorders, most of the scientific community preferred to avoid the terms "OLP with atypia" and "OLP with dysplasia" as these are misleading: in fact, most of these reactions are not OLP, but primary epithelial maturational disorders indicative of malignant potential. Therefore the terms "atypical lichenoid stomatitis" (ALS) (in case of cellular atypia in the affected epithelium) and "lichenoid dysplasia" (LD) (in case of epithelial dysplasia with lichenoid reaction) have been proposed [480]. However, the recent WHO workshop recommended that the term "lichenoid dysplasia" should not be used, and pathologists should diagnose all oral epithelial dysplastic lesions with lichenoid immune reactions as "*oral epithelial dysplasia with lichenoid features*" or "*OLP with dysplasia*," unless clinicopathological correlation produces compelling reasons to consider that OLP is present [28] (Sect. 5.5.16).

Therefore, to date, the use of the terms *non-specific lichenoid stomatitis* and *atypical lichenoid stomatitis* is no longer recommended.

- *Lichenoid and granulomatous stomatitis* (*LGS*). It is a condition characterized by the presence of lichenoid inflammation with concomitant granulomatous inflammation, rarely observed within the oral tissues. Clinically, it presents as an inflamed red patch of the labial mucosa of the upper lip [487]. But this finding is visible in many other disorders; therefore a histological investigation can clarify the nature of the disorder:
- Acute and chronic inflammation in the absence of other distinctive pathologies (non-specific stomatitis) [487]
- Granulomatous inflammation, leading to a short list of conditions or oral granulomatosis, divided into three groups: those caused by microorganisms (tuberculosis, syphilis, deep mycosis), those associated with the implanta-

tion of foreign bodies (abrasive toothpastes, dental materials, pulse granuloma), and idiopathic diseases (orofacial granulomatosis, Melkersson-Rosenthal syndrome, Crohn's disease, sarcoidosis, Wegener's granulomatosis, giant cell arteritis) [488]

- Lichenoid inflammation at the epithelial-connective tissue interface, suggesting a limited range of disorders including LP, OLL, OLCL, LE, GvHD, and lichen sclerosus et atrophicus [487]

Robinson M.C. et al. [487] report six clinical cases of subjects affected by inflammatory processes in the mucosa of the upper lip, presenting histologically both as lichenoid inflammation (with infiltrate of T lymphocytes) and as granulomatous inflammation (with few or numerous small granulomas, well formed or poorly formed) simultaneously. The deep lymphocyte infiltrate was in most cases mixed (B and T cells) with perineural distribution. When the two models are present simultaneously, there are problems in determining which represents the primary disease process or, effectively, if the coexistence of the two inflammatory models represents a distinct pathological entity. For example, it is possible that lichenoid inflammation makes the oral mucosa more sensitive to the entry of foreign material, resulting in the formation of granuloma. However, the authors systematically examined the biopsy material using careful inspection and polarized light, but no foreign material was observed [487]. However, the detection of foreign particles in biopsies can be difficult and not all extrinsic materials are detectable using polarized light [489, 490]. Interestingly, two patients were known to take drugs which have an association with lichenoid eruptions (naproxen, atenolol, and ramipril) and which have also been implicated in lichenoid and granulomatous dermatitis [487, 491]. A recent case report described a patient with nivolumab-induced lichenoid granulomatous stomatitis successfully treated for 2 weeks with topical corticosteroids in addition to doxycycline 40 mg twice a day given due to its antimicrobial and anti-inflammatory action in granulomatous inflammation [492]. Thus, it is possible that these particular lesions may also represent unusual drug eruptions. Basically, all the oral lesions described by the authors were persistent (not resolvable even with steroid treatment), but remained localized and generally showed phases of active disease followed by periods of quiescence [487]. In 1 study [493], 22 patients with lichenoid reactions of the mucous membrane of the upper lip were treated with chlorhexidine: in 80% of these patients, the lesions improved or completely healed, indicating a possible microbial association. Therefore, the lichenoid reactions present on the mucosal side of the lips might be triggered by microbial plaque precipitated on the vestibular surfaces of the anterior teeth [493]. It is therefore also necessary to pay attention to the presence of conservative/prosthetic restorations in these dental elements which could further favor the accumulation of plaque. A retrospective study of 47 LGS cases showed that the lesions were (in order) distributed to the gingiva, buccal mucosa, vestibule, tongue, lip, and palate, with occasional multifocal involvement, and that all cases were CD68 positive in the histiocytic infiltrates and were negative for microorganisms utilizing acid-fast bacilli, Grocott methenamine silver, and periodic acid-Schiff stains [494]. Hakeem et al. recently proposed a new classification system for oral LGS (Table 5.14) [494].

Table 5.14 Hakeem LGS Classification

Hakeem LGS Classification	Histologic description
Type 1	Band-like lymphocytic infiltration with superficially loose or aggregates of histiocytes and perivascular inflammatory infiltrate
Type 2	Band-like lymphocytic infiltration with superficially loose or aggregates of histiocytes and no perivascular inflammatory infiltrate
Type 3	Lichenoid infiltration with epithelioid giant cell granuloma and perivasculitis
Type 4	Lichenoid infiltration with epithelioid giant cell granuloma and no perivasculitis

- *Solitary fixed drug eruptions* (*FDE*) on the lip have also been reported rarely [96]. They are characterized by a particularly sudden onset of solitary, or occasionally multiple, well-defined erythematous lesions on the mucous membranes, which may or may not become ulcerated. Histopathology shows a lichenoid interface dermatitis which includes plasma cells and tends to surround small vessels [495]. The diagnostic hallmark is the reappearance of the lesion exactly on the previously affected site when the offending agent is reused [96].
- *Lichen sclerosus* (*LS*) is clinically characterized by the development of well-defined hyperkeratotic lesions on the skin and genitals and very rarely on the oral mucosa, followed by fibrosis/sclerosis [496, 497]. It can mimic other disorders that cause hyperkeratotic plaques including OLP [96]. The histopathology of lichen sclerosus shows epithelial atrophy, local hydropic degeneration of the basal cells, loss of epithelial ridges, and homogenization of the underlying connective tissue with reduction of the presence of elastic fibers, hyalinization, and sclerosis of the connective tissue. The lichenoid lymphocytic infiltrate is often present but does not show a distinct band of lymphocytes in the epithelial-connective tissue junction as in the OLP and other OLLs [496]. A case report showed a patient with oral LS significantly improved with perilesional 40 mg triamcinolone infiltration (Trigon depot®) (seven infiltrations: one every 10 days) [497].

5.5.16.3 Summary and Final Considerations

Table 5.15 shows a summary of the main aspects of the disorders that have been described in this chapter.

Due to the enormous overlap in the clinical and histopathological presentation of inflammatory, reactive, immune-mediated, and potentially malignant lesions affecting the oral mucosa, oral lichenoid lesions (OLLs) can represent a diagnostic challenge [65]. A complete history and clinical evaluation by a multidisciplinary team of specialists may be required to investigate oral, skin, nail, scalp, genital, esophageal, laryngeal, and conjunctival involvement [96]. The psychological profile of patients with OLP should not be underestimated. In fact, as reported in a multicenter study by the Italian Society of Oral Pathology and Medicine (SIPMO) mood disorders are frequently associated with OLP with an unexpected symptomatology correlated with the number of oral symptoms and with the extension of disease suggesting a peripheral neuropathy [498].

We have a paucity of good epidemiological studies on OLP, mainly due to the difficulty in distinguishing OLP from a number of similar lesions. Existing classifications seem unsuitable to encompass all possible OLLs and of particular concern is the lack of consideration of LE as a diagnostic alternative. The only OLL that can be easily differentiated from OLP without further investigation is cGvHD [67]. As suggested in the new textbook "Patologia e Medicina Orale" [499] written by the Italian Society of Oral Pathology and Medicine (SIPMO), although the clinical and histopathological aspects of OLP are similar to those of OLLs, the great difference in terms of pathogenesis may also change the risk of developing oral cancer. Lichenoid lesions are in fact associated with a series of factors such as direct trauma, drug intake, food intolerances and manifestations of autoimmune diseases. For this reason, with respect to OLP, given the diagnosis of OLL, it is possible to act effectively by eliminating the causal factors when it is possible to recognize them. The clinical features of OLP alone, particularly when they occur in the "classic" hyperkeratotic reticular bilateral form, often support the exclusion of other oral keratotic diseases such as leukoplakia, friction keratosis, and PVL [96]. Traditionally, the diagnosis of OLL is based on clinical/histological correlation but, in several cases, this approach does not provide a reliable diagnosis. The inclusion of molecular techniques can refine the capacity for diagnostic discrimination. In particular, immunoblotting, IP, and ELISA can aid in the diagnosis of some OLLs such as CUS, LPP, MMP, and PNP/PAMS [67]. In case of recalcitrant and atypical mucocu-

Table 5.15 Classification and characteristics of oral lichenoid lesions

Disease	Clinical appearance	Histology	DIF	IIF	Immunoblotting	ELISA	Others	Comorbidity
OLP	Bilateral, white reticular patches not always symmetrical usually on the buccal mucosa. Sometimes erosions/atrophy and rarely scarring lesions	Usually hyperkeratosis but sometimes orthokeratosis. The epithelium can be atrophic and acanthotic and have "sawtooth" epithelial ridges. Vacuolar degeneration of basal keratinocytes. Banded/irregular infiltration of lymphocytes at the level of the basement membrane. In the erosive forms, there can be subbasal separation with degeneration of the basal cells and the inflammation can contain plasma cells, as well as in the case of gingival biopsies. Any reactive, regenerative, or reparative epithelial changes depending on the degree of ulceration. Possible dysplasia in the absence of verrucous architectural changes	Commonly negative. Deposits of fibrinogen and/or C3 with a "shaggy" appearance in the bodies of Civatte and in the basement membrane. Bodies of Civatte can be IgM^+	Usually negative	Occasionally a weak band at 180 kDa	–	Association with numerous genetic polymorphisms for various cytokines	HCV. Sometimes extraoral lesions (genitals, skin, scalp, nails, esophagus, conjunctiva)
OLCL	It can be both unilateral and bilateral. Common topographical relationship with amalgam (or other) restorations and flavoring agents. Rare gingival involvement	Similar to OLP but sometimes inflammatory infiltrate mixed with plasma cells and neutrophils. Sometimes also perivascular inflammation and scattered eosinophils. Tertiary lymphoid follicles can be observed in reactions to dental materials. Acanthosis with elongated epithelial ridges in cinnamon stomatitis	Similar or identical to OLP	Usually negative	–	–	Patch test may confirm hypersensitivity to mercury but not invariably. Lymphocyte transformation test usually not helpful	Malignant potential unclear. Unlikely to cause extraoral lesions
OLDR	Similar/identical to OLP but more commonly one-sided. Sometimes a temporal relationship with taking a new drug. But possible late onset (>1 year later)	Similar to OLP but sometimes inflammatory infiltrate mixed with plasma cells and neutrophils. Sometimes the infiltrate extends into the deep stroma and may be perivascular	Similar if not identical to OLP		–	–	–	Malignant or unclear potential. Sometimes it causes extraoral lesions
GvHD	Similar/identical to OLP, especially cGvHD. Sometimes LK-like. Common scarring lesions. History of bone marrow transplant (at least 6 months previously)	Similar/identical to OLP but sometimes more scattered lymphocyte infiltrate	Similar/identical to OLP	–	–	–	–	Sjögren-type sialoadenitis. Pulmonary, gastrointestinal, cutaneous, genital involvement. Potentially malignant

PV	Multiple flaccid and erythematous vesiculo-bullous lesions. Intense burning. Desquamative gingivitis in the advanced stages. Positive Nikolsky's sign. Idiopathic but sometimes trigger factors	Acantholysis in the basal and suprabasal layer. Appearance like a "row of tombstones." Non-specific inflammatory infiltrate of the stroma	Intercellular deposits of IgG and C3 but also IgM and IgA (reticular morphology). 100% sensitivity	Positivity in 80% of cases with IgG circulating against the cell surfaces of keratinocytes	Feasible in cases of uncertain diagnosis (ditto for immunoprecipitation)	Detection of anti-Dsg1 and anti-Dsg3 antibodies in serum	Spherical acantholytic cells (Tzanck cells) observed with Tzanck cytodiagnostic examination	Oral lesions usually precede skin lesions. Sometimes involvement of conjunctival, nasal, pharyngeal, laryngeal, esophageal, genital, anal, and even bronchial and stomach mucous membranes
BP	Infrequent but possible oral lesions, smaller and less painful than PV. Blisters, erosions, vesicles	Subepidermal vesicles. Almost always inflammatory infiltrate of eosinophils in the superficial dermis	Linear deposits of C3 and IgG	Circulating IgG that binds to the basement membrane	–	–	Immunohistochemistry shows C3 and C4 confirming the diagnosis	Skin lesions with tense blisters. Itchy skin. Negative Nikolsky's sign. Rarely pharyngolaryngeal lesions
LPP	Combination of LP and BP (vesicles or blisters) in the oral mucosa, skin, or both	In the oral cavity similar/identical to OLP and having characteristics of MMP (subepithelial separation)	Linear staining in the case of IgG and C3 at the basement membrane	Circulating anti-basement membrane IgG	Positive band at 180 kDa, rarely at 230 kDa	Antibody positivity against the C-terminal portion of NC16A of BP180	–	Uncertain association with malignancy
MMP	Rarely, intact oral blisters (sometimes with blood content). Frequent erosions covered with fibrin (yellowish color, unlike PV) and desquamative gingivitis and post-inflammatory atrophy similar to OLP. Positive Nikolsky's sign (but also in bullous OLP)	Subepithelial separation (EOLP-like) with subepithelial blister formation. The clear separation of the epithelium from the lamina propria or the absence of connective tissue should be noted. Absent hydropic degeneration of basal keratinocytes with formation of cytoid bodies. Mixed inflammatory infiltrate (sometimes fewer eosinophils than BP)	A test for certainty showing linear deposits of IgG C3 (sometimes also IgM and IgA) on the basement membrane	Usually negative. IIF-SSS can detect circulating antibodies located on the roof or floor of the separation	It can help in the diagnosis	It can help in the diagnosis	–	Frequent concomitant ocular lesions up to blindness. Sometimes skin, laryngeal, esophageal, anal, genital involvement

(continued)

Table 5.15 (continued)

Disease	Clinical appearance	Histology	DIF	IIF	Immunoblotting	ELISA	Others	Comorbidity
PNP/ PAMS	Frequent extensive oral erosions typically (not exclusively) in the lips. Sometimes oral and skin pleomorphic lichenoid lesions	Sometimes similar/identical to OLP	Often equivocal (e.g., double positivity: linear to the basement membrane and intercellular within the epithelium)	Usually positive with anti-keratinocyte antibodies using rat bladder epithelium	Possible positive band 190, 210, 230, 250, and 500 kDa	Positivity to BP180, BP230, Dsg1, Dsg3, and envoplachin	Association with some HLAs. Immunoprecipitation reveals antibodies against envoplachin, periplachin, desmoplachins 1–2, BP230, plectin, A2ML1. Less common antibody detections against Dsg1 and 3, placophilin 3, and desmocollins 1–3	Almost always associated with tumors, Castleman's disease, and OLP-like lesions. Sometimes respiratory failure
CUS	Similar/identical to OLP	Similar to OLP	Anti-nucleus antibodies (SES-ANA) on the basal and lower third cell layers	IgG positivity according to a speckled and/or granular pattern (SES-ANA) on monkey esophagus	Positive band at 70 kDa	ΔNp63α positivity	–	–
EM	Spread of oral ulcers. Acute onset. Usually recurrent and rarely chronic. Target skin lesions. Oral ulcer-erosive lesions and crusted lesions of the lip	Intraepithelial edema and early spongiosis, with necrosis of satellite cells and intra- and subepithelial vesicles. Often severe stromal edema of the papillary areas and vacuolar degeneration of the basement membrane with intense lymphocytic infiltration that is also localized at the perivascular level	Commonly negative	Usually negative	Positive band at 210 and 250 kDa	DSP-I and DSP-II?	Association with several HLAs. PCR for HSV-1 in case of recurrent lesions	Systemic symptoms, particularly in the major forms
DLE	Most commonly asymmetrical lesions consisting of central atrophic areas or superficial erosions, radiating white streaks at the margins, and telangiectasias (radial rays). Typically much less clearly defined than in OLP	Similar/identical to OLP. Focal or extensive thickening of the basement membrane. Sometimes deeper and perivascular inflammatory infiltrate. Vessel walls may be prominent with endothelial swelling. Edema and variable mucin deposits may be present. Sometimes keratin plugs	Possible granular deposition of Ig and/or complement in the basement membrane (lupus band). Usually negative on oral biopsies	Usually negative in oral lesions	–	–	Association with various HLA, ITGAM, CTLA4, TYK2, IRF5	Potentially malignant disorder. Commonly skin lesions in areas exposed to sunlight

SLE	Similar to DLE and/or OLP. Oral ulcers, erythema of malar eminences in the face and bridge of the nose (butterfly erythema)	Similar/identical to DLE. Milder hyperkeratosis and focal liquefactive degeneration of the basal layers and lymphocyte infiltrate. No thickening of the basement membrane	Similar to DLE	Commonly ANA positivity. Also anti-dsDNA, anti-Sm, RNP, Ro/SSA and La/SSB, aPL, aCL	–	–	Association with various HLA, MSH5, IRF5, ITGAM, STAT4/ STAT1, FcGR2A, PTPN22. Positive test for lupus anticoagulant	Multi-organic involvement. Hematological anomalies
LK	Homogeneous form: uniform and flat white plaque with well-defined margins Non-homogeneous form: fragmented white areas, sometimes verrucous/nodular appearance	From hyperkeratosis to severe dysplasia/carcinoma in situ	–	–	–	–	–	Variable probability of malignant degeneration
EK/ ELK	Macula of red color, clear or slightly shaded margins. Sometimes mixed with white components	Moderate or severe dysplasia/ carcinoma in situ	–	–	–	–	Toluidine blue positive, but there can be false positives and negatives	Very probable neoplastic transformation
PVL	Keratosis and multifocal lesions. It can be similar to OLP. Hard palate often involved. Central area of ulceration surrounded by radiant keratotic striae	Similar to OLP, sometimes deep perivascular inflammation. Verrucous architectural change and cellular atypia/ dysplasia may not be present at an early stage	Similar to OLP	Usually negative	–	–	–	Aggressive lesion with malignant transformation in 70–100% of cases
LGS	Erythematous patches on the inside of the lips and the adjacent adherent gingiva	Lichenoid inflammation with concomitant granulomatous inflammation	–	–	–	–	–	Possible good response to antiseptics
FDE	Erythematous lesions on mucous membranes that may or may not be ulcerated	Lichenoid inflammation of the interface that includes plasma cells and tends to surround the small vessels	–	–	–	–	–	–
LS	Mostly white patches	Epithelial atrophy, hyalinization, and sclerosis of the connective tissue	–	–	–	–	–	Most often it affects the genitals

BP bullous pemphigoid; *CUS* chronic ulcerative stomatitis; *DLE* discoid lupus erythematosus; *EK/ELK* erythroplakia/erythroleukoplakia; *EM* erythema multiforme; *FDE* fixed drug eruption; *GvHD* graft-versus-host disease; *LGS* lichenoid and granulomatous stomatitis; *LPP* lichen planus pemphigoides; *LS* lichen sclerosus; *OLCL* oral lichenoid contact lesion; *OLDR* oral lichenoid drug reaction; *OLP* oral lichen planus; *MMP* mucous membrane pemphigoid; *PNP/PAMS* paraneoplastic pemphigus/paraneoplastic autoimmune multiorgan syndrome; *PV* pemphigus vulgaris; *SLE* systemic lupus erythematosus taneous manifestations, further investigations are warranted, including a PET scan to screen for total body cancer if PNP/PAMS is suspected [96]. Some genetic tests may also be of help, and new technologies and diagnostic platforms are available to detect ANA that have already shown the heterogeneity that exists within SLE cohorts [67]. When medical history, clinical features, and immunological findings (e.g., positive ANA tests) suggest SLE, tests for anti-dsDNA and other autoantibodies including anti-Sm, anti-RNP, anti-Ro/SSA and La/SSB, aPL, and aCL should be considered. For other OLLs such as DLE, OLCL, and OLDR, however, reliable diagnostic tests are lacking and further research is needed [96]. Some of the techniques mentioned above are not universally or commercially available [67].

Some OLLs such as OLP, OLCL, DLE, and CUS are more susceptible to topical therapy than PNP/PAMS, SLE, and LPP, which usually require systemic drugs and multidisciplinary management. A growing understanding of the pathogenetic mechanisms underlying OLP and other OLLs can help to better identify and distinguish these disorders. New animal or experimental models of OLL should be developed, focusing mainly on the oral cavity. Furthermore, the study of new biomarkers will allow to revolutionize the diagnostic and therapeutic decisions of these disorders [96].

References

1. Spadari F, Pallotti F, Bombeccari GP, di Patologia A, Os D. Lichen planus orale: revisione della letteratura.
2. Eisen D. The evaluation of cutaneous, genital, scalp, nail, esophageal, and ocular involvement in patients with oral lichen planus. Oral Surg Oral Med Oral Pathol Oral Radiol Endodontol. 1999;88(4):431–6.
3. Farhi D, Dupin N. Pathophysiology, etiologic factors, and clinical management of oral lichen planus, part I: facts and controversies. Clin Dermatol. 2010;28(1):100–8.
4. Parashar P. Oral lichen planus. Otolaryngol Clin N Am. 2011;44(1):89–107., vi. https://doi.org/10.1016/j.otc.2010.09.004.
5. Scully C, Carrozzo M. Oral mucosal disease: lichen planus. Br J Oral Maxillofac Surg. 2008;46(1):15–21. https://doi.org/10.1016/j.bjoms.2007.07.199.
6. Sugerman PB, Sabage N. Oral lichen planus: causes, diagnosis and management. Aust Dent J. 2002;47(4):290–7.
7. Eisen D. The clinical manifestations and treatment of oral lichen planus. Dermatol Clin. 2003;21(1):79–89. https://doi.org/10.1016/s0733-8635(02)00067-0.
8. Pelisse M, Leibowitch M, Sedel D, Hewitt J. A new vulvovaginogingival syndrome. Plurimucous erosive lichen planus. Annales de Dermatologie et de Venereologie. 1982:797–8.
9. Rogers RS, Eisen D. Erosive oral lichen planus with genital lesions: the vulvovaginal-gingival syndrome and the peno-gingival syndrome. Dermatol Clin. 2003;21(1):91–8.
10. Pelisse M. The vulvo-vaginal-gingival syndrome: a new form of erosive lichen planus. Int J Dermatol. 1989;28(6):381–4.
11. Dwyer C, Kerr R, Millan D. Squamous carcinoma following lichen planus of the vulva. Clin Exp Dermatol. 1995;20(2):171–2.
12. Franck JM, Young AW Jr. Squamous cell carcinoma in situ arising within lichen planus of the vulva. Dermatol Surg. 1995;21(10):890–4.
13. Olson MA, Rogers RS 3rd, Bruce AJ. Oral lichen planus. Clin Dermatol. 2016;34(4):495–504. https://doi.org/10.1016/j.clindermatol.2016.02.023.
14. Setterfield JF, Neill S, Shirlaw PJ, Theron J, Vaughan R, Escudier M, et al. The vulvovaginal gingival syndrome: a severe subgroup of lichen planus with characteristic clinical features and a novel association with the class II HLA DQB1∗0201 allele. J Am Acad Dermatol. 2006;55(1):98–113.
15. Cribier B, Ndiaye I, Grosshans E. Peno-gingival syndrome. A male equivalent of vulvo-vagino-gingival syndrome? Rev Stomatol Chir Maxillofac. 1993;94(3):148–51.
16. Bain L, Geronemus R. The association of lichen planus of the penis with squamous cell carcinoma in situ and with verrucous squamous carcinoma. J Dermatol Surg Oncol. 1989;15(4):413–7.
17. Harewood G, Murray J, Cameron A. Esophageal lichen planus: the Mayo Clinic experience. Dis Esophagus. 1999;12(4):309–11.
18. Abraham SC, Ravich WJ, Anhalt GJ, Yardley JH, Wu T-T. Esophageal lichen planus: case report and review of the literature. Am J Surg Pathol. 2000;24(12):1678–82.
19. Evans A, Fletcher C, Owen W, Hay R. Oesophageal lichen planus. Clin Exp Dermatol. 2000;25(1):36–7.
20. Souto P, Sofia C, Pina-Cabral J, Castanheira A, Saraiva S, Tellechea O, et al. Oesophageal lichen planus. 1997.
21. Chandan VS, Murray JA, Abraham SC. Esophageal lichen planus. Arch Pathol Lab Med. 2008;132(6):1026–9.
22. Ravi K, Codipilly DC, Sunjaya D, Fang H, Arora AS, Katzka DA. Esophageal lichen planus is associated with a significant increase in risk of squamous cell carcinoma. Clin Gastroenterol Hepatol. 2019;17(9):1902–3. e1

23. Rai P, Madi MY, Lee R, Dickstein A. A case series of Esophageal lichen planus: an underdiagnosed cause of dysphagia. The Korean J Helicobacter Upper Gastrointestinal Res. 2019;19(4):266–71.
24. Chaklader M, Morris-Larkin C, Gulliver W, McGrath J. Cyclosporine in the management of esophageal lichen planus. Can J Gastroenterol. 2009;23(10):686–8. https://doi.org/10.1155/2009/802075.
25. Keate R, Williams J, Connolly S. Lichen planus esophagitis: report of three patients treated with oral tacrolimus or intraesophageal corticosteroid injections or both. Dis Esophagus. 2003;16(1):47–53.
26. Jencks KJ, Abdulla H, Qiu S. 1825 Esophageal stricture due to Esophageal lichen planus and its successful management using local corticosteroid injection. Official J Am Coll Gastroenteroll ACG. 2019;114:S1024.
27. Ferreira KS, Bakhit M, Nam GH, Hussain Z. Esophageal lichen planus: a rare condition and a unique treatment approach. Am J Gastroenterol. 2018;113:S1025-S.
28. Warnakulasuriya S, Kujan O, Aguirre-Urizar JM, Bagan JV, González-Moles MÁ, Kerr AR, et al. Oral potentially malignant disorders: a consensus report from an international seminar on nomenclature and classification, convened by the WHO collaborating Centre for Oral Cancer. Oral Dis. 2021;27(8):1862–80.
29. Shirasuna K. Oral lichen planus: malignant potential and diagnosis. Oral Sci Int. 2014;11(1):1–7.
30. Sugerman P, Savage N, Walsh L, Zhao Z, Zhou X, Khan A, et al. The pathogenesis of oral lichen planus. Critical Rev Oral Biol Med. 2002;13(4):350–65.
31. Sugerman PB, Savage NW, Zhou X, Walsh LJ, Bigby M. Oral lichen planus. Clin Dermatol. 2000;18(5):533–9.
32. Cheng Y-SL, Gould A, Kurago Z, Fantasia J, Muller S. Diagnosis of oral lichen planus: a position paper of the American Academy of Oral and maxillofacial pathology. Oral Surg Oral Med Oral Pathol Oral Radiol. 2016;122(3):332–54.
33. Eisen D. The therapy of oral lichen planus. Crit Rev Oral Biol Med. 1993;4(2):141–58. https://doi.org/10.1177/10454411930040020101.
34. Rojo-Moreno J, Bagán J, Rojo-Moreno J, Donat JS, Milián MA, Jiménez Y. Psychologic factors and oral lichen planus: a psychometric evaluation of 100 cases. Oral Surg Oral Med Oral Pathol Oral Radiol Endodontol. 1998;86(6):687–91.
35. Ballantyne JC, Fishman SM, Rathmell JP. Bonica's management of pain. Lippincott Williams & Wilkins; 2018.
36. Kaliakatsou F, Hodgson T, Lewsey J, Hegarty A, Murphy A, Porter S. Management of recalcitrant ulcerative oral lichen planus with topical tacrolimus. J Am Acad Dermatol. 2002;46(1):35–41.
37. Malhotra AK, Khaitan BK, Sethuraman G, Sharma VK. Betamethasone oral mini-pulse therapy compared with topical triamcinolone acetonide (0.1%) paste in oral lichen planus: a randomized comparative study. J Am Acad Dermatol. 2008;58(4):596–602.
38. Escudier M, Ahmed N, Shirlaw P, Setterfield J, Tappuni A, Black M, et al. A scoring system for mucosal disease severity with special reference to oral lichen planus. Br J Dermatol. 2007;157(4):765–70.
39. Piboonniyom S-o, Treister N, Pitiphat W, Woo S-B. Scoring system for monitoring oral lichenoid lesions: a preliminary study. Oral Surg Oral Med Oral Pathol Oral Radiol Endodontol. 2005;99(6):696–703.
40. Raj A, Sreelatha K, Balan A. Dapsone in the treatment of resistant oral erosive lichen planus: a clinical study. J Ind Academy Oral Med Radiol. 2012;24(1):20.
41. Carrozzo M, Gandolfo S. The management of oral lichen planus. Oral Dis. 1999;5(3):196–205.
42. Singh A, Rai A, Aftab M, Jain S, Singh M. Efficacy of steroidal vs non-steroidal agents in oral lichen planus: a randomised, open-label study. J Laryngol Otol. 2017;131(1):69–76.
43. Santonocito S, Polizzi A, De Pasquale R, Ronsivalle V, Lo Giudice A, Isola G. Analysis of the efficacy of two treatment protocols for patients with symptomatic Oral lichen planus: a randomized clinical trial. Int J Environ Res Public Health. 2021;18(1):56.
44. Polizzi A, Santonocito S, Lo Giudice A, Alibrandi A, De Pasquale R, Isola G. Analysis of the response to two pharmacological protocols in patients with oral lichen planus: a randomized clinical trial. Oral Dis. 2021;
45. Wang J, Van der Waal I. Disease scoring systems for oral lichen planus; a critical appraisal. Med Oral, Patol Oral Cir Bucal. 2015;20(2):e199.
46. Ismail SB, Kumar SK, Zain RB. Oral lichen planus and lichenoid reactions: etiopathogenesis, diagnosis, management and malignant transformation. J Oral Sci. 2007;49(2):89–106.
47. Scully C, El-Kom M. Lichen planus: review and update on pathogenesis. J Oral Pathol Med. 1985;14(6):431–58.
48. Gümrü B. A retrospective study of 370 patients with oral lichen planus in Turkey. Med Oral Patol Oral Cir Bucal. 2013;18(3):e427.
49. Mignogna MD, Russo LL, Fedele S. Gingival involvement of oral lichen planus in a series of 700 patients. J Clin Periodontol. 2005;32(10):1029–33.
50. Eisen D, Carrozzo M, Bagan Sebastian JV, Thongprasom K. Number V Oral lichen planus: clinical features and management. Oral Dis. 2005;11(6):338–49.
51. Gupta S, Jawanda MK. Oral lichen planus: an update on etiology, pathogenesis, clinical presentation, diagnosis and management. Indian J Dermatol. 2015;60(3):222.
52. Soni AG. Nikolsky's sign-a clinical method to evaluate damage at epidermal-dermal junction. J Ind Academy Oral Med Radiol. 2018;30(1):68.

53. Channual J, Wu JJ. The Nikolskiy sign. Arch Dermatol. 2008;144(9):1140. https://doi.org/10.1001/archderm.144.9.1140.
54. Seshadri D, Kumaran MS, Kanwar AJ. Acantholysis revisited: Back to basics. Ind J Dermatol Venereol Leprol. 2013;79(1)
55. Ganapati S. Eponymous dermatological signs in bullous dermatoses. Indian J Dermatol. 2014;59(1):21.
56. Urbano FL. Nikolsky's sign in autoimmune skin disorders. Hosp Physician. 2001;37:23–4.
57. Mignogna MD, Fortuna G, Leuci S, Ruoppo E, Marasca F, Matarasso S. Nikolsky's sign on the gingival mucosa: a clinical tool for oral health practitioners. J Periodontol. 2008;79(12):2241–6.
58. Uzun S, Durdu M. The specificity and sensitivity of Nikolskiy sign in the diagnosis of pemphigus. J Am Acad Dermatol. 2006;54(3):411–5.
59. Polifka M, Krusinski PA. The Nikolsky sign. Cutis. 1980;26(5):521–6.
60. Doubleday CW. Who is Nikolsky and what does his sign mean? J Am Acad Dermatol. 1987;16(5 Pt 1):1054–5.
61. Salopek T. Nikolsky's sign: is it 'dry'or is it 'wet'? Br J Dermatol. 1997;136(5):762–7.
62. Sachdev D. Sign of Nikolskiy & related signs. Ind J Dermatol Venereol Leprol. 2003;69:243–4.
63. Grando SA, Grando AA, Glukhenky BT, Doguzovc V, Nguyen VT, Holubar K. History and clinical significance of mechanical symptoms in blistering dermatoses: a reappraisal. J Am Acad Dermatol. 2003;48(1):86–92.
64. Mergoni G, Ergun S, Vescovi P, Mete Ö, Tanyeri H, Meleti M. Oral postinflammatory pigmentation: an analysis of 7 cases. 2011.
65. Müller S. Oral lichenoid lesions: distinguishing the benign from the deadly. Mod Pathol. 2017;30(1):S54–67.
66. Jorizzo JL, Salisbury PL, Rogers RS III, Goldsmith SM, Shar GG, Callen JP, et al. Oral lesions in systemic lupus erythematosus: do ulcerative lesions represent a necrotizing vasculitis? J Am Acad Dermatol. 1992;27(3):389–94.
67. Khudhur AS, Di Zenzo G, Carrozzo M. Oral lichenoid tissue reactions: diagnosis and classification. Expert Rev Mol Diagn. 2014;14(2):169–84.
68. Carrozzo M. Lichen planus orale: quale approccio? Stomatologia dermatologica. 2014:30–5.
69. Pindborg J. World Health Organization international histological classification of tumours. Histological typing of cancer and precancer of the oral mucosa. 1997;
70. Shklar G. Lichen planus as an oral ulcerative disease. Oral Surg Oral Med Oral Pathol. 1972;33(3):376–88.
71. Gorouhi F, Davari P, Fazel N. Cutaneous and mucosal lichen planus: a comprehensive review of clinical subtypes, risk factors, diagnosis, and prognosis. Sci World J. 2014;2014
72. Arora SK, Chhabra S, Saikia UN, Dogra S, Minz RW. Lichen planus: a clinical and immuno-histological analysis. Indian J Dermatol. 2014;59(3):257.
73. Payeras MR, Cherubini K, Figueiredo MA, Salum FG. Oral lichen planus: focus on etiopathogenesis. Arch Oral Biol. 2013;58(9):1057–69.
74. Hashimoto K. Apoptosis in lichen planus and several other dermatoses. Intra-epidermal cell death with filamentous degeneration. Acta Derm Venereol. 1976;56(3):187–210.
75. Weedon D. Apoptosis in lichen planus. Clin Exp Dermatol. 1980;5(4):425–30.
76. Dekker NP, Lozada-Nur F, Lagenaur LA, MacPhail LA, Bloom CY, Regezi JA. Apoptosis-associated markers in oral lichen planus. J Oral Pathol Med. 1997;26(4):170–5.
77. Shimizu M, Higaki Y, Higaki M, Kawashima M. The role of granzyme B-expressing CD8-positive T cells in apoptosis of keratinocytes in lichen planus. Arch Dermatol Res. 1997;289(9):527–32.
78. Haapalainen T, Oksala O, Kallioinen M, Oikarinen A, Larjava H, Salo T. Destruction of the epithelial anchoring system in lichen planus. J Investig Dermatol. 1995;105(1):100–3.
79. Aguirre-Urizar JM, Alberdi-Navarro J, de Mendoza IL-I, Marichalar-Mendia X, Martínez-Revilla B, Parra-Pérez C, et al. Clinicopathological and prognostic characterization of oral lichenoid disease and its main subtypes: a series of 384 cases. Med Oral, Patol Oral Cir Bucal. 2020;25(4):e554.
80. Patterson J. The lichenoid reaction pattern ("interface dermatitis"). Weedon's Skin Pathol. 2016;4:37–80.
81. Mutafchieva MZ, Draganova-Filipova MN, Zagorchev PI, Tomov GT. Oral lichen planus–known and unknown: a review. Folia Med (Plovdiv). 2018;60(4):528–35.
82. Fitzpatrick SG, Honda KS, Sattar A, Hirsch SA. Histologic lichenoid features in oral dysplasia and squamous cell carcinoma. Oral Surg Oral Med Oral Pathol Oral Radiol. 2014;117(4):511–20.
83. Krutchkoff DJ, Eisenberg E. Lichenoid dysplasia: a distinct histopathologic entity. Oral Surg Oral Med Oral Pathol. 1985;60(3):308–15.
84. Giuliani M, Troiano G, Cordaro M, Corsalini M, Gioco G, Lo Muzio L, et al. Rate of malignant transformation of oral lichen planus: a systematic review. Oral Dis. 2019;25(3):693–709.
85. Kramer I. Definition of leukoplakia and related lesions: an aid to studies on oral precancer. Oral Surg Oral Med Oral Pathol. 1978;46:518–39.
86. Van der Meij E, Reibel J, Slootweg P, Van der Wal J, De Jong W, Van der Waal I. Interobserver and intraobserver variability in the histologic assessment of oral lichen planus. J Oral Pathol Med. 1999;28(6):274–7.
87. Van der Meij E, Schepman K, Plonait D, Axéll T, Van der Waal I. Interobserver and intraobserver variability in the clinical assessment of oral lichen planus. J Oral Pathol Med. 2002;31(2):95–8.
88. Onofre MA, Sposto M, Navarro CM, Motta M, Turatti E, Almeida R. Potentially malignant epithe-

lial oral lesions: discrepancies between clinical and histological diagnosis. Oral Dis. 1997;3(3):148–52.
89. Van der Meij E, Van der Waal I. Lack of clinico-pathologic correlation in the diagnosis of oral lichen planus based on the presently available diagnostic criteria and suggestions for modifications. J Oral Pathol Med. 2003;32(9):507–12.
90. Rad M, Hashemipoor MA, Mojtahedi A, Zarei MR, Chamani G, Kakoei S, et al. Correlation between clinical and histopathologic diagnoses of oral lichen planus based on modified WHO diagnostic criteria. Oral Surg Oral Med Oral Pathol Oral Radiol Endodontol. 2009;107(6):796–800.
91. Neville BW, Damm DD, Allen C, Chi AC. Oral and maxillofacial pathology. Elsevier Health Sciences; 2015.
92. Reibel J, Sghiödt M. Immunohistochemical studies on colloid bodies (Civatte bodies) in oral lesions of discoid lupus erythematosus. Eur J Oral Sci. 1986;94(6):536–44.
93. Joshi R. Interface dermatitis. Indian J Dermatol Venereol Leprol. 2013;79(3):349–59. https://doi.org/10.4103/0378-6323.110780.
94. Scully C, Bagan J-V. Adverse drug reactions in the orofacial region. Crit Rev Oral Biol Med. 2004;15(4):221–39.
95. Al-Hashimi I, Schifter M, Lockhart PB, Wray D, Brennan M, Migliorati CA, et al. Oral lichen planus and oral lichenoid lesions: diagnostic and therapeutic considerations. Oral Surg Oral Med Oral Pathol Oral Radiol Endodontol. 2007;103:S25.e1. S.e12
96. Carrozzo M, Porter S, Mercadante V, Fedele S. Oral lichen planus: a disease or a spectrum of tissue reactions? Types, causes, diagnostic algorhythms, prognosis, management strategies. Periodontology 2000. 2019;80(1):105–25.
97. Van der Meij E, Mast H, van der Waal I. The possible premalignant character of oral lichen planus and oral lichenoid lesions: a prospective five-year follow-up study of 192 patients. Oral Oncol. 2007;43(8):742–8.
98. Van Dis M, van der Meij E, Schepman K, Smeele L, van der Wal J, Bezemer P, et al. A review of the recent literature regarding malignant transformation of oral lichen planus. Oral Surg Oral Med Oral Pathol Oral Radiol Endodontol. 1999;88(3):307–10.
99. McParland H, Warnakulasuriya S. Oral lichenoid contact lesions to mercury and dental amalgam—a review. J Biomed Biotechnol. 2012;2012
100. Reichart PA, Warnakulasuriya S. Oral lichenoid contact lesions induced by areca nut and betel quid chewing: a mini review. J Investig Clin Dent. 2012;3(3):163–6.
101. Farah CS, Balasubramaniam R, McCullough MJ. Contemporary oral medicine: a comprehensive approach to clinical practice. Springer; 2019.
102. Mutasim DF, Adams BB. Immunofluorescence in dermatology. J Am Acad Dermatol. 2001;45(6):803–24.
103. Suresh L, Neiders ME. Definitive and differential diagnosis of desquamative gingivitis through direct immunofluorescence studies. J Periodontol. 2012;83(10):1270–8. https://doi.org/10.1902/jop.2012.110627.
104. Morrison LH. Direct immunofluorescence microscopy in the diagnosis of autoimmune bullous dermatoses. Clin Dermatol. 2001;19(5):607–13. https://doi.org/10.1016/s0738-081x(00)00179-6.
105. Helander SD, Rogers RS III. The sensitivity and specificity of direct immunofluorescence testing in disorders of mucous membranes. J Am Acad Dermatol. 1994;30(1):65–75.
106. Kulthanan K, Jiamton S, Varothai S, Pinkaew S, Sutthipinittharm P. Direct immunofluorescence study in patients with lichen planus. Int J Dermatol. 2007;46(12):1237–41.
107. Abell E, Presbury D, Marks R, Ramnarain D. The diagnostic significance of immunoglobulin and fibrin deposition in lichen planus. Br J Dermatol. 1975;93(1):17–24.
108. Crincoli V, Di Bisceglie MB, Scivetti M, Lucchese A, Tecco S, Festa F. Oral lichen planus: update on etiopathogenesis, diagnosis and treatment. Immunopharmacol Immunotoxicol. 2011;33(1):11–20.
109. Bermejo-Fenoll A, López-Jornet P. Familial oral lichen planus: presentation of six families. Oral Surg Oral Med Oral Pathol Oral Radiol Endodontol. 2006;102(2):e12–e5.
110. Sivolella S, Berengo M, Cernuschi S, Valente M. Diode laser treatment is effective for plaque-like lichen planus of the tongue: a case report. Lasers Med Sci. 2012;27(2):521–4.
111. Daniels TE, Quadra-White C. Direct immunofluorescence in oral mucosal disease: a diagnostic analysis of 130 cases. Oral Surg Oral Med Oral Pathol. 1981;51(1):38–47.
112. Laskaris G, Sklavounou A, Angelopoulos A. Direct immunofluorescence in oral lichen planus. Oral Surg Oral Med Oral Pathol. 1982;53(5):483–7.
113. Firth NA, Rich AM, Radden BG, Reade PC. Direct immunofluorescence of oral mucosal biopsies: a comparison of fresh-frozen tissue and formalin-fixed, paraffin-embedded tissue. J Oral Pathol Med. 1992;21(8):358–63.
114. Raghu AR, Nirmala NR, Sreekumaran N. Direct immunofluorescence in oral lichen planus and oral lichenoid reactions. Quintessence Int. 2002;33(3)
115. Camisa C, Neff JC, Olsen RG. Use of indirect immunofluorescence in the lupus erythematosus/lichen planus overlap syndrome: an additional diagnostic clue. J Am Acad Dermatol. 1984;11(6):1050–9.
116. Inalöz H, Chowdhury M, Motley R. Lupus erythematosus/lichen planus overlap syndrome with scarring alopecia. J Eur Acad Dermatol Venereol. 2001;15(2):171–4.
117. Montague L, Bhattacharyya I, Islam M, Cohen D, Fitzpatrick S. Direct immunofluorescence testing results in cases of premalignant and malignant oral lesions. Oral Surg Oral Med Oral Pathol Oral Radiol. 2015;119(6):675–83.

118. Watanabe C, Hayashi T, Kawada A. Immunofluorescence study of drug-induced lichen planus-like lesions. J Dermatol. 1981;8(6):473–7.
119. Aoki V, Sousa JX Jr, Fukumori LM, Périgo AM, Freitas EL, Oliveira ZN. Direct and indirect immunofluorescence. An Bras Dermatol. 2010;85: 490–500.
120. Woodley DT. Immunofluorescence on salt-split skin for the diagnosis of epidermolysis bullosa acquisita. Arch Dermatol. 1990;126(2):229–31.
121. Kneisel A, Hertl M. Autoimmune bullous skin diseases. Part 2: diagnosis and therapy. JDDG: Journal der Deutschen Dermatologischen Gesellschaft. 2011;9(11):927–47.
122. Mahoney MG, Wang Z, Rothenberger K, Koch PJ, Amagai M, Stanley JR. Explanations for the clinical and microscopic localization of lesions in pemphigus foliaceus and vulgaris. J Clin Invest. 1999;103(4):461–8.
123. Chan LS, Ahmed AR, Anhalt GJ, Bernauer W, Cooper KD, Elder MJ, et al. The first international consensus on mucous membrane pemphigoid: definition, diagnostic criteria, pathogenic factors, medical treatment, and prognostic indicators. Arch Dermatol. 2002;138(3):370–9.
124. Betts A, Yeoman C, Farthing P. Oral mucosal involvement as the sole or main manifestation of linear IgA disease: case report and review of the literature. Oral Surg. 2009;2(4):198–204.
125. Lin S-C, Sun A, Wu Y-C, Chiang C-P. Presence of anti-basal cell antibodies in oral lichen planus. J Am Acad Dermatol. 1992;26(6):943–7.
126. Van Joost T. Incidence of circulating antibodies reactive with basal cells of skin in drug reactions. Acta Derm Venereol. 1974;54(3):183–7.
127. McQueen A, Behan WM. Immunofluorescence microscopy the "string of pearls" phenomenon—an immunofluorescent serological finding in patients screened for adverse drug reactions. Am J Dermatopathol. 1982;4(2):155–60.
128. Ishii K, Amagai M, Hall RP, Hashimoto T, Takayanagi A, Gamou S, et al. Characterization of autoantibodies in pemphigus using antigen-specific enzyme-linked immunosorbent assays with baculovirus-expressed recombinant desmogleins. J Immunol. 1997;159(4):2010–7.
129. Sárdy M, Kostaki D, Varga R, Peris K, Ruzicka T. Comparative study of direct and indirect immunofluorescence and of bullous pemphigoid 180 and 230 enzyme-linked immunosorbent assays for diagnosis of bullous pemphigoid. J Am Acad Dermatol. 2013;69(5):748–53.
130. Sugerman P, Satterwhite K, Bigby M. Autocytotoxic T-cell clones in lichen planus. Br J Dermatol. 2000;142(3):449–56.
131. Shekar C, Ganesan S. Oral lichen planus: review. J Dent Sci Res. 2011;2(1):62–87.
132. Lind PO, Hurlen B, Lyberg T, Aas E. Amalgam-related oral lichenoid reaction. Eur J Oral Sci. 1986;94(5):448–51.
133. Laine J, Kalimo K, Happonen RP. Contact allergy to dental restorative materials in patients with oral lichenoid lesions. Contact Dermatitis. 1997;36(3):141–6.
134. Chang JYF, Chiang CP, Hsiao CK, Sun A. Significantly higher frequencies of presence of serum autoantibodies in Chinese patients with oral lichen planus. J Oral Pathol Med. 2009;38(1):48–54.
135. Lin HP, Wang YP, Chia JS, Chiang CP, Sun A. Modulation of serum gastric parietal cell antibody level by levamisole and vitamin B12 in oral lichen planus. Oral Dis. 2011;17(1):95–101.
136. Rai B, Kharb S, Jain R, Anand S. Salivary lipid peroxidation product malonaldehyde in various dental diseases. World J Med Sci. 2006;1(2):100–1.
137. Shirzad A, Pouramir M, Seyedmajidi M, Jenabian N, Bijani A, Motallebnejad M. Salivary total antioxidant capacity and lipid peroxidation in patients with erosive oral lichen planus. J Dent Res, Dent Clin, Dent Prospect. 2014;8(1):35.
138. Halliwell B. Free radicals and antioxidants: updating a personal view. Nutr Rev. 2012;70(5):257–65.
139. Halliwell B. Antioxidants in human health and disease. Annu Rev Nutr. 1996;16(1):33–50.
140. Dormandy T. An approach to free radicals. Lancet. 1983;322(8357):1010–4.
141. Ergun S, Troşala ŞC, Warnakulasuriya S, Özel S, Önal AE, Ofluoğlu D, et al. Evaluation of oxidative stress and antioxidant profile in patients with oral lichen planus. J Oral Pathol Med. 2011;40(4):286–93.
142. Rai B, Kaur J, Jacobs R, Singh J. Possible action mechanism for curcumin in pre-cancerous lesions based on serum and salivary markers of oxidative stress. J Oral Sci. 2010;52(2):251–6.
143. Sistig S, Vučićević-Boras V, Lukač J, Kusić Z. Salivary IgA and IgG subclasses in oral mucosal diseases. Oral Dis. 2002;8(6):282–6.
144. Ghalayani P, Razavi SM, Gholami D. Comparative study of number and distribution of IgG+ cells in oral lichen planus and oral lichenoid lesions. Dent Res J. 2009;6(1):1.
145. Sato K. Enzyme-linked immunosorbent assay of SIgA in whole saliva of healthy subjects and patients with oral diseases. Bull Tokyo Med Dent Univ. 1991;38(2):9–18.
146. Nosratzehi T, ARBABI KF, Salimi S, Honarmand E. The evaluation of psychological factor and salivary cortisol and IgA levels in patients with oral lichen planus. 2014.
147. Sontheimer RD. Lichenoid tissue reaction/interface dermatitis: clinical and histological perspectives. J Investig Dermatol. 2009;129(5):1088–99.
148. Pinkus H. Lichenoid tissue reactions: a speculative review of the clinical spectrum of epidermal basal cell damage with special reference to erythema dyschromicum perstans. Arch Dermatol. 1973;107(6):840–6.
149. Yamauchi M, Moriyama M, Hayashida J-N, Maehara T, Ishiguro N, Kubota K, et al. Myeloid dendritic cells stimulated by thymic stromal lym-

phopoietin promote Th2 immune responses and the pathogenesis of oral lichen planus. PLoS One. 2017;12(3):e0173017.
150. Carrozzo M, Thorpe R. Oral lichen planus: a review. Minerva Stomatol. 2009;58(10):519–37.
151. Fitzpatrick SG, Hirsch SA, Gordon SC. The malignant transformation of oral lichen planus and oral lichenoid lesions: a systematic review. J Am Dent Assoc. 2014;145(1):45–56.
152. Calabresi V, Carrozzo M, Cozzani E, Arduino P, Bertolusso G, Tirone F, et al. Oral pemphigoid autoantibodies preferentially target BP180 ectodomain. Clin Immunol. 2007;122(2):207–13.
153. Carrozzo M. A reappraisal of diagnostic criteria for mucous membrane pemphigoid. J Oral Pathol Med. 2009;38(1):160.
154. Handley T, Ogden G. Dyskeratosis congenita: oral hyperkeratosis in association with lichenoid reaction. J Oral Pathol Med. 2006;35(8):508–12.
155. Tsushima F, Sakurai J, Shimizu R, Kayamori K, Harada H. Oral lichenoid contact lesions related to dental metal allergy may resolve after allergen removal. J Dent Sci. 2022;17(3):1300–6. https://doi.org/10.1016/j.jds.2021.11.008.
156. Müller S. The lichenoid tissue reactions of the Oral mucosa: Oral lichen planus and other lichenoid lesions. Surg Pathol Clin. 2011;4(4):1005–26.
157. Issa Y, Duxbury A, Macfarlane T, Brunton P. Oral lichenoid lesions related to dental restorative materials. Br Dent J. 2005;198(6):361–6.
158. Thornhill MH, Sankar V, Xu XJ, Barrett AW, High AS, Odell EW, et al. The role of histopathological characteristics in distinguishing amalgam-associated oral lichenoid reactions and oral lichen planus. J Oral Pathol Med. 2006;35(4):233–40.
159. Müller S. Oral manifestations of dermatologic disease: a focus on lichenoid lesions. Head Neck Pathol. 2011;5(1):36–40.
160. Allen CM, Blozis GG. Oral mucosal reactions to cinnamon-flavored chewing gum. J Am Dent Assoc. 1988;116(6):664–7.
161. Miller RL, Gould AR, Bernstein ML. Cinnamon-induced stomatitis venenata: clinical and characteristic histopathologic features. Oral Surg Oral Med Oral Pathol. 1992;73(6):708–16.
162. Schlosser BJ. Lichen planus and lichenoid reactions of the oral mucosa. Dermatol Ther. 2010;23(3):251–67.
163. Nyfeler B, Pichler W. The lymphocyte transformation test for the diagnosis of drug allergy: sensitivity and specificity. Clin Exp Allergy. 1997;27(2):175–81.
164. Von Blomberg-Van Der Flier M, Van Der Burg CK, Pos O, Van De Plassche-Boers EM, Bruynzeel DP, Garotta G, et al. In vitro studies in nickel allergy: diagnostic value of a dual parameter analysis. J Investig Dermatol. 1987;88(4):362–8.
165. Cederbrant K, Gunnarsson L-G, Hultman P, Norda R, Tibbling-Grahn L. In vitro lymphoproliferative assays with HgCl2 cannot identify patients with systemic symptoms attributed to dental amalgam. J Dent Res. 1999;78(8):1450–8.
166. Baccaglini L, Thongprasom K, Carrozzo M, Bigby M. Urban legends series: lichen planus. Oral Dis. 2013;19(2):128–43.
167. Thornhill MH, Pemberton MN, Simmons RK, Theaker ED. Amalgam-contact hypersensitivity lesions and oral lichen planus. Oral Surg Oral Med Oral Pathol Oral Radiol Endodontol. 2003;95(3):291–9.
168. Larsson Å, Warfvinge G. Oral lichenoid contact reactions may occasionally transform into malignancy. Eur J Cancer Prev. 2005;14(6):525–9.
169. Asarch A, Gottlieb AB, Lee J, Masterpol KS, Scheinman PL, Stadecker MJ, et al. Lichen planus–like eruptions: an emerging side effect of tumor necrosis factor-α antagonists. J Am Acad Dermatol. 2009;61(1):104–11.
170. Woo V, Bonks J, Borukhova L, Zegarelli D. Oral lichenoid drug eruption: a report of a pediatric case and review of the literature. Pediatr Dermatol. 2009;26(4):458–64.
171. Yuan A, Woo SB. Adverse drug events in the oral cavity. Oral Surg Oral Med Oral Pathol Oral Radiol. 2015;119(1):35–47. https://doi.org/10.1016/j.oooo.2014.09.009.
172. Friedman RS, Bangur CS, Zasloff EJ, Fan L, Wang T, Watanabe Y, et al. Molecular and immunological evaluation of the transcription factor SOX-4 as a lung tumor vaccine antigen. J Immunol. 2004;172(5):3319–27.
173. Jacobson JJ, Lamey P, McCartan B, MacDonald D, MacKie R. Basal cell cytoplasmic autoantibodies in oral lichenoid reactions. Oral Surg Oral Med Oral Pathol Oral Radiol Endodontol. 1995;79(1):44–9.
174. Lage D, Juliano PB, Metze K, Souza EM, Cintra ML. Lichen planus and lichenoid drug-induced eruption: a histological and immunohistochemical study. Int J Dermatol. 2012;51(10):1199–205.
175. McCartan B, McCreary C. Oral lichenoid drug eruptions. Oral Dis. 1997;3(2):58–63.
176. McCartan B, Lamey P-J. Lichen planus-specific antigen in oral lichen planus and oral lichenoid drug eruptions. Oral Surg Oral Med Oral Pathol Oral Radiol Endodontol. 2000;89(5):585–7.
177. Dickinson AM, Sviland L, Wang XN, Jackson G, Taylor PR, Dunn A, et al. Predicting graft-versus-host disease in HLA-identical bone marrow transplants: a comparison of T-cell frequency analysis and a human skin explant model. Transplantation. 1998;66(7):857–63.
178. Wang X-n, Collin M, Sviland L, Marshall S, Jackson G, Schulz U, et al. Skin explant model of human graft-versus-host disease: prediction of clinical outcome and correlation with biological risk factors. Biol Blood Marrow Transplant. 2006;12(2):152–9.
179. Demarosi F, Lodi G, Carrassi A, Moneghini L, Sarina B, Sardella A. Clinical and histopathological features of the oral mucosa in allogeneic haemato-

poietic stem cell transplantation patients. Exp Oncol. 2007;29(4):304–8.
180. Roy DC, Perreault C. Major vs minor histocompatibility antigens. Blood. 2017;129(6):664–6.
181. Vincent K, Roy D-C, Perreault C. Next-generation leukemia immunotherapy. Blood. 2011;118(11):2951–9.
182. Counce S, Smith P, Barth R, Snell GD. Strong and weak histocompatibility gene differences in mice and their role in the rejection of homografts of tumors and skin. Ann Surg. 1956; 144(2):198.
183. Filipovich AH. Diagnosis and manifestations of chronic graft-versus-host disease. Best Pract Res Clin Haematol. 2008;21(2):251–7.
184. Imanguli M, Alevizos I, Brown R, Pavletic S, Atkinson J. Oral graft-versus-host disease. Oral Dis. 2008;14(5):396–412.
185. Basara N, Blau W, Römer E, Rudolphi M, Bischoff M, Kirsten D, et al. Mycophenolate mofetil for the treatment of acute and chronic GVHD in bone marrow transplant patients. Bone Marrow Transplant. 1998;22(1):61–5.
186. Woo S-B, Lee SJ, Schubert MM. Graft-vs.-host disease. Crit Rev Oral Biol Med. 1997;8(2):201–16.
187. Demarosi F, Lodi G, Carrassi A, Soligo D, Sardella A. Oral malignancies following HSCT: graft versus host disease and other risk factors. Oral Oncol. 2005;41(9):865–77.
188. Kruse AL, Grätz KW. Oral carcinoma after hematopoietic stem cell transplantation–a new classification based on a literature review over 30 years. Head Neck Oncol. 2009;1(1):1–6.
189. Treister N, Duncan C, Cutler C, Lehmann L. How we treat oral chronic graft-versus-host disease. Blood. 2012;120(17):3407–18. https://doi.org/10.1182/blood-2012-05-393389.
190. Imanguli MM, Pavletic SZ, Guadagnini J-P, Brahim JS, Atkinson JC. Chronic graft versus host disease of oral mucosa: review of available therapies. Oral Surg Oral Med Oral Pathol Oral Radiol Endodontol. 2006;101(2):175–83.
191. Johnston LJ, Brown J, Shizuru JA, Stockerl-Goldstein KE, Stuart MJ, Blume KG, et al. Rapamycin (sirolimus) for treatment of chronic graft-versus-host disease. Biol Blood Marrow Transplant. 2005;11(1):47–55.
192. Dall'Amico R, Messina C. Extracorporeal photochemotherapy for the treatment of graft-versus-host disease. Ther Apher. 2002;6(4):296–304. https://doi.org/10.1046/j.1526-0968.2002.00448.x.
193. Parker PM, Chao N, Nademanee A, O'Donnell MR, Schmidt GM, Snyder DS, et al. Thalidomide as salvage therapy for chronic graft-versus-host disease. 1995.
194. Elad S, Or R, Garfunkel AA, Shapira MY. Budesonide: a novel treatment for oral chronic graft versus host disease. Oral Surg Oral Med Oral Pathol Oral Radiol Endodontol. 2003;95(3): 308–11.
195. Wolff D, Anders V, Corio R, Horn T, Morison W, Farmer E, et al. Oral PUVA and topical steroids for treatment of oral manifestations of chronic graft-vs.-host disease. Photodermatol Photoimmunol Photomed. 2004;20(4):184–90.
196. Epstein J, Reece D. Topical cyclosporin a for treatment of oral chronic graft-versus-host disease. Bone Marrow Transplant. 1994;13(1):81–6.
197. Epstein J, Nantel S, Sheoltch S. Topical azathioprine in the combined treatment of chronic oral graft-versus-host disease. Bone Marrow Transplant. 2000;25(6):683–7.
198. Epstein J, Gorsky M, Epstein M, Nantel S. Topical azathioprine in the treatment of immune-mediated chronic oral inflammatory conditions: a series of cases. Oral Surg Oral Med Oral Pathol Oral Radiol Endodontol. 2001;91(1):56–61.
199. Choi CJ, Nghiem P. Tacrolimus ointment in the treatment of chronic cutaneous graft-vs-host disease: a case series of 18 patients. Arch Dermatol. 2001;137(9):1202–6.
200. Lodi G, Scully C, Carrozzo M, Griffiths M, Sugerman PB, Thongprasom K. Current controversies in oral lichen planus: report of an international consensus meeting. Part 2. Clinical management and malignant transformation. Oral Surg Oral Med Oral Pathol Oral Radiol Endodontol. 2005;100(2):164–78.
201. Scully C, Eisen D, Carrozzo M. Management of oral lichen planus. Am J Clin Dermatol. 2000;1(5):287–306.
202. Lindelöf B, Sigurgeirsson B, Tegner E, Larkö O, Johannesson A, Berne B, et al. PUVA and cancer: a large-scale epidemiological study. Lancet. 1991;338(8759):91–3.
203. Bandow GD, Koo J. Narrow-band ultraviolet B radiation: a review of the current literature. Int J Dermatol. 2004;43(8):555–61.
204. Elad S, Or R, Shapira M, Haviv A, Galili D, Garfunkel A, et al. CO2 laser in oral graft-versus-host disease: a pilot study. Bone Marrow Transplant. 2003;32(10):1031–4.
205. Epstein JB, Raber-Durlacher JE, Lill M, Linhares YP, Chang J, Barasch A, et al. Photobiomodulation therapy in the management of chronic oral graft-versus-host disease. Support Care Cancer. 2017;25(2):357–64.
206. Picardi A, Ferraro A, Miranda M, Meconi F, Lanti A, Adorno G, et al. Therapeutic efficiency of platelet gel for the treatment of oral ulcers related to chronic graft versus host disease after allogeneic haematopoietic stem cell transplantation. Oral Implantol. 2017;10(4):398.
207. Thongprasom K, Carrozzo M, Furness S, Lodi G. Interventions for treating oral lichen planus. Cochrane Database Syst Rev. 2011;7
208. Holmstrup P, Schiøtz AW, Westergaard J. Effect of dental plaque control on gingival lichen planus. Oral Surg Oral Med Oral Pathol. 1990;69(5):585–90.
209. Modica R, Preti G, Defabianis P. Trattato di odontoiatria clinica. Minerva Med. 2004;

210. Hammers CM, Stanley JR. Mechanisms of disease: pemphigus and bullous pemphigoid. Ann Rev Pathol. 2016;11:175–97.
211. Bascones-Martinez A, Munoz-Corcuera M, Bascones-Ilundain C, Esparza-Gómez G. Oral manifestations of pemphigus vulgaris: clinical presentation, differential diagnosis and management. J Clin Exp Dermatol Res. 2010;1(112):2.
212. Budimir J, Lugović Mihić L, Šitum M, Bulat V, Peršić S, Tomljanović-Veselski M. Oral lesions in patients with pemphigus vulgaris and bullous pemphigoid. Acta Clin Croat. 2008;47(1):18.
213. Waschke J. The desmosome and pemphigus. Histochem Cell Biol. 2008;130(1):21–54.
214. Black M, Mignogna M, Scully C. Number II pemphigus vulgaris. Oral Dis. 2005;11(3):119–30.
215. Ariyawardana A, Tilakaratne W, Dissanayake M, Vitanaarachchi N, Basnayake L, Sitheeque M, et al. Oral pemphigus vulgaris in children and adolescents: a review of the literature and a case report. Int J Paediatr Dent. 2005;15(4):287–93.
216. Shamim T, Varghese VI, Shameena PM, Sudha S. Pemphigus vulgaris in oral cavity: clinical analysis of 71 cases. 2008.
217. Cekić-Arambašin A, Vidas I, Topić B, Alajbeg I, Boras VV, Biočina-Lukenda D, et al. Oralna medicina. Školska knjiga. 2005;
218. Dagistan S, Goregen M, Miloglu O, Çakur B. Oral pemphigus vulgaris: a case report with review of the literature. J Oral Sci. 2008;50(3):359–62.
219. Scully C, Mignogna M. Oral mucosal disease: pemphigus. Br J Oral Maxillofac Surg. 2008;46(4):272–7.
220. Lagha NB, Poulesquen V, Roujeau J-C, Alantar A, Maman L. Pemphigus vulgaris: a case-based update. J Can Dent Assoc. 2005;71(9)
221. Suárez-Fernández R, España-Alonso A, Herrero-González J, Mascaró-Galy J. Manejo práctico de las enfermedades ampollosas autoinmunes más frecuentes. Actas Dermosifiliogr. 2008;99(6):441–55.
222. Prajapati V, Mydlarski P. Advances in pemphigus therapy. Skin. 2008;25
223. Ruocco E, Baroni A, Wolf R, Ruocco V. Life-threatening bullous dermatoses: Pemphigus vulgaris. Clin Dermatol. 2005;23(3):223–6.
224. Bystryn J-C, Rudolph JL. Pemphigus. Lancet. 2005;366(9479):61–73.
225. Mutasim DF, Pelc NJ, Anhalt GJ. Drug-induced pemphigus. Dermatol Clin. 1993;11(3):463–71.
226. Brenner S, Wolf R. Possible nutritional factors in induced pemphigus. Dermatology. 1994;189(4):337–9.
227. Da Silva K, Mandel L. Early manifestation of pemphigus vulgaris: a case report. N Y State Dent J. 2007;73(3):42.
228. Camacho-Alonso F, López-Jornet P, Bermejo-Fenoll A, Pemphigus vulgaris. A presentation of 14 cases and review of the literature. Med Oral Patol Oral Cir Bucal. 2005;10(4):282–8.
229. Bascones-Martínez A, Figuero-Ruiz E, Esparza-Gómez GC. Oral ulcers. Med Clin. 2005;125(15):590–7.
230. Dadras MS, Qeisari M, Givrad S. Pemphigus vulgaris manifesting as a sole persistent lesion on the lower lip: a case report. Dermatol Online J. 2009;15(6)
231. Braun-Falco O, Plewig G, Wolff HH, Burgdorf WH. Blistering diseases. Dermatol Springer. 2000:649–95.
232. Durdu M, Seçkin D, Baba M. The Tzanck smear test: rediscovery of a practical diagnostic tool. Skinmed. 2011;9(1):23–32.
233. Mehrotra R, Gupta A, Singh M, Ibrahim R. Application of cytology and molecular biology in diagnosing premalignant or malignant oral lesions. Mol Cancer. 2006;5(1):1–9.
234. Hammers CMLL, Schmidt E, Zillikens D. Contemporary management of pemphigus. Orphan Drugs: Expert Opin; 2013.
235. Almugairen N, Hospital V, Bedane C, Duvert-Lehembre S, Picard D, Tronquoy A-F, et al. Assessment of the rate of long-term complete remission off therapy in patients with pemphigus treated with different regimens including medium-and high-dose corticosteroids. J Am Acad Dermatol. 2013;69(4):583–8.
236. Beissert S, Mimouni D, Kanwar AJ, Solomons N, Kalia V, Anhalt GJ. Treating pemphigus vulgaris with prednisone and mycophenolate mofetil: a multicenter, randomized, placebo-controlled trial. J Investig Dermatol. 2010;130(8): 2041–8.
237. Progression NLR, Pacients L-R. Treatment of pemphigus and pemphigoids. Med Oral Patol Oral Cir Bucal. 2005;10:410–1.
238. Murrell DF, Dick S, Ahmed A, Amagai M, Barnadas MA, Borradori L, et al. Consensus statement on definitions of disease, end points, and therapeutic response for pemphigus. J Am Acad Dermatol. 2008;58(6):1043–6.
239. Turner MS, Sutton D, Sauder DN. The use of plasmapheresis and immunosuppression in the treatment of pemphigus vulgaris. J Am Acad Dermatol. 2000;43(6):1058–64.
240. Kasperkiewicz M, Shimanovich I, Meier M, Schumacher N, Westermann L, Kramer J, et al. Treatment of severe pemphigus with a combination of immunoadsorption, rituximab, pulsed dexamethasone and azathioprine/mycophenolate mofetil: a pilot study of 23 patients. Br J Dermatol. 2012;166(1):154–60.
241. Colliou N, Picard D, Caillot F, Calbo S, Le Corre S, Lim A, et al. Long-term remissions of severe pemphigus after rituximab therapy are associated with prolonged failure of desmoglein B cell response. Sci Transl Med. 2013;5(175):175ra30-ra30.
242. Mouquet H, Musette P, Gougeon M-L, Jacquot S, Lemercier B, Lim A, et al. B-cell depletion immunotherapy in pemphigus: effects on cellular and humoral immune responses. J Investig Dermatol. 2008;128(12):2859–69.
243. Ahmed AR, Spigelman Z, Cavacini LA, Posner MR. Treatment of pemphigus vulgaris with ritux-

imab and intravenous immune globulin. N Engl J Med. 2006;355(17):1772–9.
244. Joly P, Mouquet H, Roujeau J-C, D'Incan M, Gilbert D, Jacquot S, et al. A single cycle of rituximab for the treatment of severe pemphigus. N Engl J Med. 2007;357(6):545–52.
245. Ahmed AR, Maize JC, Provost TT. Bullous pemphigoid: clinical and immunologic follow-up after successful therapy. Arch Dermatol. 1977;113(8):1043–6.
246. Liu HNH, Su WD, Rogers RS III. Clinical variants of pemphigoid. Int J Dermatol. 1986;25(1):17–27.
247. Goodman SR. Chapter 6–cell adhesion and the extracellular matrix. In: Goodman SR, editor. Medical Cell Biology. 3rd ed. San Diego: Academic Press; 2008. p. 191–225.
248. Zhang J, Wang G. Genetic predisposition to bullous pemphigoid. J Dermatol Sci. 2020;100(2):86–91. https://doi.org/10.1016/j.jdermsci.2020.05.010.
249. Lever W. Medicine (Baltimore). Pemphigus. 1953;32:1–123.
250. Schmidt E, Zillikens D. Pemphigoid diseases. Lancet. 2013;381(9863):320–32.
251. Korman NJ. Bullous pemphigoid: the latest in diagnosis, prognosis, and therapy. Arch Dermatol. 1998;134(9):1137–41.
252. Lever WF. Pemphigus and pemphigoid. A review of the advances made since 1964. J Am Acad Dermatol. 1979;1(1):2–31. https://doi.org/10.1016/s0190-9622(79)80050-x.
253. Ohki M, Kikuchi S, Ohata A, Baba Y, Ishikawa J, Sugimoto H. Features of oral, pharyngeal, and laryngeal lesions in bullous pemphigoid. ENT: Ear, Nose Throat J. 2016:95.
254. Pfaltz K, Mertz K, Rose C, Scheidegger P, Pfaltz M, Kempf W. C3d immunohistochemistry on formalin-fixed tissue is a valuable tool in the diagnosis of bullous pemphigoid of the skin. J Cutan Pathol. 2010;37(6):654–8.
255. Kwon EJ, Ntiamoah P, Shulman KJ. The utility of C4d immunohistochemistry on formalin-fixed paraffin-embedded tissue in the distinction of polymorphic eruption of pregnancy from pemphigoid gestationis. Am J Dermatopathol. 2013;35(8):787–91.
256. Hall RP 3rd, Streilein RD, Hannah DL, McNair PD, Fairley JA, Ronaghy A, et al. Association of serum B-cell activating factor level and proportion of memory and transitional B cells with clinical response after rituximab treatment of bullous pemphigoid patients. J Invest Dermatol. 2013;133(12):2786–8.
257. Kenneth KY, Crew AB, Messingham KA, Fairley JA, Woodley DT. Omalizumab therapy for bullous pemphigoid. J Am Acad Dermatol. 2014;71(3):468–74.
258. Zaraa I, Mahfoudh A, Sellami MK, Chelly I, El Euch D, Zitouna M, et al. Lichen planus pemphigoides: four new cases and a review of the literature. Int J Dermatol. 2013;52(4):406–12.
259. Papara C, Danescu S, Sitaru C, Baican A. Challenges and pitfalls between lichen planus pemphigoides and bullous lichen planus. Australas J Dermatol. 2022;
260. Solomon LW, Helm TN, Stevens C, Neiders ME, Kumar V. Clinical and immunopathologic findings in oral lichen planus pemphigoides. Oral Surg Oral Med Oral Pathol Oral Radiol Endodontol. 2007;103(6):808–13.
261. Washio K, Nakamura A, Fukuda S, Hashimoto T, Horikawa T. A case of lichen planus pemphigoides successfully treated with a combination of cyclosporine a and prednisolone. Case Rep Dermatol. 2013;5(1):84–7.
262. Cohen DM, Ben-Amitai D, Feinmesser M, Zvulunov A. Childhood lichen planus pemphigoides: a case report and review of the literature. Pediatr Dermatol. 2009;26(5):569–74.
263. Sultan A, Stojanov IJ, Lerman MA, Kabani S, Haber J, Freedman J, et al. Oral lichen planus pemphigoides: a series of four cases. Oral Surg Oral Med Oral Pathol Oral Radiol. 2015;120(1):58–68.
264. Mignogna MD, Fortuna G, Leuci S, Stasio L, Mezza E, Ruoppo E. Lichen planus pemphigoides, a possible example of epitope spreading. Oral Surg Oral Med Oral Pathol Oral Radiol Endodontol. 2010;109(6):837–43.
265. Ben Salem C, Chenguel L, Ghariani N, Denguezli M, Hmouda H, Bouraoui K. Captopril-induced lichen planus pemphigoides. Pharmacoepidemiol Drug Saf. 2008;17(7):722–4.
266. Shah RR, Bhate C, Hernandez A, Ho CH. Lichen planus Pemphigoides: a unique form of bullous and lichenoid eruptions secondary to nivolumab. Dermatol Ther. 2022:e15432.
267. Zhu YI, Fitzpatrick JE, Kornfeld BW. Lichen planus pemphigoides associated with ramipril. Int J Dermatol. 2006;45(12):1453–5. https://doi.org/10.1111/j.1365-4632.2006.02711.x.
268. Stoebner PE, Michot C, Ligeron C, Durand L, Meynadier J, Meunier L. Simvastatin-induced lichen planus pemphigoides. Ann Dermatol Venereol. 2003;130(2 Pt 1):187–90.
269. Xu HH, Xiao T, He CD, Jin GY, Wang YK, Gao XH, et al. Lichen planus pemphigoides associated with Chinese herbs. Clin Exp Dermatol. 2009;34(3):329–32. https://doi.org/10.1111/j.1365-2230.2008.02900.x.
270. Kuramoto N, Kishimoto S, Shibagaki R, Yasuno H. PUVA-induced lichen planus pemphigoides. Br J Dermatol. 2000;142(3):509–12. https://doi.org/10.1046/j.1365-2133.2000.03366.x.
271. İlknur T, Akarsu S, Uzun S, Özer E, Fetil E. Heterogeneous disease: a child case of lichen planus pemphigoides triggered by varicella. J Dermatol. 2011;38(7):707–10. https://doi.org/10.1111/j.1346-8138.2011.01220.x.
272. Hamada T, Fujimoto W, Okazaki F, Asagoe K, Arata J, Iwatsuki K. Lichen planus pemphigoides and multiple keratoacanthomas associated with colon adenocarcinoma. Br J Dermatol. 2004;151(1):252–4. https://doi.org/10.1111/j.1365-2133.2004.06074.x.
273. Maoz KB, Brenner S. Lichen planus pemphigoides triggered by narrowband UVB, paracetamol,

and ibuprofen, with autoantibodies to 130kDa antigen. Skinmed. 2008;7(1):33–6. https://doi.org/10.1111/j.1540-9740.2007.07667.x.
274. Noël B. Lupus erythematosus and other autoimmune diseases related to statin therapy: a systematic review. J Eur Acad Dermatol Venereol. 2007;21(1):17–24. https://doi.org/10.1111/j.1468-3083.2006.01838.x.
275. Tamada Y, Yokochi K, Nitta Y, Ikeya T, Hara K, Owaribe K. Lichen planus pemphigoides: identification of 180 kd hemidesmosome antigen. J Am Acad Dermatol. 1995;32(5 Pt 2):883–7. https://doi.org/10.1016/0190-9622(95)91554-0.
276. Zillikens D, Caux F, Mascaro JM, Wesselmann U, Schmidt E, Prost C, et al. Autoantibodies in lichen planus pemphigoides react with a novel epitope within the C-terminal NC16A domain of BP180. J Invest Dermatol. 1999;113(1):117–21. https://doi.org/10.1046/j.1523-1747.1999.00618.x.
277. Genovese G, Di Zenzo G, Cozzani E, Berti E, Cugno M, Marzano AV. New insights into the pathogenesis of bullous pemphigoid: 2019 update. Front Immunol. 2019;10:1506.
278. Sekiya A, Kodera M, Yamaoka T, Iwata Y, Usuda T, Ohzono A, et al. A case of lichen planus pemphigoides with autoantibodies to the NC 16a and C-terminal domains of BP 180 and to desmoglein-1. Br J Dermatol. 2014;171(5):1230–5.
279. Chan WMM, Lee JSS, Theng CST, Chua SH, Oon HHB. Narrowband UVB-induced lichen planus pemphigoide. Dermatol Rep. 2011;3(3)
280. Yoon KH, Kim SC, Kang DS, Lee IJ. Lichen planus pemphigoides with circulating autoantibodies against 200 and 180 kDa epidermal antigens. Eur J Dermatol. 2000;10(3):212–4.
281. Lee JB, Liu Y, Hashimoto T. Cicatricial pemphigoid sera specifically react with the most C-terminal portion of BP180. J Dermatol Sci. 2003;32(1):59–64.
282. Vanderlugt CL, Miller SD. Epitope spreading in immune-mediated diseases: implications for immunotherapy. Nat Rev Immunol. 2002;2(2):85–95.
283. Vanderlugt CJ, Miller SD. Epitope spreading. Curr Opin Immunol. 1996;8(6):831–6.
284. Chan LS, Vanderlugt CJ, Hashimoto T, Nishikawa T, Zone JJ, Black MM, et al. Epitope spreading: lessons from autoimmune skin diseases. J Investig Dermatol. 1998;110(2):103–9.
285. Salato VK, Hacker-Foegen MK, Lazarova Z, Fairley JA, Lin M-S. Role of intramolecular epitope spreading in pemphigus vulgaris. Clin Immunol. 2005;116(1):54–64.
286. Li N, Aoki V, Hans-Filho G, Rivitti EA, Diaz LA. The role of intramolecular epitope spreading in the pathogenesis of endemic pemphigus foliaceus (fogo selvagem). J Exp Med. 2003;197(11):1501–10.
287. You S, Chatenoud L. Proinsulin: a unique autoantigen triggering autoimmune diabetes. J Clin Invest. 2006;116(12):3108–10.
288. Herrero-González JE, Parera Amer E, Segura S, Mas Bosch V, Pujol RM, Martinez Escala ME. Epithelial antigenic specificities of circulating autoantibodies in mucosal lichen planus. Int J Dermatol. 2016;55(6):634–9.
289. Baldo M, Bailey A, Bhogal B, Groves R, Ogg G, Wojnarowska F. T cells reactive with the NC16A domain of BP180 are present in vulval lichen sclerosus and lichen planus. J Eur Acad Dermatol Venereol. 2010;24(2):186–90.
290. Schmidt T, Solimani F, Pollmann R, Stein R, Schmidt A, Stulberg I, et al. TH1/TH17 cell recognition of desmoglein 3 and bullous pemphigoid antigen 180 in patients with lichen planus. J Allergy Clin Immunol. 2018;142(2):669–72. e7
291. Sapadin AN, Phelps RG, Fellner MJ, Kantor I. Lichen planus pemphigoides presenting with a strikingly unilateral distribution. Int J Dermatol. 1998;37(12):934–48.
292. Barnadas M, Roé E, Dalmau J, Alomar A, Martínez L, Gelpí C. Lichen planus pemphigoides: detection of anti-BP 180 antibodies by ELISA and immunoblotting tests. J Eur Acad Dermatol Venereol. 2010;24(11):1360–1.
293. Scully C, Muzio LL. Oral mucosal diseases: mucous membrane pemphigoid. Br J Oral Maxillofac Surg. 2008;46(5):358–66.
294. Du G, Patzelt S, van Beek N, Schmidt E. Mucous membrane pemphigoid. Autoimmun Rev. 2022;21(4):103036. https://doi.org/10.1016/j.autrev.2022.103036.
295. Zillikens D. Acquired skin disease of hemidesmosomes. J Dermatol Sci. 1999;20(2):134–54.
296. Hayakawa T, Furumura M, Fukano H, Li X, Ishii N, Hamada T, et al. Diagnosis of oral mucous membrane pemphigoid by means of combined serologic testing. Oral Surg Oral Med Oral Pathol Oral Radiol. 2014;117(4):483–96.
297. Buijsrogge J, Hagel C, Duske U, Kromminga A, Vissink A, Kloosterhuis A, et al. IgG antibodies to BP180 in a subset of oral lichen planus patients. J Dermatol Sci. 2007;47(3):256–8.
298. Abbas AK, Lichtman AH, Pillai S. Immunologia cellulare e molecolare 9 ed. Edra; 2018.
299. Anhalt GJ, Kim S, Stanley JR, Korman NJ, Jabs DA, Kory M, et al. Paraneoplastic pemphigus: an autoimmune mucocutaneous disease associated with neoplasia. N Engl J Med. 1990;323(25):1729–35.
300. Sehgal VN, Srivastava G. Paraneoplastic pemphigus/paraneoplastic autoimmune multiorgan syndrome. Int J Dermatol. 2009;48(2):162–9.
301. Czernik A, Camilleri M, Pittelkow MR, Grando SA. Paraneoplastic autoimmune multiorgan syndrome: 20 years after. Int J Dermatol. 2011;50(8):905–14.
302. Wong KC, Ho KK. Pemphigus with pemphigoid-like presentation, associated with squamous cell carcinoma of the tongue. Australas J Dermatol. 2000;41(3):178–80.
303. Su Z, Liu G, Liu J, Fang T, Zeng Y, Zhang H, et al. Paraneoplastic pemphigus associated with follicular dendritic cell sarcoma: report of a case and review of literature. Int J Clin Exp Pathol. 2015;8(10):11983.

304. Basir N, Telisinghe PU, Chong VH. Gastric cancer and paraneoplastic pemphigus. Ind J Surg. 2015;77(6):545–6.
305. Bazarbachi A, Bachelez H, Dehen L, Delmer A, Zittoun R, Dubertret L. Lethal paraneoplastic pemphigus following treatment of chronic lymphocytic leukaemia with fludarabine. Ann Oncol. 1995;6(7):730–1.
306. Higo T, Miyagaki T, Nakamura F, Shinohara A, Asano H, Abe H, et al. Paraneoplastic pemphigus occurring after bendamustine and rituximab therapy for relapsed follicular lymphoma. Ann Hematol. 2015;94(4):683–5.
307. Sinha A. Paraneoplastic pemphigus: autoimmune-cancer nexus in the skin. Anticancer Agents Med Chem. 2015;15(10):1215–23.
308. Mimouni D, Anhalt G, Lazarova Z, Aho S, Kazerounian S, Kouba D, et al. Paraneoplastic pemphigus in children and adolescents. Br J Dermatol. 2002;147(4):725–32.
309. Nguyen VT, Ndoye A, Bassler KD, Shultz LD, Shields MC, Ruben BS, et al. Classification, clinical manifestations, and immunopathological mechanisms of the epithelial variant of paraneoplastic autoimmune multiorgan syndrome: a reappraisal of paraneoplastic pemphigus. Arch Dermatol. 2001;137(2):193–206.
310. Nikolskaia O, Nousari C, Anhalt G. Paraneoplastic pemphigus in association with Castleman's disease. Br J Dermatol. 2003;149(6):1143–51.
311. Reich K, Brinck U, Letschert M, Blaschke V, Dames K, Braess J, et al. Graft-versus-host disease-like immunophenotype and apoptotic keratinocyte death in paraneoplastic pemphigus. Br J Dermatol. 1999;141(4):739–46.
312. Taintor AR, Leiferman KM, Hashimoto T, Ishii N, Zone JJ, Hull CM. A novel case of IgA paraneoplastic pemphigus associated with chronic lymphocytic leukemia. J Am Acad Dermatol. 2007;56(5):S73–S6.
313. Yashiro M, Nakano T, Taniguchi T, Katsuoka K, Tadera N, Miyazaki K, et al. IgA paraneoplastic pemphigus in angioimmunoblastic T-cell lymphoma with antibodies to desmocollin 1, type VII collagen and laminin 332. Acta Derm Venereol. 2014;94(2):235–6.
314. Kiyokawa C, Ruhrberg C, Nie Z, Karashima T, Mori O, Nishikawa T, et al. Envoplakin and periplakin are components of the paraneoplastic pemphigus antigen complex [4]. J Investig Dermatol. 1998;111(6):1236–8.
315. Oursler JR, Labib RS, Ariss-Abdo L, Burke T, O'Keefe EJ, Anhalt GJ. Human autoantibodies against desmoplakins in paraneoplastic pemphigus. J Clin Invest. 1992;89(6):1775–82.
316. Amagai M, Nishikawa T, Nousari HC, Anhalt GJ, Hashimoto T. Antibodies against desmoglein 3 (pemphigus vulgaris antigen) are present in sera from patients with paraneoplastic pemphigus and cause acantholysis in vivo in neonatal mice. J Clin Invest. 1998;102(4):775–82.
317. Lambert J, Bracke S, Van Roy F, Pas H, Bonné S, De Schepper S. Serum plakophilin-3 autoreactivity in paraneoplastic pemphigus. Br J Dermatol. 2010;163(3):630–2.
318. Zimmermann J, Bahmer F, Rose C, Zillikens D, Schmidt E. Clinical and immunopathological spectrum of paraneoplastic pemphigus. JDDG. J Dtsch Dermatol Ges. 2010;8(8):598–605.
319. Schepens I, Jaunin F, Begre N, Läderach U, Marcus K, Hashimoto T, et al. The protease inhibitor alpha-2-macroglobuline-like-1 is the p170 antigen recognized by paraneoplastic pemphigus autoantibodies in human. PLoS One. 2010;5(8):e12250.
320. Numata S, Teye K, Tsuruta D, Sogame R, Ishii N, Koga H, et al. Anti-alpha-2-macroglobulin-like-1 autoantibodies are detected frequently and may be pathogenic in paraneoplastic pemphigus. J Investig Dermatol. 2013;133(7):1785–93.
321. Martel P, Loiseau P, Joly P, Busson M, Lepage V, Mouquet H, et al. Paraneoplastic pemphigus is associated with the DRB1∗ 03 allele. J Autoimmun. 2003;20(1):91–5.
322. Liu Q, Bu DF, Li D, Zhu XJ. Genotyping of HLA-I and HLA-II alleles in Chinese patients with paraneoplastic pemphigus. Br J Dermatol. 2008;158(3):587–91.
323. Bialy-Golan A, Brenner S, Anhalt G. Paraneoplastic pemphigus: oral involvement as the sole manifestation. Acta Derm Venereol. 1996;76(3):253–4.
324. Broussard KC, Leung TG, Moradi A, Thorne JE, Fine J-D. Autoimmune bullous diseases with skin and eye involvement: Cicatricial pemphigoid, pemphigus vulgaris, and pemphigus paraneoplastica. Clin Dermatol. 2016;34(2):205–13.
325. Meyers SJ, Varley GA, Meisler DM, Camisa C, Wander AH. Conjunctival involvement in paraneoplastic pemphigus. Am J Ophthalmol. 1992;114(5):621–4.
326. Anhalt GJ. Paraneoplastic pemphigus. Journal of Investigative Dermatology Symposium Proceedings: Elsevier; 2004. pp. 29–33.
327. Sticherling M, Erfurt-Berge C. Autoimmune blistering diseases of the skin. Autoimmun Rev. 2012;11(3):226–30.
328. Yong AA, Tey HL. Paraneoplastic pemphigus. Australas J Dermatol. 2013;54(4):241–50.
329. Wade MS, Black MM. Paraneoplastic pemphigus: a brief update. Australas J Dermatol. 2005;46(1):1–8.
330. Maldonado F, Pittelkow MR, Ryu JH. Constrictive bronchiolitis associated with paraneoplastic autoimmune multi-organ syndrome. Respirology. 2009;14(1):129–33.
331. McNally MA, Vangipuram R, Campbell MT, Nagarajan P, Patel AB, Curry JL, et al. Paraneoplastic pemphigus manifesting in a patient treated with pembrolizumab for urothelial carcinoma. JAAD Case Rep. 2021;10:82–4. https://doi.org/10.1016/j.jdcr.2021.02.012.
332. Joly P, Richard C, Gilbert D, Courville P, Chosidow O, Roujeau J, et al. Sensitivity and specificity of

clinical, histologic, and immunologic features in the diagnosis of paraneoplastic pemphigus. J Am Acad Dermatol. 2000;43(4):619–26.
333. Helou J, Allbritton J, Anhalt GJ. Accuracy of indirect immunofluorescence testing in the diagnosis of paraneoplastic pemphigus. J Am Acad Dermatol. 1995;32(3):441–7.
334. Liu AY, Valenzuela R, Helm TN, Camisa C, Melton AL, Bergfeld WF. Indirect immunofluorescence on rat bladder transitional epithelium: a test with high specificity for paraneoplastic pemphigus. J Am Acad Dermatol. 1993;28(5):696–9.
335. Probst C, Schlumberger W, Stöcker W, Recke A, Schmidt E, Hashimoto T, et al. Development of ELISA for the specific determination of autoantibodies against envoplakin and periplakin in paraneoplastic pemphigus. Clin Chim Acta. 2009;410(1–2):13–8.
336. Powell JG, Grover RK, Plunkett RW, Seiffert-Sinha K, Sinha AA. Evaluation of a newly available ELISA for Envoplakin autoantibodies for the diagnosis of paraneoplastic Pemphigus. J Drug Dermatol: JDD. 2015;14(10):1103–6.
337. Poot A, Diercks G, Kramer D, Schepens I, Klunder G, Hashimoto T, et al. Laboratory diagnosis of paraneoplastic pemphigus. Br J Dermatol. 2013;169(5):1016–24.
338. Frew JW, Murrell DF. Current management strategies in paraneoplastic pemphigus (paraneoplastic autoimmune multiorgan syndrome). Dermatol Clin. 2011;29(4):607–12.
339. Pablo MIMD, Iranzo P, Mascaro JM, Llambrich A, Baradad M, Herrero C. Paraneoplastic pemphigus associated with non-Hodgkin B-cell lymphoma and good response to prednisone. Acta Dermato Venereologica. 2005;85(3):233–5.
340. Vezzoli P, Berti E, Marzano AV. Rationale and efficacy for the use of rituximab in paraneoplastic pemphigus. Expert Rev Clin Immunol. 2008;4(3):351–63.
341. Gergely L, Váróczy L, Vadász G, Remenyik É, Illés Á. Successful treatment of B cell chronic lymphocytic leukemia-associated severe paraneoplastic pemphigus with cyclosporin a. Acta Haematol. 2003;109(4):202–5.
342. Izaki S, Yoshizavva Y, Kitamura K, Kato H, Hashimoto H, Korman N, et al. Paraneoplastic pemphigus: potential therapeutic effect of plasmapheresis. Br J Dermatol. 1996;134(5):987–9.
343. Hainsworth JD, Burris HA III, Morrissey LH, Litchy S, Scullin DC Jr, Bearden JD III, et al. Rituximab monoclonal antibody as initial systemic therapy for patients with low-grade non-Hodgkin lymphoma. Blood. 2000;95(10):3052–6.
344. Vassileva S, Drenovska K, Manuelyan K. Autoimmune blistering dermatoses as systemic diseases. Clin Dermatol. 2014;32(3):364–75.
345. Wang L, Bu D, Yang Y, Chen X, Zhu X. Castleman's tumours and production of autoantibody in paraneoplastic pemphigus. Lancet. 2004;363(9408): 525–31.
346. Zhang B, Zheng R, Wang J, Bu D, Zhu X. Epitopes in the linker subdomain region of envoplakin recognized by autoantibodies in paraneoplastic pemphigus patients. J Investig Dermatol. 2006;126(4):832–40.
347. Jaremko WM, Beutner EH, Kumar V, Kipping H, Condry P, Zeid MY, et al. Chronic ulcerative stomatitis associated with a specific immunologic marker. J Am Acad Dermatol. 1990;22(2):215–20.
348. Wörle B, Wollenberg A, Schaller M, Kunzelmann KH, Plewig G, Meurer M. Chronic ulcerative stomatitis. Br J Dermatol. 1997;137(2):262–5.
349. Chorzelski TP, Olszewska M, Jarzabek-Chorzelska M. Is chronic ulcerative stomatitis an entity? Clinical and immunological findings in 18 cases. Eur J Dermatol. 1998;8(4):261–5.
350. Solomon LW, Aguirre A, Neiders M, Costales-Spindler A, Jividen GJ Jr, Zwick MG, et al. Chronic ulcerative stomatitis: clinical, histopathologic, and immunopathologic findings. Oral Surg Oral Med Oral Pathol Oral Radiol Endodontol. 2003;96(6):718–26.
351. Islam M, Cohen D, Ojha J, Stewart C, Katz J, Bhattacharyya I. Chronic ulcerative stomatitis: diagnostic and management challenges—four new cases and review of literature. Oral Surg Oral Med Oral Pathol Oral Radiol Endodontol. 2007;104(2):194–203.
352. Islam MN, Alramadhan S, Solomon L. Chronic ulcerative stomatitis 14. Diseases of the oral Mucosa: study guide and review. 151.
353. Cozzani E, Cacciapuoti M, Di Marco E, Zerega B, Descalzi Cancedda F, Parodi A. Patients with oral erosive and cutaneous lichen planus may have antibodies directed against the chronic ulcerative stomatitis protein antigen of 70-kDa. Acta Dermatovenerol Alp Pannonica Adriat. 2008;17(3):120–4.
354. Solomon L, Stark P, Winter L, Kumar V, Sinha S. ELISA test for p63 antibodies in chronic ulcerative stomatitis. Oral Dis. 2010;16(2):151–5.
355. Carlson MW, Garlick JA, Solomon LW. Chronic ulcerative stomatitis: evidence of autoimmune pathogenesis. Oral Surg Oral Med Oral Pathol Oral Radiol Endodontol. 2011;111(6):742–8.
356. Fourie J, Van Heerden WFP, McEachen SC, Van Zyl A. Chronic ulcerative stomatitis: a distinct clinical entity? S Afr Dent J. 2011;66(3):119–21.
357. Qari H, Villasante C, Richert J, Rees T, Kessler H. The diagnostic challenges of separating chronic ulcerative stomatitis from oral lichen planus. Oral Surg Oral Med Oral Pathol Oral Radiol. 2015;120(5):622–7.
358. Herzum A, Burlando M, Cozzani E, Parodi A. The 30th birthday of chronic ulcerative stomatitis: a systematic review. Int J Immunopathol Pharmacol. 2021;35:20587384211052437.
359. Rinaggio J, Crossland DM, Zeid MY. A determination of the range of oral conditions submitted for microscopic and direct immunofluorescence analysis. J Periodontol. 2007;78(10):1904–10.
360. Parodi A, Cozzani E, Chorzelski TP, Beutner EH, Rebora A. A molecule of about 70 kd is the immuno-

logic marker of chronic ulcerative stomatitis. J Am Acad Dermatol. 1998;38(6 I):1005–6.
361. Vassileva S. Drug-induced pemphigoid: bullous and cicatricial. Clin Dermatol. 1998;16(3):379–87.
362. Carrizosa AM, Elorza FL, Camacho FM. Antinuclear antibodies in patients with lichen planus. Exp Dermatol. 1997;6(1):54–6.
363. Cacciapuoti M, Di Marco E, Cozzani E, Zerega B, Cancedda FD, Parodi A. The antibody to the 70-kd antigen in chronic ulcerative stomatitis and lichen planus. J Am Acad Dermatol. 2004; 50(3):486.
364. Parodi A, Cozzani E, Massone C, Rebora A, Priano L, Ghigliotti G, et al. Prevalence of stratified epithelium-specific antinuclear antibodies in 138 patients with lichen planus. J Am Acad Dermatol. 2007;56(6):974–8.
365. Lee LA, Walsh P, Prater CA, Su L-J, Marchbank A, Egbert TB, et al. Characterization of an autoantigen associated with chronic ulcerative stomatitis: the CUSP autoantigen is a member of the p53 family. J Investig Dermatol. 1999;113(2):146–51.
366. Choi H-R, Batsakis JG, Zhan F, Sturgis E, Luna MA, El-Naggar AK. Differential expression of p53 gene family members p63 and p73 in head and neck squamous tumorigenesis. Hum Pathol. 2002;33(2):158–64.
367. Ebrahimi M, Nylander E, Bäcklund B, Wahlin YB, Coates PJ, Nylander K. The use of a novel ELISA method for detection of antibodies against p63 in sera from patients diagnosed with oral and/or genital and skin lichen planus. J Oral Pathol Med. 2010;39(6):486–90.
368. Mockenhaupt M. The current understanding of Stevens–Johnson syndrome and toxic epidermal necrolysis. Expert Rev Clin Immunol. 2011;7(6):803–15.
369. Leaute-Labreze C, Lamireau T, Chawki D, Maleville J, Taieb A. Diagnosis, classification, and management of erythema multiforme and Stevens–Johnson syndrome. Arch Dis Child. 2000;83(4):347–52.
370. Carrozzo M, Togliatto M, Gandolfo S. Erythema multiforme. A heterogeneous pathologic phenotype Minerva stomatologica. 1999;48(5):217–26.
371. Dumas V, Thieulent N, Souillet A, Jullien D, Faure M, Claudy A. Recurrent erythema multiforme and chronic hepatitis C: efficacy of interferon alpha. Br J Dermatol. 2000;142(6):1248–9.
372. Özkaya E. Oral mucosal fixed drug eruption: characteristics and differential diagnosis. J Am Acad Dermatol. 2013;69(2):e51–e8.
373. Webster K, Godbold P. Nicorandil induced oral ulceration. Br Dent J. 2005;198(10):619–21.
374. Oyama N, Setterfield JF, Gratian MJ, Bhogal BS, Shirlaw P, Challacombe SJ, et al. Oral and genital lichenoid reactions associated with circulating autoantibodies to desmoplakins I and II: a novel target antigen or example of epitope spreading? J Am Acad Dermatol. 2003;48(3):433–8.
375. Farthing P, Bagan JV, Scully C. Number IV erythema multiforme. Oral Dis. 2005;11(5):261–7.
376. Scully C, Bagan J. Oral mucosal diseases: erythema multiforme. Br J Oral Maxillofac Surg. 2008;46(2):90–5.
377. Williams PM, Conklin RJ. Erythema multiforme: a review and contrast from Stevens-Johnson syndrome/toxic epidermal necrolysis. Dent Clin. 2005;49(1):67–76.
378. Maxfield L, Gaston D, Peck A, Hansen K. Topical imiquimod and subsequent erythema multiforme. J Osteopathic Med. 2020;120(1):45–8.
379. Yanes DA, Kaffenberger JA, Carr DR. Erythema multiforme as a reaction to imiquimod 5% cream. Dermatol Online J. 2017;23(2)
380. Yavuz İH, Yavuz GÖ, Bilgili SG, Bayram İ, Savaş H. Erythema multiforme; sixty six case series with review of literature. Eastern J Med. 2018;23(4):308.
381. Khalil I, Lepage V, Douay C, Morin L, Al-Daccak R, Wallach D, et al. HLA DQB1* 0301 allele is involved in the susceptibility to erythema multiforme. J Investig Dermatol. 1991;97(4):697–700.
382. Profaizer T, Eckels D. HLA alleles and drug hypersensitivity reactions. Int J Immunogenet. 2012;39(2):99–105.
383. de Roux SC, Serratrice J, Granel B, Weiller-Merli C, Rey J, Lepidi H, et al. Stevens-Johnson syndrome followed by Gougerot-Sjögren syndrome. Presse Med. 2001;30(11):531–2.
384. Nazir A, Ali K. Drug induced erythema multiforme-oral variant: a case report. Oral Maxillofac Surg Case. 2022;8(1):100241. https://doi.org/10.1016/j.omsc.2021.100241.
385. Foedinger D, Anhalt GJ, Boecskoer B, Elbe A, Wolff K, Rappersberger K. Autoantibodies to desmoplakin I and II in patients with erythema multiforme. J Exp Med. 1995;181(1):169–79.
386. Hinterhuber G, Binder M, Marquardt Y, Cauza K, Riedl E, Rappersberger K, et al. Enzyme-linked immunosorbent assay for detection of peptide-specific human antidesmoplakin autoantibodies. Br J Dermatol. 2005;153(2):413–6.
387. Cozzani E, Di Zenzo G, Calabresi V, Caproni M, Schena D, Quaglino P, et al. Anti-desmoplakin antibodies in erythema multiforme and Stevens-Johnson syndrome sera: pathogenic or epiphenomenon? Eur J Dermatol. 2011;21(1):32–6.
388. Johnson SM, Smoller BR, Horn TD. Erythema multiforme associated human autoantibodies against desmoplakin I and II. J Invest Dermatol. 1999;112(3):395–6.
389. Oke V, Wahren-Herlenius M. Cutaneous lupus erythematosus: clinical aspects and molecular pathogenesis. J Intern Med. 2013;273(6):544–54.
390. Järvinen TM, Hellquist A, Koskenmies S, Einarsdottir E, Koskinen LL, Jeskanen L, et al. Tyrosine kinase 2 and interferon regulatory factor 5 polymorphisms are associated with discoid and subacute cutaneous lupus erythematosus. Exp Dermatol. 2010;19(2):123–31.
391. Järvinen TM, Hellquist A, Koskenmies S, Einarsdottir E, Panelius J, Hasan T, et al. Polymorphisms of the ITGAM gene confer higher

risk of discoid cutaneous than of systemic lupus erythematosus. PLoS One. 2010;5(12):e14212.
392. Namjou B, Kothari PH, Kelly JA, Glenn SB, Ojwang JO, Adler A, et al. Evaluation of the TREX1 gene in a large multi-ancestral lupus cohort. Genes Immunity. 2011;12(4):270–9.
393. Jessop S, Whitelaw DA, Grainge MJ, Jayasekera P. Drugs for discoid lupus erythematosus. Cochrane Database Syst Rev. 2017;5
394. Walling HW, Sontheimer RD. Cutaneous lupus erythematosus. Am J Clin Dermatol. 2009;10(6):365–81.
395. Callen JP. Cutaneous lupus erythematosus: a personal approach to management. Australas J Dermatol. 2006;47(1):13–27.
396. Merola JF, Prystowsky SD, Iversen C, Gomez-Puerta JA, Norton T, Tsao P, et al. Association of discoid lupus erythematosus with other clinical manifestations among patients with systemic lupus erythematosus. J Am Acad Dermatol. 2013;69(1):19–24.
397. Uva L, Miguel D, Pinheiro C, Freitas JP, Marques Gomes M, Filipe P. Cutaneous manifestations of systemic lupus erythematosus. Autoimmune Dis 2012;2012.
398. Werth VP. Clinical manifestations of cutaneous lupus erythematosus. Autoimmun Rev. 2005;4(5):296–302.
399. Thorne JE, Jabs DA, Nikolskaia O, Anhalt G, Nousari HC. Discoid lupus erythematosus and cicatrizing conjunctivitis: clinicopathologic study of two cases. Ocul Immunol Inflamm. 2002;10(4):287–92.
400. Rothfield N, Sontheimer RD, Bernstein M. Lupus erythematosus: systemic and cutaneous manifestations. Clin Dermatol. 2006;24(5):348–62.
401. Chong B, Song J, Olsen N. Determining risk factors for developing systemic lupus erythematosus in patients with discoid lupus erythematosus. Br J Dermatol. 2012;166(1):29–35.
402. Tan EM, Cohen AS, Fries JF, Masi AT, Mcshane DJ, Rothfield NF, et al. The 1982 revised criteria for the classification of systemic lupus erythematosus. Arthritis Rheumatism. 1982;25(11):1271–7.
403. Nico MMS, Vilela MAC, Rivitti EA, Lourenço SV. Oral lesions in lupus erythematosus: correlation with cutaneous lesions. Eur J Dermatol. 2008;18(4):376–81.
404. Tao D, Shangwu L, Qun W, Yan L, Wei J, Junyan L, et al. CD226 expression deficiency causes high sensitivity to apoptosis in NK T cells from patients with systemic lupus erythematosus. J Immunol. 2005;174(3):1281–90.
405. Savage NW, Boras VV, Zaini ZM. Oral squamous cell carcinoma with discoid lupus erythematosus. Oral Oncol Extra. 2006;42(1):32–5. https://doi.org/10.1016/j.ooe.2005.08.006.
406. Nagao K, Chen KR. A case of lupus erythematosus/lichen planus overlap syndrome. The. J Dermatol. 2006;33(3):187–90.
407. Hung T, Crawford RI, Martinka M. Degree of histologic inflammation in lupus erythematosus and direct immunofluorescence results: red and inflamed lesions do not increase the chances of getting a bright band. J Cutan Med Surg. 2013;17(1):22–6.
408. Nieboer C. The reliability of immunofluorescence and histopathology in the diagnosis of discoid lupus erythematosus and lichen planus. Br J Dermatol. 1987;116(2):189–98.
409. Lee JS, Haug BL, Sibley JT. Decreased mRNA levels coding for poly (ADP-ribose) polymerase in lymphocytes of patients with SLE. Lupus. 1994;3(2):113–6.
410. Chong BF, Tseng L-c, Lee T, Vasquez R, Li QZ, Zhang S, et al. IgG and IgM autoantibody differences in discoid and systemic lupus patients. J Investig Dermatol. 2012;132(12):2770–9.
411. Fernando MMA, Stevens CR, Sabeti PC, Walsh EC, McWhinnie AJM, Shah A, et al. Identification of two independent risk factors for lupus within the MHC in United Kingdom families. PLoS Genet. 2007;3(11):e192.
412. Harley JB, Alarcón-Riquelme ME, Criswell LA, Jacob CO, Kimberly RP, Moser KL, et al. Genome-wide association scan in women with systemic lupus erythematosus identifies susceptibility variants in ITGAM, PXK, KIAA1542 and other loci. Nat Genet. 2008;40(2):204–10.
413. Harley IT, Kaufman KM, Langefeld CD, Harley JB, Kelly JA. Genetic susceptibility to SLE: new insights from fine mapping and genome-wide association studies. Nat Rev Genet. 2009;10(5):285–90.
414. Nath SK, Kilpatrick J, Harley JB. Genetics of human systemic lupus erythematosus: the emerging picture. Curr Opin Immunol. 2004;16(6):794–800.
415. Cervera R, Khamashta M, Font J, Hughes GR, Erythematosus EWPSL. European working party on systemic lupus erythematosus: a 10 year report. Lupus. 2001;10(12):892–4.
416. Estes D, Christian CL. The natural history of systemic lupus erythematosus by prospective analysis. Medicine. 1971;50(2):85–96.
417. Gladman DD, Urowitz MB, Esdaile JM, Hahn BH, Klippel J, Lahita R, et al. Guidelines for referral and management of systemic lupus erythematosus in adults. Arthritis Rheum. 1999;42(9):1785–96.
418. Jonsson R, Heyden G, Westberg N, Nyberg G. Oral mucosal lesions in systemic lupus erythematosus–a clinical, histopathological and immunopathological study. J Rheumatol. 1984;11(1):38–42.
419. McCauliffe DP. Cutaneous lupus erythematosus. Semin Cutan Med Surg. 2001;20(1):14–26. https://doi.org/10.1053/sder.2001.23091.
420. Aringer M, Costenbader K, Daikh D, Brinks R, Mosca M, Ramsey-Goldman R, et al. 2019 European league against rheumatism/American College of Rheumatology classification criteria for systemic lupus erythematosus. Arthritis Rheumatol. 2019;71(9):1400–12.
421. Brennan MT, Valerin MA, Napeñas JJ, Lockhart PB. Oral manifestations of patients with lupus erythematosus. Dent Clin. 2005;49(1):127–41.

422. Farthing PM, Speight PM. Problems and pitfalls in oral mucosal pathology. Curr Diagn Pathol. 2006;12(1):66–74.
423. Rodsaward P, Prueksrisakul T, Deekajorndech T, Edwards SW, Beresford MW, Chiewchengchol D. Oral ulcers in juvenile-onset systemic lupus erythematosus: a review of the literature. Am J Clin Dermatol. 2017;18(6):755–62.
424. Fritzler MJ. Toward a new autoantibody diagnostic orthodoxy: understanding the bad, good and indifferent. Autoimmunity Highlights. 2012;3(2):51–8.
425. Cervera R, Khamashta MA, Font J, Sebastiani GD, Gil A, Lavilla P, et al. Morbidity and mortality in systemic lupus erythematosus during a 10-year period: a comparison of early and late manifestations in a cohort of 1,000 patients. Medicine. 2003;82(5):299–308.
426. Lam DK, Clokie CM, Sándor GK. Systemic lupus erythematosus: a review for dentists. J Can Dent Assoc. 2007;73(9)
427. Goldsmith LA, Katz SI, Gilchrest BA, Paller AS, Leffell DJ, Wolff K. Fitzpatrick's dermatology in general medicine, 8e. McGrawHill Medical. 2012:2421–9.
428. Burge S, Frith P, Juniper R, Wojnarowska F. Mucosal involvement in systemic and chronic cutaneous lupus erythematosus. Br J Dermatol. 1989;121(6):727–41.
429. Fessler BJ, Alarcón GS, McGwin G Jr, Roseman J, Bastian HM, Friedman AW, et al. Systemic lupus erythematosus in three ethnic groups: XVI. Association of hydroxychloroquine use with reduced risk of damage accrual. Arthritis Rheum. 2005;52(5):1473–80.
430. Lander S, Wallace D, Weisman M. Celecoxib for systemic lupus erythematosus: case series and literature review of the use of NSAIDs in SLE. Lupus. 2002;11(6):340–7.
431. Reich A, Werth V, Furukawa F, Kuhn A, Szczęch J, Samotij D, et al. Treatment of cutaneous lupus erythematosus: current practice variations. Lupus. 2016;25(9):964–72.
432. Glick M. Burket's Oral medicine. 12th ed. Shelton: People's Medical Publishing House-USA; 2015.
433. Lee L. Cutaneous lupus in infancy and childhood. Lupus. 2010;19(9):1112–7.
434. Thorbinson C, Oni L, Smith E, Midgley A, Beresford MW. Pharmacological management of childhood-onset systemic lupus erythematosus. Pediatr Drugs. 2016;18(3):181–95.
435. Fessler BJ, Boumpas DT. Severe major organ involvement in systemic lupus erythematosus: diagnosis and management. Rheum Dis Clin N Am. 1995;21(1):81–98.
436. Chong BF, Werth VP. Management of cutaneous lupus erythematosus. Dubois' lupus Erythematosus and related syndromes. Elsevier; 2019. p. 719–26.
437. David M, Hodak E, Lowe NJ. Adverse effects of retinoids. Med Toxicol Adverse Drug Exp. 1988;3(4):273–88.
438. Werth VP, Fiorentino D, Sullivan BA, Boedigheimer MJ, Chiu K, Wang C, et al. Brief report: pharmacodynamics, safety, and clinical efficacy of AMG 811, a human anti–interferon-γ antibody, in patients with discoid lupus Erythematosus. Arthritis Rheumatol. 2017;69(5):1028–34.
439. Schiødt M. Oral manifestations of lupus erythematosus. Int J Oral Surg. 1984;13(2):101–47.
440. Reddy JS. Systemic lupus Erythematosus presenting with Oral mucosal lesions-a case report. J Clin Pediatr Dent. 2009;33(3)
441. Wang X, Zhang L, Luo J, Wu Z, Mei Y, Wang Y, et al. Tacrolimus 0.03% ointment in labial discoid lupus erythematosus: a randomized, controlled clinical trial. J Clin Pharmacol. 2015;55(11):1221–8.
442. Merola JF, Moschella S. Overview of cutaneous lupus erythematosus. UpToDate UpToDate, Waltham, MA (Accessed on September 20, 2015). 2016.
443. Muñoz-Corcuera M, Esparza-Gómez G, González-Moles M, Bascones-Martínez A. Oral ulcers: clinical aspects. A tool for dermatologists. Part I. Acute ulcers. Clin Exp Dermatol: Clin Dermatol. 2009;34(3):289–94.
444. Weening JJ, D'agati VD, Schwartz MM, Seshan SV, Alpers CE, Appel GB, et al. The classification of glomerulonephritis in systemic lupus erythematosus revisited. Kidney Int. 2004;65(2):521–30.
445. Saccucci M, Di Carlo G, Bossù M, Giovarruscio F, Salucci A, Polimeni A. Autoimmune diseases and their manifestations on oral cavity: diagnosis and clinical management. J Immunol Res 2018;2018.
446. Carroll CL, Fleischer J, Alan B. Tacrolimus ointment: the treatment of atopic dermatitis and other inflammatory cutaneous disease. Expert Opin Pharmacother. 2004;5(10):2127–37.
447. Walker S, Kirby B, Chalmers R. Use of 0.1% tacrolimus ointment in patients with various forms of lupus erythematosus. Eur J Dermatol: EJD. 2002;12(4):387–8. author reply 9
448. Walker S, Kirby B, Chalmers R. Topical tacrolimus for cutaneous lupus erythematosus. J Dermatol. 2002;147:405–6.
449. Axéll T, Pindborg J, Smith C, Van der Waal I, Lesions aICGoOW. Oral white lesions with special reference to precancerous and tobacco-related lesions: conclusions of an international symposium held in Uppsala, Sweden, may 18–21 1994. J Oral Pathol Med. 1996;25(2):49–54.
450. Villa A, Sonis S. Oral leukoplakia remains a challenging condition. Oral Dis. 2018;24(1–2):179–83.
451. Villa A, Woo SB. Leukoplakia—a diagnostic and management algorithm. J Oral Maxillofac Surg. 2017;75(4):723–34.
452. Van der Waal I. Oral leukoplakia, the ongoing discussion on definition and terminology. Med Oral, Patol Oral Cir Bucal. 2015;20(6):e685.
453. Schepman K, Van der Waal I. A proposal for a classification and staging system for oral leukoplakia: a preliminary study. Eur J Cancer B Oral Oncol. 1995;31(6):396–8.

454. Sen S. Aneuploidy and cancer. Curr Opin Oncol. 2000;12(1):82–8. https://doi.org/10.1097/00001622-200001000-00014.
455. Oulton R, Harrington L. Telomeres, telomerase, and cancer: life on the edge of genomic stability. Curr Opin Oncol. 2000;12(1):74–81.
456. Siebers TJ, Bergshoeff VE, Otte-Höller I, Kremer B, Speel E-JM, Van Der Laak J, et al. Chromosome instability predicts the progression of premalignant oral lesions. Oral Oncol. 2013;49(12):1121–8.
457. Kulkarni V, Saranath D. Concurrent hypermethylation of multiple regulatory genes in chewing tobacco associated oral squamous cell carcinomas and adjacent normal tissues. Oral Oncol. 2004;40(2):145–53.
458. Kato K, Hara A, Kuno T, Mori H, Yamashita T, Toida M, et al. Aberrant promoter hypermethylation of p16 and MGMT genes in oral squamous cell carcinomas and the surrounding normal mucosa. J Cancer Res Clin Oncol. 2006;132(11):735–43.
459. Brito JA, Gomes CC, Guimarães AL, Campos K, Gomez RS. Relationship between micro RNA expression levels and histopathological features of dysplasia in oral leukoplakia. J Oral Pathol Med. 2014;43(3):211–6.
460. Nasser W, Flechtenmacher C, Holzinger D, Hofele C, Bosch FX. Aberrant expression of p53, p16INK4a and Ki-67 as basic biomarker for malignant progression of oral leukoplakias. J Oral Pathol Med. 2011;40(8):629–35.
461. Angiero F, Berenzi A, Benetti A, Rossi E, Del Sordo R, Sidoni A, et al. Expression of p16, p53 and Ki-67 proteins in the progression of epithelial dysplasia of the oral cavity. Anticancer Res. 2008;28(5A):2535–9.
462. Pitiyage G, Tilakaratne W, Tavassoli M, Warnakulasuriya S. Molecular markers in oral epithelial dysplasia. J Oral Pathol Med. 2009;38(10):737–52.
463. Graveland AP, Bremmer JF, De Maaker M, Brink A, Cobussen P, Zwart M, et al. Molecular screening of oral precancer. Oral Oncol. 2013;49(12):1129–35.
464. Vogelstein B, Kinzler KW. The path to cancer—three strikes and you're out. N Engl J Med. 2015;373(20):1895–8.
465. Ferris RL. Immunology and immunotherapy of head and neck cancer. J Clin Oncol. 2015;33(29):3293.
466. Chow LQ, Haddad R, Gupta S, Mahipal A, Mehra R, Tahara M, et al. Antitumor activity of pembrolizumab in biomarker-unselected patients with recurrent and/or metastatic head and neck squamous cell carcinoma: results from the phase Ib KEYNOTE-012 expansion cohort. J Clin Oncol. 2016;34(32):3838.
467. Ferris RL, Blumenschein G Jr, Fayette J, Guigay J, Colevas AD, Licitra L, et al. Nivolumab for recurrent squamous-cell carcinoma of the head and neck. N Engl J Med. 2016;375:1856–67.
468. Yagyuu T, Hatakeyama K, Imada M, Kurihara M, Matsusue Y, Yamamoto K, et al. Programmed death ligand 1 (PD-L1) expression and tumor microenvironment: implications for patients with oral precancerous lesions. Oral Oncol. 2017;68:36–43.
469. Lodi G, Franchini R, Warnakulasuriya S, Varoni EM, Sardella A, Kerr AR, et al. Interventions for treating oral leukoplakia to prevent oral cancer. Cochrane Database Syst Rev. 2016;7(7):Cd001829. https://doi.org/10.1002/14651858.CD001829.pub4.
470. Farah CS, Woo SB, Zain RB, Sklavounou A, McCullough MJ, Lingen M. Oral cancer and oral potentially malignant disorders. Int J Dent. 2014;2014:853479. https://doi.org/10.1155/2014/853479.
471. Ribeiro AS, Salles PR, da Silva TA, Mesquita RA. A review of the nonsurgical treatment of oral leukoplakia. Int J Dent. 2010;2010
472. Mogedas-Vegara A, Hueto-Madrid J-A, Chimenos-Küstner E, Bescós-Atín C. Oral leukoplakia treatment with the carbon dioxide laser: a systematic review of the literature. J Cranio-Maxillofac Surg. 2016;44(4):331–6.
473. Vohra F, Al-Kheraif AA, Qadri T, Hassan MIA, Ahmed A, Warnakulasuriya S, et al. Efficacy of photodynamic therapy in the management of oral premalignant lesions. A systematic review. Photodiagn Photodyn Ther. 2015;12(1):150–9.
474. Berlin JM. Current and emerging treatment strategies for the treatment of actinic keratosis. Clin Cosmetic Investig Dermatol: CCID. 2010;3:119.
475. Rahvar M, Lamel SA, Maibach HI. Randomized, vehicle-controlled trials of topical 5-fluorouracil therapy for actinic keratosis treatment: an overview. Immunotherapy. 2012;4(9):939–45.
476. Chau L, Jabara JT, Lai W, Svider PF, Warner BM, Lin H-S, et al. Topical agents for oral cancer chemoprevention: a systematic review of the literature. Oral Oncol. 2017;67:153–9.
477. Gillenwater AM, Vigneswaran N, Fatani H, Saintigny P, El-Naggar AK. Proliferative verrucous leukoplakia: recognition and differentiation from conventional leukoplakia and mimics. Head Neck. 2014;36(11):1662–8.
478. Gillenwater AM, Vigneswaran N, Fatani H, Saintigny P, El-Naggar AK. Proliferative verrucous leukoplakia (PVL): a review of an elusive pathologic entity! Adv Anat Pathol. 2013;20(6):416–23.
479. van der Waal I, Reichart PA. Oral proliferative verrucous leukoplakia revisited. Oral Oncol. 2008;44
480. Eisenberg E. Oral lichen planus: a benign lesion. J Oral Maxillofac Surg. 2000;58(11):1278–85.
481. Zhang L, Cheng X, Li Y-h, Poh C, Zeng T, Priddy R, et al. High frequency of allelic loss in dysplastic lichenoid lesions. Lab Investig. 2000;80(2):233–7.
482. Mignogna M, Muzio LL, Russo LL, Fedele S, Ruoppo E, Bucci E. Clinical guidelines in early detection of oral squamous cell carcinoma arising in oral lichen planus: a 5-year experience. Oral Oncol. 2001;37(3):262–7.
483. Mignogna MD, Fedele S, Russo LL. Dysplasia/neoplasia surveillance in oral lichen planus patients: a

description of clinical criteria adopted at a single Centre and their impact on prognosis. Oral Oncol. 2006;42(8):819–24.
484. Mignogna M, Fedele S, Russo LL, Mignogna C, De Rosa G, Porter S. Field cancerization in oral lichen planus. Eur J Surg Oncol (EJSO). 2007;33(3):383–9.
485. Odell E, Kujan O, Warnakulasuriya S, Sloan P. Oral epithelial dysplasia: recognition, grading and clinical significance. Oral Dis. 2021;
486. Eisenberg E, Krutchkoff DJ. Lichenoid lesions of oral mucosa: diagnostic criteria and their importance in the alleged relationship to oral cancer. Oral Surg Oral Med Oral Pathol. 1992;73(6):699–704.
487. Max Robinson C, Oxley JD, Weir J, Eveson JW. Lichenoid and granulomatous stomatitis: an entity or a non-specific inflammatory process? J Oral Pathol Med. 2006;35(5):262–7.
488. Eveson JW. Granulomatous disorders of the oral mucosa. Semin Diagn Pathol. 1996;13(2):118–27.
489. Daley TD, Wysocki GP. Foreign body gingivitis: an iatrogenic disease? Oral Surg Oral Med Oral Pathol. 1990;69(6):708–12.
490. Gordon SC, Daley TD. Foreign body gingivitis: identification of the foreign material by energy-dispersive x-ray microanalysis. Oral Surg Oral Med Oral Pathol Oral Radiol Endodontol. 1997;83(5):571–6.
491. Magro CM, Crowson AN. Lichenoid and granulomatous dermatitis. Int J Dermatol. 2000;39(2):126–33.
492. Gouveris P, Georgakopoulou E, Grigoraki A, Zouki D, Kardara V, Ioannou S, et al. Nivolumab-induced lichenoid granulomatous stomatitis in a patient with advanced melanoma: a case report. Mol Clin Oncol. 2022;16(4):1–6.
493. Bäckman K, Jontell M. Microbial-associated oral lichenoid reactions. Oral Dis. 2007;13(4):402–6.
494. Hakeem A, Bhattacharyya I, Aljabri M, Bindakhil M, Pachigar K, Islam MN, et al. Lichenoid reaction with granulomatous stomatitis: a retrospective histologic study of 47 patients. J Oral Pathol Med. 2019;48(9):846–54.
495. Pemberton MN, Yar R, Sloan P. Fixed drug eruption to oxybutynin. Oral Surg Oral Med Oral Pathol Oral Radiol Endodontol. 2008;106(3):e19–21.
496. Azevedo RS, Romañach MJ, de Almeida OP, Mosqueda-Taylor A, Vega-Memije ME, Carlos-Bregni R, et al. Lichen sclerosus of the oral mucosa: clinicopathological features of six cases. Int J Oral Maxillofac Surg. 2009;38(8):855–60.
497. Jiménez Y, Gavaldá C, Carbonell E, Margaix M, Sarrión G. Lichen sclerosus of the oral mucosa: a case report. Med Oral Patol Oral Cir Bucal. 2008;13(7):E403–6.
498. Adamo D, Calabria E, Coppola N, Lo Muzio L, Giuliani M, Bizzoca ME, ... & SIPMO (Italian Society of Oral Pathology, Medicine) a. Psychological profile and unexpected pain in oral lichen planus: A case–control multicenter SIPMO studya. Oral Diseases. 2022:28(2):398–414.
499. Biasotto M, Campisi G, Lodi G, Lo Muzio L, Mignogna MD, Montebugnoli e L, Sardella A. Patologia e Medicina Orale - SIPMO. Edra, 1° Edition. 2022.

6 Therapy

Small white OLP lesions are predominantly asymptomatic and, generally, do not require local drug therapy but careful planning of clinical checks and observations only to assess the possible morphological changes that are quite common in the various types of OLP [1]. The main aim of therapy is symptomatic control [2]. Furthermore, the dentist must identify and eliminate potential precipitating and irritating factors (fractured or malpositioned teeth, incongruous dental prostheses, consumption of alcohol and tobacco, or spicy, flavored, and/or acidic foods): this can lead to an improvement in symptoms and represents thus an important initial step in the management of symptomatic OLP. It is also important to maintain good oral, home, and professional hygiene, which sometimes associated with the use of alcohol-free chlorhexidine-based mouthwashes, can have beneficial effects on lesions and must always be recommended, especially in those forms with gingival involvement [1–3]. In these cases, the so-called occlusal therapy can also be adopted, in which the drug is administered locally through individual silicone splints or acrylic labial veneers; this method allows to overcome the main drawback of conventional topical therapy: the inability to provide continuous contact between the agent and the treated areas [4, 5]. In the red forms of OLP, the goal of local therapy is to alleviate symptoms and immune-inflammatory reactions but also reduce the potential for neoplastic degeneration. Finally, before the therapeutic approach, a careful drug history must be integrated to intercept possible molecules or drug interactions with xerostomic potential [1].

The management of symptomatic OLP can make use of many therapeutic approaches, but a permanent cure is not yet available. Topical treatment is generally preferable given the fewer side effects, but in the case of lesions resistant to topical agents or spread over multiple districts, systemic drugs may be necessary [2]. In fact, among the various immunosuppressive drugs commonly used for OLP/OLL, few have been developed specifically for oral disease, and consequently there is a lack of adequate studies to determine their efficacy [6]. Furthermore, many aspects of therapy such as optimal dose, duration of treatment, safety, and true efficacy remain largely unknown [7]. Therefore, the clinician must warn all patients about the off-label use (administration outside the conditions authorized by the appropriate bodies) of most of the compounds used to treat OLP, especially with regard to the instructions for use that contain the words "for external use only" [2]. Usually off-label use concerns molecules already known and used for some time, for which there is considerable scientific evidence that would allow their rational use even in clinical situations and in ways not provided for in the technical data sheet and in the package leaflet.

G. Isola et al., *Oral Lichen Planus and Lichenoid Lesions*,
https://doi.org/10.1007/978-3-031-29765-6_6

In this chapter, the main therapeutic approaches available and some more recent ones under evaluation will be discussed.

6.1 Glucocorticoids

The adrenal cortex secretes sex steroids and corticosteroids, the latter divided into mineralocorticoids (aldosterone) and glucocorticoids (cortisol). The synthesis of cortisol is modulated and controlled by the hypothalamic CRF (corticotrophin-releasing factor) which induces the production of corticotrophin or ACTH by the adenohypophysis which in turn stimulates the synthesis of cortisol. There are two feedback mechanisms that regulate the release of CRF and ACTH:

- A short circuit with negative feedback controls the release of CRF as a function of the blood levels of ACTH.
- A long negative feedback circuit in which blood levels of the glucocorticoid (both endogenous and exogenous) control the release of CRF and ACTH.

Cortisol has metabolic effects (mainly concerning glucose and protein metabolism through gluconeogenesis and protein catabolism but also lipid metabolism) and an anti-inflammatory and immunosuppressive action (inhibition of all events of the inflammatory process). Cortisol enters the target cell in free form and performs a dual action:

- Genomic mechanism of action. Cortisol binds to a cytoplasmic receptor (activated by dissociation from a heat shock protein (HSP)), and the hormone-receptor complex formed migrates to the nucleus where it binds to specific DNA sequences known as HRE (hormone response elements) inducing the production of specific functional proteins. The genomic mechanism of action is responsible for all the metabolizing effects and partly for the anti-inflammatory and immunosuppressive effects, the latter due to the production of various anti-inflammatory proteins such as:

  Lipocortin 1: it inhibits phospholipase A2 (PLA2) and consequently the production of PAF and eicosanoids (prostanoids, leukotrienes, 12-HETE, lipoxins).
  Vasocortin: it reduces vascular permeability and inhibits the release of histamine on mast cells and basophils.
  IkB: in the cytoplasm it binds and inhibits the nuclear factor κB (NF-κB) blocking its effects on inflammation and immunity.

The genomic mechanism of action occurs at least 30 min after binding to the receptor sites of the DNA, and therefore the effect is not immediate.

- Non-genomic mechanism of action. In addition to the genomic mechanism of action, high-dose glucocorticoids have a powerful anti-inflammatory and immunosuppressive action that develops within a few minutes, through the non-genomic mechanism of action. It consists in the direct inhibition, in the cytosol and in the nucleus, of pro-inflammatory transcription factors, such as NF-κB: in the cytosol the hormone-receptor complex blocks the NF-κB/IkB dissociation, and in the nucleus it hinders the interaction of NF-κB with DNA.

Cortisol possesses mineralocorticoid properties (water and sodium retention, potassium expulsion, and blood pressure increase) which, at the doses necessary to obtain the anti-inflammatory and immunosuppressive effects, lead to unacceptable side effects. Thanks to the insertion in the hormone molecule of a double bond in position 1–2 (or delta-1), prednisolone was obtained which, compared to cortisol, has greater anti-inflammatory activity and less mineralocorticoid effect. Numerous delta-derivatives were then obtained from prednisolone characterized by further increases in immunosuppressive activity and duration of action and lower mineralocorticoid effects. However, as the anti-inflammatory power of these synthetic analogues increases, the hormonal and metabolic effects that cannot be separated also increase [8].

6.1.1 Systemic Glucocorticoids

Systemic glucocorticoids may be needed in recalcitrant lesions with severe signs and symptoms. Their role seems to be limited to three main clinical indications: (1) initial OLP with severe and/or diffuse ulcer-erosive lesions, (2) treatment of resistant/recalcitrant forms, or (3) treatment of resistant/recalcitrant LP involving, beyond the oral cavity, also different districts of the body [3]. The characteristics of the main molecules derived from cortisol are listed below, some of which (prednisone, prednisolone, methylprednisolone, betamethasone) can also be used in the systemic treatment of OLP:

- *Hydrocortisone* (or *cortisol*). It is the drug of choice in replacement therapy (intravenously) of acute adrenal insufficiency and in the treatment of anaphylactic shock, etc.
- *Cortisone*. It is the natural precursor of cortisol used (orally) in the replacement therapy of adrenal insufficiency (Addison's disease) and in some rheumatological diseases [8].
- *Prednisone* and *prednisolone*. They are the delta-1 analogues of cortisone and hydrocortisone, respectively (prednisolone is the active metabolite following hepatic transformation). It is the most used molecule in the oral therapy of chronic inflammatory processes, allergies, and autoimmune diseases and in the prevention of rejection of organ transplants [8]. It has an anti-inflammatory activity four to five times higher than cortisol and less mineralocorticoid activity [9]. Prednisone is the main systemic corticosteroid treatment in OLP. Systemically administered corticosteroids are sometimes considered the most effective treatment for OLP [2]. However, a prospective comparative study involving a total of 49 patients with OLP with a mean follow-up of 36 months reported no differences in clinical response between the use of systemic prednisone (1 mg/kg/day) and topical clobetasol on an adhesive basis [10]. A study by Kuo et al. [11] showed complete response in 90% of a sample of 50 EOLP patients after a combination of locally injected triamcinolone acetonide and oral prednisolone for 2 weeks. Systemic corticosteroids are indicated in patients with severe painful OLP/OLL lesions who have not responded to topical therapy or have oral-genital, cutaneous, esophageal, and skin adnexal involvement [12]. Doses of prednisolone of 40 to 80 mg/day for 1–4 weeks are usually sufficient to achieve a response, either when taken for short periods (5–7 days) and stopped abruptly or if gradually reduced to 5–10 mg/day over 2–4 weeks [2, 13]. Other authors report doses of 30–60 mg per day for 2–3 weeks as the most effective treatment [14] or 0.5 to 1.0 mg per kg of the patient's body weight until therapeutic response is achieved [3], but in general it is always a short-term and high-dose treatment.
- *Methylprednisolone*. It is a methylated derivative of prednisolone and has the same action and indications [8].
- *Betamethasone* [15] (see later).

Relapses are not uncommon, and therefore systemic corticosteroids do not represent a reasonable therapeutic option in chronic OLP/OLL lesions [16] due to the toxic effects associated with long-term therapy [13]. The major undesirable effects are given by iatrogenic Cushing's syndrome (metabolic effects from glucocorticoids) and suppression of the hypothalamus-pituitary-adrenal axis. Iatrogenic Cushing's syndrome is characterized by impaired glucose metabolism (hyperglycemia and risk of diabetes), protein (decreased muscle mass, skin thinning, capillary fragility, impaired wound healing, osteoporosis, growth inhibition in children), lipid (lipogenesis and redistribution of fat in the abdomen, in the face with "full moon face," and in the back with "buffalo hump"), and hydrosaline (modest mineralocorticoid effects with water and sodium retention, hypokalemia, alkalosis, and arterial hypertension). The systemic administration of these molecules for several weeks or months can also result in the suppression of the hypothalamic-pituitary-adrenal axis with a reduction in ACTH secretion and atrophy of the adrenal cortex. Following the discontinuation of chronic therapy, the gland can take several months to resume its function; therefore abrupt cessation of therapy (rather than gradual cessation, based on the duration of therapy) will result in an acute adrenal crisis which can be fatal. Other complications from systemic and prolonged use of glucocorticoids can be susceptibility to infections, ulcerative or peptic pathologies (due to prostaglandin inhibition), cataracts, glaucoma, dermatological changes (acneiform eruptions and hair growth), and neurological disorders (behavioral changes, anxiety, insomnia, mood alterations) [8].

6.1.2 Topical Glucocorticoids

Topical corticosteroids are universally recognized as first-line treatment of symptomatic OLP/OLL [13] and may be useful in the initial treatment and also for maintenance [3]. The response to treatment with medium-potency steroids such as 0.1% triamcinolone acetonide and betamethasone, high-potency fluorates such as 0.1% fluocinolone acetonide and 0.05% fluocinonide, and super potent halogenates such as clobetasol propionate at 0.05% reported therapeutic success rates in the order of 30% to 100% [2, 13, 17, 18]. Among the topical steroids, the high therapeutic efficacy of clobetasol propionate [3] is highlighted. The general characteristics of topical glucocorticoids used in the treatment of OLP are listed individually below:

- *Triamcinolone acetonide*. It is a derivative of prednisolone, with less mineralocorticoid effects. It is indicated in allergic diseases (asthma, rhinitis, dermatitis) and osteoarticular inflammations and is available in different formulations (in addition to the topical one, also for oral and intramuscular administration); systemic therapy often leads to the onset of myopathy [8]. Esterification in C-17 (e.g., triamcinolone acetonide, betamethasone valerate/benzoate/dipropionate) increases the lipophilicity of the molecule making it easier for local administration of high doses of the active ingredient with negligible systemic absorption [9]. Intralesional injections of triamcinolone acetonide (10 mg/ml) in lidocaine have been found to be effective in the treatment of refractory EOLP; however this type of application involves the risk of area atrophy and adverse effects from systemic absorption [19, 20]. Topical applications in the form of oral suspensions with a concentration of 0.1–0.2% have been proven effective in reducing erythema and ulceration of the mucous membranes; the suspension is prepared by a clinical pharmacologist using injectable triamcinolone acetonide and distilled water [20]. A double-blind randomized clinical study showed comparable efficacy between an aloe vera mouthwash and a 0.1% triamcinolone acetonide-based paste in determining an improvement in the signs and symptoms of OLP [21].
- *Betamethasone*. It is a methylated derivative (in C16-trans) of triamcinolone, used in the treatment of inflammatory and allergic processes [8]. Similar to dexamethasone, it has an anti-inflammatory activity that is about 25 times higher and a half-life 3–4 times longer; however the increase in anti-inflammatory power also leads to an increase in toxicity [9]. In a basic form, it can be administered orally, while as sodium phosphate (which confers water solubility), it can be used orally (as effervescent tablets) and parenteral (im, iv); in addition, numerous preparations for topical use are available in the form of valerate, benzoate, dipropionate, and valeroacetate which increase their lipophilicity allowing local administration of high doses with negligible systemic absorption [8, 9]. The topical application of betamethasone valerate can be useful in the initial and maintenance therapy of OLP [2, 3, 22, 23].
- *Dexamethasone*. It is an isomer of betamethasone (methylated in C16-bis) and has similar pharmacokinetic and pharmacodynamic characteristics [8, 9]. In a basic form, it can be administered orally, while as sodium phosphate, it can be administered parenterally (im, iv) [8]. In case of widespread OLP lesions in the oral cavity, the oral solution formulation

may be useful [24]. A study on 13 patients showed that topical application of 0.1% dexamethasone for 6 weeks resulted in a significant reduction in OLP-related symptoms and in the salivary concentration of some cytokines [25]. A pilot study showed comparable efficacy in reducing the symptoms and signs of EOLP between amlexanox and dexamethasone paste [26].

- *Fluticasone propionate*. It is an ester of glucocorticoids carboxylated in C-21 whose characteristic is that it is rapidly metabolized after absorption in an inactive compound; this allows to obtain a local glucocorticoid activity with minimized systemic effects [9]. Fluticasone propionate can also be used in the local treatment of OLP [3].
- *Fluocinolone acetonide*. It is a synthetic derivative of hydrocortisone that has 1/24 of the solubility of dexamethasone in an aqueous solution, allowing the release of the steroid for a much longer period of time [27]. A clinical study by Thongprasom et al. [18] showed the efficacy of 0.1% fluocinolone acetonide both in solution and especially in Orabase in inducing complete remission of OLP lesions after a 2-year follow-up. It has also been reported that 0.1% fluocinolone acetonide gel is an equally effective alternative to the 0.1% Orabase form in the treatment of OLP [28]. The same study group also showed that 0.1% fluocinolone acetonide in Orabase is more effective than 0.05% retinoic acid in Orabase in the treatment of atrophic-erosive OLP [29]. It also appears that 0.1% fluocinolone acetonide in Orabase is relatively more effective and rapid than 0.1% triamcinolone acetonide in Orabase in inducing an improvement in OLP lesions [30]. The topical application of 0.1% fluocinolone acetonide in Orabase is able to reduce the high expression of TNF-α in OLP lesions [31].
- *Fluocinonide*. It is a high-potency glucocorticoid with anti-inflammatory and vasoconstrictive properties [32]. Already some time ago, the good efficacy of topical application of 0.025% fluocinonide in the treatment of OLP was shown by a double-blind randomized controlled clinical trial [33]; however it was found that 0.05% fluocinonide is less effective than 0.05% clobetasol in the treatment of the signs and symptoms of OLP and vesiculo-erosive oral disorders [17, 34].
- *Clobetasol propionate*. It is a more recent compound that has a chlorine atom in place of the hydroxyl group (OH) in C-21 and a strong local anti-inflammatory activity [9]. It is 1600 times more powerful than fluocinolone and has proven to be reliable in the treatment of oral diseases [35]. 0.05% clobetasol propionate is one of the most effective and first choice topical therapeutic protocols in the treatment of symptomatic OLP [2, 3, 36], since, as already mentioned, its activity stands out compared to that of other topical glucocorticoids such as fluocinonide, fluticasone, betamethasone, and triamcinolone [3, 10, 17, 23, 35, 37]. However a recent Cochrane review concluded that there is no consistent evidence that any particular corticosteroid was better than any other [38]. It was observed that, after 6 months of follow-up without therapy, 65% of patients treated for 6 months with 0.05% clobetasol maintained the improvements [17]. A concentration of 0.025% has also been shown to be effective [3]. According to a group of researchers, however, a concentration of 0.05% would not lead to a further improvement in clinical parameters compared to 0.025% clobetasol [39]. A comparative prospective study with a mean follow-up of 36 months reported comparable efficacy between topical clobetasol and systemic prednisone (1 mg/kg/day) [10], and a systematic review and meta-analysis of the literature concluded that topical tacrolimus (0.01%) and clobetasol propionate (0.05%) have comparable effects in the treatment of OLP [40]. A recent Cochrane review reported that there is low-certainty evidence that topical tacrolimus may be more effective in the management of OLP compared to corticosteroids [38]. Ciclosporin in the form of a mouthwash is expensive and less effective than topical clobetasol in inducing healing of OLP lesions, although the two active ingredients have com-

parable effects on symptoms and clobetasol can cause more side effects than cyclosporine [41]. A pilot study has shown that the formulation of clobetasol in adhesive paste induces a more rapid remission of pain than the ointment or a formulation with an analgesic oral base [42]. Campisi G. et al. [43] observed that a lipid microsphere formulation loaded with 0.025% clobetasol propionate can increase the efficacy of the corticosteroid, at least in terms of symptom remission and compliance, compared to a more commonly used formulation (a kind of dispersion of a lipophilic ointment in the hydrophilic phase). A study group successfully treated small and accessible erosive lesions localized on the gingiva and palate through the use of a clobetasol-based adherent paste placed in an individual tray, achieving contact time control over the entire surface of the lesions [44]. Even the 0.05% clobetasol-based mouthwash formulation is effective in the treatment of severe EOLP [45]. Especially when used over a long period of time, superpotent steroids such as clobetasol can induce potential adrenal insufficiency and tachyphylaxis [32] (a form of tolerance characterized by early and noticeable loss of the molecule's effect due to administration in small amounts but with rather short time intervals between one application and another).

Topical corticosteroids can be used in conjunction with adhesive vehicles or in the form of oral rinses. Topical corticosteroids in the form of oral rinses seem to have good efficacy in forms of multifocal diffusion OLP, where the lesions are difficult to access from the outside for the placement of a gel or ointment [1]. Commonly, ointments and suspensions are preferred, while creams may taste bitter and not melt well with adhesive pastes, and gels almost invariably contain alcohol and can cause burning; however, gels and creams are usually well accepted by patients. Sprays, commonly used for nasal allergies and asthma, can also be used intraorally [13]. The biggest problem in the use of topical corticosteroids in the oral cavity is related to the difficult adhesion to the mucosa for a sufficient time [2]. To overcome this problem, the use of adhesive mediums has been proposed, such as sodium carboxymethylcellulose (Orabase, ConvaTec Ltd., Reading, UK) and hydroxyethyl cellulose, as well as the use of special release systems, such as microspheres loaded with lipids [2, 13]. Oral solutions based on dexamethasone, triamcinolone, and clobetasol can be used for oral rinses in cases of widespread oral involvement or in elderly patients who may find it technically difficult to apply a gel or ointment to the sites of active oral lesions, however there is a potentially increased risk of systemic absorption and candida infection with oral corticosteroid rinses; there is no definitive evidence that topical corticosteroids combined with an adhesive paste (such as Orabase), despite widely used, are more effective than other preparations [24, 28, 46, 47].

Side effects resulting from the use of topical steroids are limited and generally well tolerated [1]. Adverse reactions include secondary candidiasis, nausea, mucosal/skin atrophy (based on application site), xerostomia, dysgeusia, delayed oropharyngeal wound healing during treatment, telangiectasia, and acne (in case of skin application) [8, 12, 48]. The trans-mucosal systemic absorption of topical molecules is modest [12]. A useful indicator for evaluating systemic absorption during long-term topical treatment is represented by a reduced elimination of cortisol in the urine in the last 24 h (due to hypothalamic-pituitary-adrenal suppression) [8]. Although there are some data report cases of adrenal suppression induced by the systemic absorption of very potent topical corticosteroids used in the treatment of chronic skin diseases, these effects are unusual when these drugs are used in the oral district, provided that patients are adequately educated on the correct use [2]. In this regard, when a topical product is prescribed for the oral cavity, the patient must be instructed to apply a small amount of the product to the affected mucosa (in the case of corticosteroids one to three times a day) avoiding drinking, talking, and eating for at least 30–60 min. After this time interval, it will be possible to rinse to avoid swallowing the medication.

In any case, clinical experience and laboratory studies have not shown significant systemic effects in almost all cases [12]. The most commonly observed adverse effect is acute pseudomembranous candidiasis [13]. This can be prevented with the use of antifungals (miconazole gel) or chlorhexidine-based mouthwashes [17, 49]. When OLP/OLL lesions are exclusively gingival, topical steroids can best be applied using individual soft resin or silicone trays to create a sort of oral occlusive dressing [2, 44].

6.2 Immunomodulating Agents

6.2.1 Calcineurin Inhibitors

Calcineurin inhibitors are immunosuppressive drugs with inhibitory activity against calcineurin, a calcium-dependent protein with phosphatase activity, responsible for the immune response: in particular, calcineurin dephosphorylates the transcription factor NF-AT (nuclear factor of activated T cells) which, at the nuclear level, binds to various genes, including the promoter of the IL-2 gene, inducing its transcription, a cytokine essential for the activation of T lymphocytes [9, 50, 51].

- *Cyclosporine*. It is a cyclic peptide composed of 11 amino acids and is the cornerstone of immunosuppressive therapy, essential in the prevention of organ transplant rejection [9]. Cyclosporin, by binding with a cytosolic protein, cyclophilin, inhibits the activity of calcineurin, resulting in a deficiency of IL-2 in the cytoplasm of T lymphocytes, resulting in a lack of proliferation and activation [9, 23]. In addition to immunosuppression in transplant patients, cyclosporine is indicated in various rheumatological and inflammatory diseases such as methotrexate-resistant rheumatoid arthritis, Behçet's syndrome, SLE, inflammatory bowel diseases (IBD), nephrotic syndrome, psoriasis, and severe atopic dermatitis. Among the side effects, dose-dependent, the main one is given by renal toxicity which is reversible if detected and managed early; the intake of this medication is not recommended during pregnancy and breastfeeding [9]. Systemically administered cyclosporine may be indicated in severe forms of OLP refractory to topical treatment, although the risk of adverse effects must be considered [2]. Side effects of topical cyclosporine administration are minimal; despite the significant improvement in oral symptoms, rinses with cyclosporine solution do not produce results superior to those obtained with a 0.1% triamcinolone paste [52, 53]. Many studies have shown the efficacy of cyclosporine in OLP, a drug that affects Th lymphocytes in a T-cell-mediated disorder, but as previously mentioned, this type of therapy is expensive and less effective than topical clobetasol in inducing healing of OLP lesions, and the benefits have only been demonstrated in some cases and are dose-dependent [41, 52, 54–56]; therefore cyclosporine cannot represent a first-line therapy [57]. The oral formulation of 5-ml cyclosporine solution (50–1500 mg/ml) can be used as a mouthwash, or the drug may be applied through an adhesive base (26–128 mg up to three times a day), although if cyclosporine is characterized by a high molecular mass which interferes with the penetration of the mucosa. Therefore, the efficacy of this immunosuppressive agent could be related to its systemic absorption (although it is modest) which can cause nephrotoxic effects, hypertension, and neurological dysfunction [2, 3, 15, 58, 59]. Another known dose-related effect is gingival hyperplasia which is reduced when the drug is stopped [23]. Low doses of cyclosporine combined with systemic prednisolone have been effective in the treatment of one case of LPP [60]. This drug can also be used in the treatment of cGvHD [3]. According to a 2011 Cochrane review, however, there is a weak and unreliable evidence that cyclosporine can reduce the pain and clinical signs of OLP [6]. A recent systematic review and meta-analysis of the literature states that cyclosporine does not induce a statistically significant improvement in the clinical signs, symptoms, and scores of OLP compared to topical glucocorticoids [61].

- *Tacrolimus*. It is a macrolide antibiotic with a mechanism of action similar to cyclosporine (it does not bind to cyclophilin but to a different cytoplasmic immunophylline, Fkb12, or macrophylline-12) but with a much more powerful action increases plasma concentration with grapefruit juice. Like cyclosporine, it is indicated in the prophylaxis of organ transplant rejection and in various other disorders. It can cause nephrotoxic and neurotoxic effects, hyperglycemia, but unlike cyclosporine tacrolimus does not induce dyslipidemia and gingival hyperplasia [9]. Several articles document the effectiveness of tacrolimus in concentrations of 0.03–0.1% [62–68]. For example, a literature review [69] reports strong evidence that supports the use of tacrolimus ointment in OLP, with an efficacy at least equivalent to that of 0.05% clobetasol. Furthermore, the study showed that topical application of tacrolimus results in an increase in its plasma concentrations but without clinically significant adverse effects. Azizi et al. [70] found that 0.1% tacrolimus was as effective as 0.1% topical triamcinolone acetonide in reducing the signs and symptoms associated with lesions. Singh et al. [71] also showed the efficacy of 0.1% tacrolimus comparable to that of other corticosteroid and non-corticosteroid topical agents. Hodgson et al. [64] reported a 14% complete and 80% partial success rate in the use of 0.1% tacrolimus in ulcer-erosive lesions resistant to corticosteroid treatment, while 6% of patients did not report clinical benefits. Furthermore, the patients underwent an average treatment lasting 19.8 months, and the most commonly reported adverse effects were the burning sensation (16%) and a transient alteration of the sensation of taste (8%), while not long-lasting hepatic or renal biochemical changes were observed. Polizzi et al. [72] reported a complete success rate of about 1/3 of treated patients and partial success rate of about 2/3 with a 3-month treatment protocol, but not all cases were ulcer-erosive lesions. A survey by Morrison et al. [66] also showed the efficacy of 0.1% tacrolimus in the treatment of EOLP lesions unresponsive to topical corticosteroids. A systematic review and meta-analysis of the literature confirms the possible role of topical tacrolimus as an alternative to topical clobetasol in the treatment of OLP [40]. A review by Ribero S. et al. [73] also concludes that topical tacrolimus may represent a valid therapeutic option in severe treatment-resistant OLP. However, a more recent systematic review and meta-analysis of the literature reports that tacrolimus does not induce a statistically significant improvement in the clinical signs, symptoms, and scores of OLP compared to topical glucocorticoids [61]. In this regard, a recent Cochrane review concluded that there is very low evidence that topical tacrolimus may improve pain control in symptomatic OLP lesions compared to clobetasol [38]. Kaliakatsou et al. [62] conducted a non-comparative open-label study submitting patients with ulcer-erosive OLP treatment with 0.1% tacrolimus for 8 weeks and following them for a 22-week follow-up period after the end of treatment. Also in this case, the efficacy of tacrolimus has been documented, and the adverse effect reported in 35% of patients was local irritation. But the most interesting fact is that in as many as 13 out of 17 patients there was a recurrence of the lesion from 2 to 15 weeks after the cessation of therapy. The same recent systematic review cited above [61] reports that the range of time to relapse after discontinuation of therapy would be between 2 weeks and 6 months and these periods would not differ significantly from those related to treatment with topical corticosteroids. Arduino et al. [74] found longer-lasting long-term benefits with the topical use of pimecrolimus compared to tacrolimus. Furthermore, tacrolimus, although very effective, is hypothesized to favor the development of OSCC in OLP lesions [1, 75, 76], and by inducing local immunosuppression, it can cause the appearance of superinfections. Therefore, topical tacrolimus is not suitable as long-term maintenance therapy in those patients who do not experience complete remission of signs and symptoms, and even in cases of complete but momentary remission, the risk of relapse after discontinuation of therapy appears to be probable according to the literature, although few studies have been conducted in this regard.

- *Pimecrolimus*. It is the most recent calcineurin inhibitor used in the treatment of OLL/OLP, with action similar to that of tacrolimus and fewer side effects: in fact, it exerts its action by binding to Fkb12 and inducing a reduction in the cytokine production of T lymphocytes (both of type Th1 such as IL-12, IFN-γ, and TNF-α and type Th2 such as IL-4 and IL-10); however it is more selective as it has no effect on Langerhans cells [2, 13, 22, 61, 77, 78]. Pimecrolimus prevents the release of cytokines and mastocellular mediators, and topical use seems to have little systemic immunosuppressive effects [23]. It is also believed that the immunosuppressive potency of pimecrolimus is weaker than cyclosporine and tacrolimus and has less permeation through the skin than topical steroids or topical tacrolimus [13]. Like 0.1% tacrolimus, 1% pimecrolimus represents an alternative for patients refractory to glucocorticoid therapy [57]. Topical pimecrolimus reduced Fas expression on oral keratinocytes of OLP patients [79] and appears to have comparable efficacy to medium potent topical steroids such as triamcinolone acetonide [80]. A recent randomized controlled trial comparing 1% pimecrolimus with 0.1% tacrolimus in adhesive ointment in the management of symptomatic OLP/OLL showed no difference in clinical efficacy, although it appears that treatment with pimecrolimus tends to guarantee results more stable over time, with a lower risk of relapse [74]. Although four small randomized placebo-controlled trials have suggested that 1% pimecrolimus cream may be an effective and well-tolerated treatment for EOLP/OLL [81–84], a Cochrane meta-analysis reported that there is no concrete evidence that 1% pimecrolimus is more effective than placebo in the treatment of EOLP [6]. A recent meta-analysis showed that pimecrolimus does not induce a greater improvement in clinical scores and symptoms than topical glucocorticoids [61].

The most reported local side effects from treatment with calcineurin inhibitors are the transient burning sensation, altered taste, xerostomia, and hyperpigmentation of the mucous membranes [57, 61]. These adverse effects in patients treated with cyclosporine and pimecrolimus are not more frequent than in those treated with topical glucocorticoids, while the incidence is higher in those treated with tacrolimus. Furthermore, treatment with tacrolimus and cyclosporine has been reported to induce several non-severe side effects such as nausea, headache, gastrointestinal upset, and dizziness within 2 weeks/3 months, while no systemic adverse effects have been reported with pimecrolimus [61]. The US Food and Drug Administration (FDA) has warned about an increased theoretical risk of malignancy (lymphomas and squamous carcinomas) in patients using topical tacrolimus/pimecrolimus for the treatment of skin psoriasis [2]. The decision was heavily criticized in the medical community as concerns stemmed from case reports and animal data [85]. A "deductive meta-analysis" found no evidence of an increased risk of skin cancer associated with the use of topical calcineurin inhibitors, but this study presents conflicts of interest [86]. The issue remains controversial, as two separate case reports reported the development of OSCC in two patients with OLP/OLL and with a history of 0.1% topical tacrolimus application [75, 76]. The topic therefore remains debated.

6.2.2 Analogues of the Synthesis of Purine and Pyrimidine Bases

- *Mycophenolate mofetil* (MMF). It is a derivative of mycophenolic acid isolated from a fungus, initially studied for its antibiotic and antiviral properties, but known above all for its immunosuppressive effects. MMF is a prodrug that is converted in the body into mycophenolic acid which, by inhibiting the enzyme inosine monophosphate dehydrogenase (IMPDH), causes an accumulation of 6-thionosinic acid; through a negative feedback mechanism, this determines a depletion of purines, in particular of guanethidine but not of adenine, thus stopping the S phase and the proliferation of T and B lymphocytes which, unlike other proliferating cells, do not possess a alternative route to synthesize guanethidine. This explains why mycophenolic acid acts less critically on proliferating cells than lymphocytes and is not a cytotoxic agent [9]. MMF is indicated in the prevention of organ transplant rejection and in the treatment of SLE, rheumatoid arthritis, cGvHD, and other disorders [9, 22]. It is a well-tolerated drug, and the main toxic effects consist of leukopenia, increase in liver enzymes, and gastrointestinal disorders; therefore a monthly monitoring of blood counts and liver function is recommended in these patients [9]. Some studies have shown the efficacy of systemic MMF in the management of EOLP, refractory and recalcitrant to topical corticosteroids [87, 88]. In the first case report study [87], clinicians successfully treated a woman with EOLP resistant to topical treatment based on clobetasol and tacrolimus with MMF (2000 mg/day) first associated with systemic cyclosporine and then individually, gradually lowering the dosage up to 100 mg/day. The second study is a retrospective review that reported the positive effects of MMF in patients with severe forms of ulcerative mucocutaneous LP [88]. MMF has been used successfully, up to complete remission, also for the treatment of severe ulcer-erosive forms of oral and genital LP resistant to other systemic therapies; no exacerbations were observed during the subsequent 4 years of follow-up, although improvement in lesions was observed only after 4–6 weeks of therapy, possibly due to the drug's mechanism of action [89]. A study showed that in patients with EOLP treated with MMF and topical pimecrolimus there was a reduction in serum levels of IL-6 and a lack of resistance to therapy, while patients treated with topical methotrexate and pimecrolimus did not show a significant reduction in serum levels of IL-6, and resistance to therapy has been observed in some of these, especially in the plaque forms; this could indicate that elevated levels of IL-6 in EOLP reflect the chronic inflammatory nature of the disease [77]. MMF and azathioprine are usually required for long-term therapy as corticosteroid-sparing agents [15]. Although its potency is similar to that of azathioprine, MMF, in moderate doses, appears to be more effective than azathioprine in the treatment of cutaneous LP [90]; this is probably due to the fact that in addition to its cytostatic effect on lymphocytes, MMF is able to inhibit leukocyte recruitment and adhesion to endothelial cells [22]. Mycophenolate is quite expensive and effective with long-term use [91]. MMF has shown a promise as an alternative to azathioprine as an immunomodulating agent with a better safety profile in managing graft rejection in organ transplant recipients and GvHD and therefore may be a candidate for use in recalcitrant OLP [92]. The MMF in topical formulation of 2% adhesive paste is effective in reducing the symptoms and size of OLP ulcerative lesions, although these effects were obtained starting from the fourth week of treatment [93].

- *Azathioprine*. It hinders leukocyte proliferation (S phase) by inhibiting the synthesis of purines followed by apoptotic death. It is indicated in organ transplants and in autoimmune diseases (lupus, rheumatoid arthritis, psoriatic arthritis, ulcerative colitis, Crohn's disease, etc.), although it currently tends to be replaced by mycophenolate mofetil. Due to a polymorphism of the gene encoding the thiopurine S-methyltransferase (TPMT) enzyme (present in 10% of the population, of which 0.5% are homozygous), some patients have little or no activity of the enzyme with the risk of toxic effects of acute myelosuppression from 6-thioguanine (6-TG) accumulation [9]. Blood monitoring of 6-TG and TPMT allows to maintain myelotoxic effects (leukopenia, thrombocytopenia, and anemia) within acceptable limits. The association of azathioprine with allopurinol (xanthine oxidase inhibitor used in hyperuricemia) is not recommended as this enzyme inhibits the active metabolites of azathioprine: the consequence is an increase in the toxic effects of azathioprine [3, 9]. In addition to the effects on the bone marrow, azathioprine causes gastrointestinal toxicity (usually mild) and can increase the risk of the onset of infections and neoplasms, especially in the case of a long-term therapy. Its use is not recommended during pregnancy and breastfeeding [9]. Azathioprine can be indicated as a systemic therapy in cases of severe forms of OLP refractory to topical treatment [2, 18]. Treatment with azathioprine has been shown to be effective in patients with severe and generalized forms of LP, although MMF seems more effective [90, 94–97]. Azathioprine is a steroid-sparing agent useful in the treatment of cutaneous LP, but there is less evidence of its effectiveness in the management of recalcitrant OLP. In general, the starting dose should be approximately 1.0 mg/kg/day (50 to 100 mg) gradually increasing in increments of 0.5 mg/kg/day over several weeks, if needed up to a maximum dose of 2 mg/kg/day. Careful monitoring of patients' complete blood counts (ideally weekly) is essential for the first 8 weeks of therapy, to reduce the frequency thereafter (but it is recommended to repeat it at least three times a month). If the patient's clinical condition does not improve within 3 months, azathioprine should be discontinued [3]. Topical azathioprine (5–25 mg/ml oral suspension three to four times a day or 5 mg/ml gel) has been used in the treatment of oral cGvHD (OLL-cGvHD) lesions [98, 99].

- *Methotrexate (MTX)*. It is an antimetabolite analogue of folic acid with a dose-dependent mechanism of action: at high doses (antiblastic therapy), it inhibits the activity of dihydrofolate reductase (DHFR) and other folate-dependent enzymes causing a lack of purine synthesis, while a low dose inhibits IL-1 activity. It is indicated in the treatment of rheumatoid arthritis, polymyositis, dermatomyositis, and LE, with a dosage of 7.5–12 mg per week, orally or intramuscularly administered in one or three doses spaced 12 h apart. MTX causes hepatic toxicity (increased transaminases) and in 10–20% of patients, if the therapy is long-lasting, hepatic fibrosis, gastrointestinal toxicity (nausea, vomiting, diarrhea), and hematological toxicity (leukopenia and thrombocytopenia), mucocutaneous disorders such as rash, alopecia, and stomatitis may rarely be reported. Frequent checks of blood counts and liver and kidney function are therefore recommended [9]. The use of low doses of oral methotrexate (2.5–15 mg per week, with or without folic acid 1 mg/day) is effective in the treatment of aggressive forms of EOLP and resistant to other topical or systemic treatments [100, 101]. MTX is well tolerated and effective for severe EOLP; however, clinical benefits are obtained after several weeks of therapy; therefore patients must be motivated to continue treatment until signs and symptoms have completely improved [102]. MTX at 7.5 mg/week for 7–9 months was less effective than MMF (1 g/day for 3–4 months) in reducing serum IL-6 levels, and some patients have showed resistance to therapy compared to those treated with MMF [77].

6.2.3 mTOR Inhibitors

- *Sirolimus (rapamycin)*. It is a macrolide antibiotic with immunosuppressive and antiproliferative properties. Similar to tacrolimus, it inhibits the immune response of B and T lymphocytes; in activated T cells, it binds to immunophylline FKBP-12, and the complex formed inhibits a kinase called mTOR (mammalian target of rapamycin) involved in the progression of the cell cycle (G1-S) and in the synthesis of IL-2 resulting in a blocking of proliferation and immune activity. Side effects include infections, lymphomas, thrombosis, gastrointestinal disturbances, delayed wound healing, and mixed dyslipidemia [9]. Sirolimus can be used in the treatment of recalcitrant EOLP and be administered together with MMF when steroid-sparing agents are to be used [22]. Soria et al. [103] observed that topical application of sirolimus (1 mg/ml, twice a day for 3 months) in seven patients with recalcitrant EOLP resulted in complete remission in four out of seven and in two out of seven a partial remission with minimal side effects. Furthermore, sirolimus also possesses antitumor properties and could theoretically control painful symptoms and at the same time reduce the risk of OSCC in patients with OLP/OLL [15].

6.2.4 NF-κB Inhibitors

- *Thalidomide*. It is a drug with a powerful teratogenic effect and immunomodulatory properties. Thalidomide favors the link between the transcription factor NF-κB and its cytoplasmic inhibitor IkB, causing a block of the actions of the former: inflammation, organogenesis, angiogenesis, cell survival, and metastasis; in addition, thalidomide interferes with the function of various growth factors and with the expression of adhesion molecules [9]. Thalidomide is used in the management of aphthous stomatitis, leprosy, erythema nodosum, atrophic arthritis, myelodysplastic syndromes, and Crohn's disease because it has the potential to reduce the formation of TNF-α [104, 105]. The systemic use of thalidomide (50–200 mg/day) has been proven effective in the treatment of EOLP [106, 107]. It has been observed that 1% topical thalidomide paste has the same efficacy as 0.043% dexamethasone paste in the treatment of EOLP [108], but it would be useful to make comparisons with stronger topical therapies [78].
- *Amlexanox*. It is an immunomodulatory, anti-inflammatory, and anti-allergic agent, inhibitor of protein kinase IKK-ε and TBK1 (TANK-binding kinase 1) used in the treatment of recurrent aphthous ulcers (5% oral paste), allergic rhinitis (spray nasal), conjunctivitis (eye drops), and bronchial asthma (oral tablets) [109, 110]. Amlexanox potently inhibits the release of histamine and leukotrienes from mast cells, basophils, and neutrophils, possibly through the increase of intracellular cyclic AMP in inflammatory cells, a stabilizing effect of the membrane, or the inhibition of calcium influx [111]. When administered orally, in animal models, amlexanox has been shown to suppress both immediate and delayed hypersensitivity reactions; however, the clinical relevance of these actions in recurrent aphthous stomatitis is unknown [109]. Furthermore, it has recently been shown that amlexanox is able to block the RANKL-induced activation of NF-κB, MAPK, c-Fos, and NFATc1 and that in animal models it can suppress osteoclastogenesis and prevent bone loss induced by ovariectomy; therefore, amlexanox could be considered a new therapeutic candidate for osteoclast-related diseases, such as osteoporosis and rheumatoid arthritis [110]. This drug is also a new agent under study for the management of OLP [112]. A single randomized controlled clinical trial [26] found the equal efficacy of amlexanox (5%) in paste with dexamethasone (0.043%) in the treatment of EOLP; the latter, however, is a corticosteroid with very moderate potency. Therefore it will be necessary to compare the effectiveness of amlexanox with more effective agents such as clobetasol and fluocinolone acetonide [78].

6.2.5 Antibiotics

- *Dapsone*. It is an antibiotic with an antimetabolite effect and a mechanism of action similar to sulfonamides: it competes with PABA in binding with the enzyme dihydropteroate synthase, thus inhibiting the synthesis of dihydrofolic acid, and therefore is used in the treatment of leprosy [23]. It also has anti-inflammatory and immunomodulating effects (inhibition of the release of mastocellular chemotactic factors [113]) and may be indicated for some mucocutaneous disorders [114]. Due to these properties, dapsone can also be used in the treatment of OLP and severe EOLP [113, 115]. A recent open-label randomized clinical trial showed that oral dapsone (100 mg twice daily, combined with iron and folic acid tablets) was the most effective treatment in treating patients with OLP com-

pared to 0.1% triamcinolone acetonide in paste and 0.1% tacrolimus and topical retinoids, but the only statistically significant difference was observed between dapsone and retinoids, while this did not occur compared to the other treatments [71]. Dapsone causes hemolysis of varying degrees in a dose-dependent manner and develops in nearly every individual given 200–300 mg of oral dapsone per day. Deficiency of glucose-6-phosphate dehydrogenase (G6PD) may increase the risk of hemolytic anemia or methemoglobinemia; therefore screening for G6PD deficiency is required before prescribing dapsone. In addition, patients treated with many drugs can develop dapsone-induced hypersensitivity syndrome (DHS) which causes rash, fever, and jaundice usually within the first 6 weeks of therapy, symptoms that can be improved with corticosteroid treatment [116].
- *Other antibiotics*. Other antibiotics that some authors have employed to treat patients with OLP are some penicillins and tetracyclines, including doxycycline [7], but these therapies have never been definitively validated, and it is important to consider the phenomenon of antibiotic resistance in these patients which would require prolonged therapy.

6.2.6 Antimicotics

- *Amphotericin B*. Amphotericin B is an antifungal drug with the broadest spectrum of action: it performs a fungicidal action by complexing with ergosterol in the plasma membrane of the fungus (which causes the formation of pores) and causing oxidative damage [9]. It has shown positive effects in patients with OLP and candidiasis [117], although a controlled clinical study has suggested that this therapy plays a marginal role in the management of OLP [118].
- *Griseofulvin*. It is a mycostatic agent that interferes with the synthesis of chitin and with the polymerization of microtubules, preventing the formation of the mitotic spindle. Concentrating in the keratinized layers of the epithelia, it is indicated in the management of superficial and cutaneous mycoses; furthermore, being an inducer of CYP450, griseofulvin reduces the activity of oral anticoagulants, barbiturates, and all drugs metabolized by this enzyme complex [9]. It has been proposed in the treatment of OLP and LP [115, 119], and some efficacy has been shown (e.g., with doses of 500 mg/day) [120–123], but in larger studies no significant benefits [124–126].

6.2.7 Antiprotozoals

- *Metronidazole*. Belonging to the class of nitroimidazoles, it is one of the most effective agents against anaerobic bacteria and protozoa, thanks to the formation, after reduction reactions, of anionic nitro radicals which damage the DNA of sensitive organisms [9]. Metronidazole also possesses immunomodulatory properties, and these may have contributed to an improvement in patients with oral and generalized LP undergoing oral treatment with a dosage of 500 mg twice a day or 250 mg three times a day [127, 128].
- *Chloroquine and hydroxychloroquine*. They are antimalarial drugs that bind to heme, released during the breakdown of hemoglobin by parasites, preventing its seizure; the heme-chloroquine bond is responsible for oxidative damage to membranes and digestive proteases [9]. In addition to this, the immunomodulating effect is known: these molecules are weak lipophilic bases that accumulate in cellular lysosomes, raising their pH [129]. This leads to an inhibition of lysosomal acid proteases, a reduction in glycosylation, and secretion of proteins, with various immunological consequences such as a reduced functioning of immune cells, chemotaxis, phagocytosis, and the production of superoxide by neutrophils [130–132]. Hydroxychloroquine, in addition to malaria, is indicated as a first-choice treatment in SLE and DLE and can also be used in rheumatoid arthritis, cutaneous porphyria, chronic ulcerative stomatitis (CUS), and vari-

ous other disorders [15, 133, 134]. Chloroquine and hydroxychloroquine may be indicated in severe forms of OLP resistant to topical treatment [135]. Semi-annual treatment based on 400 mg hydroxychloroquine proved to be relatively more effective than 500 mg griseofulvin in the treatment of LP [136]. An open-label study found an excellent response in 9/10 patients with OLP treated with hydroxychloroquine 200–400 mg/day [137]. But it is not always effective, and it may take several months for improvement to occur [3]. A similar and more recent study obtained a complete response in 5/21 patients with EOLP and a partial response in 12/21 after treatment with hydroxychloroquine sulfate 400 mg/day, but the response to therapy was observed after 2–4 months [138]. In addition, hydroxychloroquine has several side effects, and, before starting therapy, it is advisable to perform and repeat the basic visual acuity test every 6–12 months to check for ocular toxicity. Sun UV-induced skin lichenoid reactions have also been reported with this agent, as well as hematological abnormalities and altered liver function tests; therefore regular monitoring of complete blood counts and liver function tests is also recommended [3]. Finally, hydroxychloroquine (which can be administered not only in OLP and CUS but also in Sjogren's syndrome) at high doses causes prolongation of the QT tract with possible secondary arrhythmias [139]. A research group has demonstrated the success of a gel formulation based on hydroxychloroquine niosomes, i.e., nano-sized vesicles used as carriers of the drug [140].

6.2.8 Anti-Welmintics

- *Levamisole*. It is an anthelmintic agent, effective in humans as an adjuvant in the oncological field, as, through its immunomodulatory action on B and T lymphocytes and macrophages, it promotes a more efficient elimination of neoplastic cells. Usually the toxic effects are on the gastrointestinal level, but the rarest and most fearful is the severe agranulocytosis (especially in HLA-B27-positive patients) of autoimmune origin, a complication that strongly limits the therapeutic indications of this medication. Furthermore, corticosteroids antagonize the effects of levamisole [9]. The use of levamisole in the management of the OLP has been reported [115]. In one study, 23 patients with recalcitrant OLP were treated with levamisole 150 mg/day and prednisolone 15 mg/day for three consecutive days per week; 12/21 showed complete remission of signs and symptoms in the first 2 weeks, while 11/21 showed partial remission; therefore it is possible that adding levamisole to prednisolone treatment may produce improved outcomes in EOLP management [141], but no comparison was made with prednisolone treatment alone. Furthermore, levamisole may occasionally induce lichenoid lesions [142].

6.2.9 Other Immunomodulating Agents

- *Mesalazine*. It is an NSAID belonging to salicylates, which acts by causing a reduction in the production of leukotrienes and inhibiting IL-1, with limited action to the gastrointestinal tract, used in the management of IBD, but also to some oral conditions such as Behçet's syndrome, recurrent oral aphthosis, and ulcerative mucositis in bone marrow transplant patients [143]. Topical application of 5% mesalamine has shown effects similar to 0.05% clobetasol in the management of patients with OLP [142]. But this drug has been associated with the onset of lichenoid reactions that can only be resolved by discontinuing therapy [144].
- *Enoxaparin*. It is a low-molecular-weight heparin which, by binding to antithrombin, increases the reaction rate with thrombin by about 1000 times, thus determining an anticoagulant effect [9]. Low-dose heparin without anticoagulant activity inhibits the activity of heparinase of T lymphocytes, an enzyme cru-

cial in the migration of these cells to target tissues. Some patients with generalized LP were treated with 3 mg of enoxaparin subcutaneously once a week, and within 4–10 weeks, complete regression of the eruptions was achieved in 8/10 patients, but of the four patients also affected by OLP, only one showed improvements [145]. The forms of cutaneous LP and reticular OLP seem to have the best response to this type of approach [146]. A more recent study has shown that weekly treatment with enoxaparin 5 mg, while providing benefits in patients with disseminated LP, is less effective than oral prednisone 0.5 mg/kg [147]. Therefore, while representing an alternative treatment, especially in generalized LP, without side effects, however enoxaparin is less effective than glucocorticoids.

- *Interferons (IFNs) and direct-acting antivirals (DAAs) without IFN.* Interferons have antiviral, immunomodulatory, and antiproliferative activity; IFN-α and IFN-β have superimposable effects and modulate the cytotoxic activity of lymphocytes, NK cells, and macrophages, while IFN-γ has fewer antiviral effects but greater immunomodulatory action through the activation of macrophages with production of ROS and the expression of MHC-II antigens for antigen presentation by the macrophage to the lymphocyte and by modulating local inflammatory responses [9]. Patients with OLP can be treated with IFN-α [148]. Two small uncontrolled studies have suggested that the topical application of a gel containing IFN-β and a cream based on IFN-α can improve EOLP [149, 150]. Systemic IFN-α (3–10 million IU three times a week) can be used successfully in the treatment of OLP patients with and without HCV infection [151–153]. But, despite these successes, interferon can also cause or worsen LP lesions [154–156], and anti-IFN-γ antibodies were able to resolve experimentally induced lichenoid reactions [157]. Furthermore, subjects treated with interferons may present severe signs of toxicity such as myelosuppression, autoimmune thyroiditis, infertility, hypotension and tachycardia, depression, paraesthesia, pain, mental confusion, and sleep disturbances [9]. It is interesting to note that recently some studies have shown that IFN-free direct-acting antiviral (DAA) therapy (in particular the combination of daclatasvir (DCV)/asunaprevir (ASV)) is effective and without relevant side effects in the treatment of patients with OLP and HCV-associated cutaneous LP, although the long-term efficacy of this type of approach is not yet known [158, 159] (see also Sect. 6.4.7). Instead, following treatment with interferons, there is often an exacerbation of the HCV-associated OLP [154, 160, 161].
- *Amitriptyline.* It is a tertiary amine belonging to the class of tricyclic antidepressants (TCAs) which inhibit the reuptake of norepinephrine (NE), serotonin (5-HT), and dopamine (DA) by non-specific blocking of the amine transporters themselves. Today they no longer represent as first-choice drugs in the treatment of depression because there are categories of drugs with fewer side effects such as SSRIs (selective serotonin reuptake inhibitors) [9]. Amitriptyline possesses local anesthetic properties [78], and on the basis of this, in theory, it could prove useful in treating symptomatic OLP in depressed patients. In a poor-quality randomized clinical trial [162] patients were treated with a ketoconazole, clobetasol, and amitriptyline solution or with a 0.5-mg dexamethasone tablet, 30 drops of mycostatin, and a 5 ml diphenhydramine syrup (antihistamine). The combination was effective; however it is not possible to establish the role of amitriptyline in obtaining these results, and it is possible that the main improvements in the two groups were obtained through clobetasol and dexamethasone.

6.3 Vitamin Complexes

6.3.1 Retinoids (Vitamin A)

Vitamin A is a fat-soluble vitamin, which occurs in the human body in three different forms: alcohol (retinol), aldehyde (retinaldehyde), and acid (retinoic acid). The term vitamin A also indicates the natural and synthetic analogues of retinol, called retinoids. Carotenoids containing at least one unsubstituted β-ionic ring (such as β-carotene) are also considered precursors of vitamin A [163].

Topical and systemic retinoids have been extensively studied for the treatment of OLP, are generally less effective than topical corticosteroids, and are more likely to cause negative side effects [1, 3, 15, 22, 115, 119, 164]. Topical retinoids can cause a transient burning sensation, while their systemic administration is associated with numerous serious side effects that prohibit their routine use in OLP: hypertransaminemia, hyperlipidemia, cheilitis, alopecia, dystrophic nail formation, and teratogenic effects. Therefore, topical retinoids are considered a second-choice therapy for OLP, while systemic retinoids are not recommended [3].

- *Retinoic acid (tretinoin and isotretinoin).* When administered as a drug, retinoic acid is called tretinoin (all-trans retinoic acid), while isotretinoin is a stereoisomer (cis form) of retinoic acid. The usefulness of 0.1% topical tretinoin and isotretinoin in the management of various forms of OLP has been known for some time [165, 166]. It has been observed that 0.18% isotretinoin is able to induce more significant histological improvements than the 0.05% concentration in patients with EOLP, and the disappearance of dysplastic phenomena has been observed with the 0.018% formulation [167]. Tretinoin (0.1%) induced histologically significant disappearance/decrease of keratinization and concentration of various cytokeratins in patients with OLP or LK [168]. Similar results were obtained with the use of 0.1% retinaldehyde and isotretinoin gel [169, 170]. However, it has been shown that fluocinolone acetonide (0.1%) in Orabase is more effective than retinoic acid 0.05% in Orabase in the treatment of atrophic-erosive OLP [29]. A clinical study by Singh et al. [71] found oral dapsone (100 mg twice daily, combined with iron and folic acid tablets) to be more effective than topical treatment with a retinoid, while the latter did not show significant differences with therapy based on 0.1% triamcinolone acetonide paste or 0.1% tacrolimus in the management of patients with OLP. The immunomodulatory effects of topical tretinoin and isotretinoin may favor the disappearance of white streaks although these effects are temporary, while the positive effects of the systemic use of these agents should be well evaluated taking into account the toxic effects [23].
- *Lycopene.* It is an antioxidant carotenoid (synergistic with vitamins C and E) that provides red color to tomatoes and various fruits. In addition to the antioxidant activity, it has various effects in the body: inhibition of the proliferation of neoplastic cells, induction of phase II enzymes, interference with protein stimulation, regulation of transcription, and restoration of communicating junctions [171–173]. Lycopene has shown some beneficial effects in the treatment of LK, OSCC, and oral submucosal fibrosis (OSMF) [78, 173]. Low serum levels of lycopene have been found in LK and OLP patients [174, 175]. Saawarn et al. [176] observed that lycopene 8 mg/day reduced the symptoms of OLP, although the placebo group showed a similar response.
- *Astaxanthin.* It is a carotenoid with anti-inflammatory and antioxidant activity. An in vitro study showed inhibitory activity against NF-κB and inflammatory cytokines IL-6 and TNF-α, and for this reason, the authors of this research hypothesized that astaxanthin may be useful in improving chronic inflammation, such as those from OLP [177].
- *Fenretinide.* It can be used in the treatment of OLP [15, 23]. Tradati et al. [178] have shown its efficacy as a topical application in patients suffering from widespread forms of LK and OLP.
- *Etretinate.* It is a synthetic retinoid; administered orally (75 mg/day), it resulted in an improvement of symptoms in patients with severe forms of OLP, although side effects were common and forced treatment to be stopped in 6/28 patients [179].

- *Acitretin.* A double-blind controlled study showed remission or marked improvement in LP patients treated with acitretin 30 mg/day for 8 weeks, a systemic treatment that may be acceptable in severe cases of LP [180]. Several cases of OLP patients have also been reported successfully treated with acitretin 25 mg/day [181].
- *Tazarotene.* It has regulatory effects on the growth and differentiation of keratinocytes and on inflammation; 0.1% tazarotene gel has been used successfully in 12 patients with hyperkeratotic OLP [182].
- *Temarotene.* Systemic treatment with temarotene (1046–4800 mg) resulted in a complete response in 6/9 patients with OLP and partial response in 2/9 with few adverse effects [183].

6.3.2 Group B Vitamins

They are a group of water-soluble vitamins that perform numerous functions in the body.

A variety of hematological abnormalities have been observed in patients with OLP, including deficiencies in vitamins B1, B6, B12, iron, and folate [184]. In a study conducted in 352 patients with OLP, an elevated serum level of homocysteine was found attributed to deficiencies in folic acid and vitamins B12 and B6, and a close relationship was shown between elevated levels of homocysteine in the blood and the severity of OLP [185]. The authors therefore suggested that supplementing hematin or multiple B vitamins including B1, B2, B6, and B12 may be beneficial for this specific group of patients with OLP.

- *Vitamin B12.* It has been observed that the treatment of OLP patients with levamisole and vitamin B12 has shown a significant reduction in serum levels of antibodies to gastric parietal cells (GPCA) and this is associated with an improvement in oral lesions [186]. Levamisole treatment also induced a reduction in serum levels of IL-6, IL-8, and TNF-α [187, 188]. However, treatment with levamisole alone did not significantly decrease serum levels of GPCA and did not lead to an improvement in oral signs and symptoms of pernicious anemia in patients with OLP, which showed that it may not be effective enough to promote healing of autoimmune atrophic gastritis [189]. This finding indicated the significant role of vitamin B12 in the healing of OLP [164].

6.3.3 Vitamin D

Vitamin D is involved in the pathogenesis of OLP and has been discussed in Sect. 4.4.2.

Recently Ahmed et al. [190] found a deficiency of vitamin D in 60% of patients with OLP and in 22.5% of healthy patients, but the latter showed more insufficient values than the sick; the authors therefore found that the deficiency in the serum level of vitamin D was not simply related to the development of OLP, but was also related to the symptoms and clinical forms of the disease. A single study evaluated the integration of vitamin D in the treatment of patients with OLP. The authors found that normalizing vitamin D levels in patients with deficiency and OLP improves the clinical course of the disease, just as it does in other autoimmune diseases. Thus, the marked improvement and long-term remission of symptoms in patients with vitamin D deficiency after restoration of its normal levels further support its role in the pathogenesis of OLP as well as other autoimmune diseases [191].

6.3.4 Tocopherol (Vitamin E)

The term vitamin E indicates eight compounds (four tocopherols and four tocotrienols) of which the most important is α-tocopherol. It is a powerful antioxidant capable of removing free radicals and has inhibitory activity against protein kinase C and phospholipase A2. High doses of vitamin E (> 800 mg/day) reduce platelet aggregation and interfere with the metabolism of vitamin K [9].

Compared to healthy subjects, in patients with OLP, there is an increase in the levels of lipid peroxidation products, including malondialdehyde (MDA) and 8-hydroxyhemoxyguanosine (8-OHdG), and a decrease in the levels of some antioxidants such as vit. C and vit. E. After treatment with curcumin for over 200 days, the level of lipid peroxidation products (oxidants) decreased and that of antioxidants increased [192].

The level of antioxidants influences the susceptibility to OLP, and oxidative stress could be a trigger of OLP [193, 194]. Therefore, antioxidant agents such as vitamins can be useful, because vitamins A and E inhibit lipid peroxidation and contribute to the integrity of cell membranes, while vitamin C acts as a cofactor of many enzymes, stabilizes the collagen structure, and also promotes reproduction of vitamin E [57, 195]. According to a cross-sectional study conducted by Bacci et al. [196], tocopherol could significantly reduce the extent of lesions in OLP, without, however, leading to an improvement in symptoms.

6.3.5 Flavonoids (Vitamin P)

Flavonoids or bioflavonoids are a class of secondary plant phenols, which include anthocyanins and anthoxanthins, with significant antioxidant and chelating properties. In the human diet, they are most concentrated in fruits, vegetables, wine, tea, and cocoa. Their cardioprotective effects derive from the ability to inhibit lipid peroxidation, chelate redox-active metals, and attenuate other processes involving ROS [197]. Flavonoids are sometimes grouped together as "vitamin P."

- *Anthocyanins*. A prospective non-randomized study showed good efficacy of local treatment with anthocyanins (100 mg/dose diluted in 5 ml of water, three times a day) extracted from grape skin in patients with OLP and EOLP, with an equal or better than treatment with a cream based on 0.05% clobetasol, 0.35% neomycin, and 100,000 UI/g nystatin [198].

6.4 Nutraceuticals

They are active substances contained in food or found in nature. They usually come from plants, foods, and microbial sources. Examples of nutraceuticals are probiotics, antioxidants, polyunsaturated fatty acids (omega-3, omega-6), vitamins, and enzyme complexes [199].

6.4.1 Oral Curcuminoids

Curcuminoids are anti-inflammatory active substances derived from *Curcuma longa*, an element of Ayurvedic medicine for hundreds of years in ancient India, because it is non-toxic and has various healing properties along with inhibitory, analgesic, antiseptic, and anticarcinogenic activities. Curcumin is the main curcuminoid extracted from the plant and is an antioxidant that has been used as a chemopreventive agent in various types of cancers, as well as in the inhibition of viral and bacterial growth [200]. It has also been shown to have an immunomodulatory effect that involves the activation of macrophages and NK cells and the modulation of lymphocyte activity [201]. It has analgesic, antiseptic, and anti-tumor effects (inhibition of cyclin D1, E, and CD4 and stimulation of p53, pRb, p21, p27, Fas, FasL, procaspase 3, 8, and 9) and inhibits various enzymes such as COX-1, COX-2, LOX (lipoxygenase), iNOS (inducible nitric oxide synthase), the protein kinase C (PKC) pathway, factor NF-κB, and several cytokines such as IL-1β, IL-2, IL-5, IL-6, IL-8, IL-12, IL-18, TNF-α, IFN-γ, and MCP-1 [104, 173]. In addition, the curcumin tablets (900 mg + 80 mg of desmethoxy curcumin +20 mg of bis-desmethoxy curcumin) resulted in an improvement in clinical parameters (pain, appearance of lesions, and degree of mouth opening) and an increase in salivary and serum levels. Antioxidants (such as vitamins C and E) in patients with OLP, LK, and OSMF have prevented lipid peroxidation and DNA damage; the increase in vitamins A, E, and C occurs through the activation of mitochondrial enzymes [192, 202, 203]. After treatment with curcumin for over 200 days, the level of lipid peroxidation products (oxidants) decreased and that of antioxidants increased in patients with OLP [192]. A curcuminoid dosage of 2000 mg/day was no more effective than placebo in the management of patients with OLP [204, 205]. On the other hand, higher doses of curcuminoids (6000 mg/day in three divided doses, standardized supplement "Curcumin C3 Complex" with at least 95% curcumin) have shown benefits in the management of OLP, especially during follow-up, but according to some researchers, 40% of patients experience side effects, including liver dysfunction [15, 206]. Side effects of treated patients included mainly abdominal discomfort and diarrhea; however the occurrence was dose-related, and the reported discomfort was mild [207]. Four clinical studies have shown that the topical application of curcumin (in the form of ointment, gel, or paste with a concentration of 1–5% 2–3 applications/day) is effective in the management of symptoms and lesions of OLP, with activity less than or equal to that of 0.1% triamcinolone acetonide in paste [201, 208–210]. Therefore, curcumin cannot be used as a first-choice active substance but rather as a maintenance drug after the patient has been treated with an initial course of corticosteroids [210]. A recent systematic review [211] found that topically applied curcumin shows promising preliminary data even though it probably cannot be considered a substitute for topical corticosteroids in most patients. Another recently conducted systematic review suggests that curcumin is safe and can be used as an adjunct in combination with corticosteroids to reduce pain, burning, and the clinical appearance of oral lesions in patients with OLP [212].

6.4.2 Aloe Vera (AV)

Aloe vera (AV) is a cactus-like plant that belongs to the Liliaceae family. AV species contain over 200 biologically active substances such as anthraquinones, vitamins, minerals, enzymes, polysaccharides, phenolic compounds, and organic acids. AV, given its complex and heterogeneous composition, has numerous pharmacological actions: it promotes cell proliferation, the production of hyaluronic acid, and tissue healing; has immunomodulatory, anti-inflammatory, antioxidant, and anti-tumor effects [173]. It inhibits inflammation by reducing TNF-α levels and interfering with the arachidonic acid pathway via COX [213]. Aloe vera gel has antifungal, antiviral, and hypoglycemic effects [214, 215]. Some cosmetic and medicinal products are made from the mucilaginous tissue in the center of the AV leaf, which is called aloe vera gel (AV gel). AV gel does not contain anthraquinones, which are responsible for the strong laxative effects of aloe vera [214–217]. AV has been used for various dermatological diseases including radiodermatitis, psoriasis, and genital herpes, with good results [216, 218]. The activity of AV has also been extensively studied in the oral field: in OLP, radio-mucositis, burning mouth syndrome, xerostomia, and recurrent aphthous ulcers [219]. A clinical case of LP has successfully responded to topical and systemic treatment with AV [220]. According to a not-very-recent Cochrane review [6], there is weak evidence from two placebo-controlled RCTs [221, 222], using different formulations (e.g., 70% AV gel: 70% AV mucilage, sorbitol, potassium sorbate, sodium metabisulfite, and hydroxyethyl cellulose), that AV may lead to pain reduction in OLP; however two more recent randomized clinical trials have reported comparable efficacy between an aloe vera mouthwash and a triamcinolone acetonide-based paste (0.1%) and a higher efficacy of AV gel than triamcinolone in bringing about an improvement in the signs and symptoms of OLP [21, 223]. To date, there are different formulations of AV, and the amount of active substance can vary considerably depending on the age of the plant, the conditions of growth and harvest, the parts of the plant, and the extraction methods used [15]. These variations may have influenced the results published by the various authors, and this represents a challenge for future research [78].

6.4.3 Hyaluronic Acid (HA)

The polymerization of the N-acetylglucosamine disaccharide and glucuronic acid forms hyaluronic acid (HA), which is a hygroscopic macromolecule [112] and one of the main components of connective tissue. HA forms a protective coating on the oral mucosa, improving its hydration and accelerating its healing by activating and modulating the response of inflammatory cells, and promoting cell proliferation, angiogenesis, and migration [224, 225]. Topical application of a 0.2% HA gel showed a reduction in pain up to 4 h after application compared to placebo and a significant reduction in the size of eroded or ulcerated areas after 28 days of treatment; therefore its use seems to bring some benefit in the management of EOLP, but the action is not of long duration [226]; therefore it could be useful to increase the frequency of application to obtain better results [112]. According to the data obtained by Hashem et al. [227], it seems instead that0.2% HA (three times a day for 4 weeks) has the same effectiveness as 0.1% triamcinolone acetonide (same frequency and duration of application) in determining a reduction in the VAS score, erythema, and extent of OLP lesions. Similar results were observed by Shetty et al. [228] which showed the effectiveness of 0.2% HA compared to placebo.

6.4.4 Green Tea

Tea is a product made from leaves and buds derived from *Camellia sinensis* [229]. It is an important source of polyphenols (such as epicatechin-3-gallate, epicatechin, epigallocatechin-3-gallate, and epigallocatechin [230]) with renowned antioxidant, anti-inflammatory, chemopreventive, and bactericidal effects [112, 231] and of flavonoids such as the catechins that have evidenced bactericidal effects in a clinical study on periodontal disease [232]. Caffeine (a natural alkaloid) contained in tea, coffee, and coconut has anti-inflammatory and antioxidant effects, protecting DNA from oxidative damage [233, 234]. Beneficial effects of green tea have also been reported in oral candidiasis, LK, and OSCC [173]. Green tea in particular inhibits the migration, activation, and proliferation of T lymphocytes and also controls various inflammatory mediators, thus regulating the non-specific and antigen-specific mechanisms involved in the etiopathogenesis of OLP [235, 236]. Zhang et al. [237] hypothesized that tea consumption could reduce the incidence of OLP and provide non-harmful and cost-effective medical help for OLP.

6.4.5 Propolis

Propolis or "bee glue" is a plant resinous substance that bees collect from the buds and bark of plants and which they process with the addition of wax, pollen, and enzymes produced by their own organism. It consists of numerous components including minerals (Mg, Ca, I, K, Na, Cu, Zn, Mn, and Fe), vitamins (B1, B2, B6, C, E, P), amino acids, and fatty acids [238]. It has been used for centuries in Ayurvedic medicine and has numerous properties: antibiotic, anti-inflammatory, antiviral, antifungal, antioxidant, anesthetic, restorative, immunomodulating, and anticancer properties [239–245]. These properties prompted researchers to test its effectiveness on OLP. It has been proven that the administration of propolis (500 mg/day capsules) causes a significant reduction in serum levels of IL-17, the VAS score, and the size of the lesions in symptomatic OLP [246]. Topical treatment with a gel containing propolis has also shown antiproliferative and anti-inflammatory effects on OLP lesions [247]. The 20% propolis gel showed effects comparable to 0.1% triamcinolone acetonide in the management of OLP [248].

6.4.6 Chamomile

Chamomile (*Matricaria recutita L.* or *Matricaria chamomilla* L.) is a plant belonging to the Asteraceae family containing flavonoids, coumarins, and essential oils with antiseptic, carminative, sedative, antioxidant, and antimicrobial effect and protector against mucous ulcers [249–253]. Furthermore, there is a growing interest in the use of apigenin, the main chemical compound of chamomile, as it has recently been recognized as a chemoprotective agent, thanks to its powerful antioxidant and anti-inflammatory effects. Therefore, chamomile may be useful in the management of radio- and chemotherapy-induced oral ulcers and mucositis [173]. A clinical study showed that a gel based on chamomile, lidocaine, and dexamethasone (0.75 mg) produces good clinical effects in NEOLP, but the gel containing only dexamethasone resulted in a greater reduction of erosion areas [254]. A recent double-blind randomized controlled clinical trial demonstrated that topical application of a 2% *Chamaemelum nobile* (chamomile) gel (0.5 ml, three times a day) is effective in reducing symptoms and lesions from OLP [255].

6.4.7 Glycyrrhizin

Glycyrrhizin is an active ingredient extracted from licorice (*Glycyrrhiza glabra*) [256]. It is an established treatment to improve liver function in patients with viral hepatitis and is used in Japan to treat patients with chronic hepatitis C. The mechanism of glycyrrhizin is not fully understood, but its metabolite, glycyrrhetinic acid, has anti-inflammatory and antiviral activities and promotes the production of IFN, which activates NK cells [257]. The anti-inflammatory mechanism of licorice includes inhibition of glucocorticoid metabolism and complement [258]. A case of a patient with HCV and OLP whose mucosal symptoms improved significantly after systemic treatment with glycyrrhizin was reported [259]. Another study reports that glycyrrhizin 40 ml/day intravenously (0.2% solution) for 4 consecutive weeks resulted in clinical improvement in OLP-HCV patients compared to untreated ones, suggesting that this compound could be useful in the treatment of OLP [260]. However, the use of glycyrrhizin is not a radical treatment of OLP, as it relapses as soon as its administration is stopped; instead IFN-free DAAs (direct-acting antivirals without interferons) such as ledipasvir and sofosbufir may have been effective in the management of a patient with HCV, hepatocellular carcinoma, and EOLP that arose during IFN treatment, although it is not possible to determine whether the OLP was due to HCV eradication or immunosuppressive therapy (given for liver transplantation) [261]. In another study of 40 patients with OLP, the first group was treated with a bioadhesive paste containing 5% licorice extract and the second group with 0.1% triamcinolone bioadhesive paste: the first group showed improvements greater than those of the second group, but not in a statistically significant way [258].

6.4.8 Eiconol

Eiconol is a complex of unsaturated fatty acids derived from sea fish oil capable of reducing excess triglycerides and cholesterol in the blood [262, 263]. Systemic administration of eiconol 6 g/day resulted in clinical improvement in 69% of patients with OLP and 18% with EOLP [264].

6.4.9 Selenium

Selenium is a naturally occurring mineral that is an essential nutrient involved in numerous biological functions [265]. It is used to eliminate free radicals in synergy with vitamin E and in many antioxidant enzymes and also plays an important role in the functioning of the thyroid gland, where it is a necessary factor for the functioning of the 5-deiodinase enzyme, responsible for the conversion of the hormone T4 in T3. Furthermore, selenium acts on the NF-κB factor, on signal transduction, and on cyclocellular checkpoints and has pro-apoptotic effects; therefore its preventive role of the tumor is not limited to its antioxidant effects [266]. In fact, although selenium is not an antioxidant per se, it is considered an essential component of the antioxidant enzyme glutathione peroxidase [267]. It has been observed that serum selenium levels decrease in patients with OLP and psoriasis [268]. Belal et al. [269] noted that EOLP was better managed by combining selenium and vitamins A, C, and E (SE-ACE) (capsules with vitamin A (β-carotene and retinol, 1500 IU), vitamin E (30 mg), vitamin C (90 mg), and selenium 100 μg, once daily) to dexamethasone and itraconazole, compared to corticosteroid alone with the antifungal. However, it is not possible to establish whether this additional effect is attributable to the selenium rather than the vitamins used. In a recent controlled and randomized study by Qataya et al. [270], however, patients with OLP were treated for 6 weeks only with selenium (systemically in the form of oral capsules of 200 μg or topically as a topical hydrogel): patients treated with 0.1% triamcinolone acetonide or systemic selenium showed greater reduction in salivary levels of MDA (malondialdehyde), while those treated with topical selenium at 12 weeks had a lower pain score than those treated with the glucocorticoid. Therefore, even selenium individually could be proposed as a treatment for OLP.

6.4.10 Ignatia

Ignatia (also called *Ignatia amara*, IA) is obtained from *Strychnos ignatii* seed extract. *Strychnos ignatii* is a plant belonging to the Loganiaceae family and is recognized as poisonous due to the high content of strychnine (a very toxic alkaloid). However, small doses of strychnine were once used medicinally as a stimulant, as a laxative, and as a treatment for other stomach ailments. IA is also one of the most commonly used homeopathic remedies for patients with anxiety and depression [271]. Given that psychosocial factors could play a role in the development of OLP, IA could be useful as a supportive treatment; a single randomized controlled clinical trial of questionable quality has suggested the potential benefit of IA in the management of OLP [6, 272].

6.4.11 *Portulaca* Extract

Purslane is an herbaceous plant from the Portulacaceae family that contains numerous biologically active compounds including omega-3 fatty acids, minerals, β-carotene, melatonin (which stimulates antioxidant enzymes and also acts as a free radical scavenger), and vitamins A, C, and E. This herbal medicament has anti-inflammatory, anti-ulcerogenic, antifungal, and antioxidant properties and has been shown to be useful in cases of infections, hypercholesterolemia, and affections of the urinary and digestive tract [112, 273]. A single, double-blind, randomized controlled trial found that patients treated with purslane (capsules with 235 mg extract) showed a significant decrease in symptoms compared to placebo, and 83% of these also had partial or complete clinical improvement, without the appearance of side effects [274]. However, the study has some methodological flaws [6].

6.4.12 Total Glucosides of Paeony (TGP)

Total glucosides of paeony (TGP) are powdered substances extracted from the roots of *Paeonia lactiflora* Pall. and are a traditional Chinese herbal medicine [275]. TGPs contain paeoniflorin (main component >90%), hydroxy-paeoniflorin, paeonine, albiflorine, and benzoylpaeoniflorin [276]. TGPs have been reported to have anti-inflammatory, immunoregulatory, antioxidant, and hepatoprotective activities and are effective in the management of rheumatoid arthritis (e.g., minimizing damage through inhibition of Th1/Th17 lymphocyte differentiation), Sjogren's syndrome, chronic urticaria, and SLE [277–282]. TGPs could also modulate serum levels of cholesterol and triglycerides and suppress the expression of TNF-α and IL-6, thus attenuating the development of atherosclerosis [276]. An in vitro study showed that TGPs are able to inhibit the production of inflammatory cytokines (such as TNF-α and IL-6) in OLP by suppressing the NF-κB signaling pathway and therefore could constitute a new potential candidate therapeutic agent [283]. Furthermore, TGPs activate the immunomodulatory functions of mesenchymal stem cells (MSCs) in OLP through the inhibition of TNF-α and IL-6 and the stimulation of TGF-β and IL-10 and through the inhibition of the expression of p-STAT3 through the upregulation of miR-124; in this way, MSCs, through the benefits of TGPs, could alleviate OLP as it occurs in other severe immune diseases [284]. A clinical study showed that, compared to 0.1% dexamethasone alone, the combined treatment of glucocorticoid with TGP capsules (400 mg, three times daily) resulted in a longer lasting maintenance of the improvements obtained in patients with reticular OLP and a major decrease in pain and injury in EOLP patients; however the effects of TGP treatment are likely to be achieved after at least 4 months of therapy [285]. The combination of TGPs with Nd:YAG laser treatment has also been proven effective and safe in the management of EOLP [286].

6.4.13 Piperine

Black pepper (*Piper nigrum* L., Piperaceae family) is one of the most widely used spices in the world in the human diet and also for medical research purposes and is well known for its main alkaloid constituent, piperine [287]. It possesses immunomodulatory, anti-inflammatory, antitumor, and antidepressant properties, potentially useful in OLP [287–291]. Piperine has shown suppressive effects on DC maturation, T-cell proliferation and activation, and the NF-κB signaling pathway but also can repress COX-2 overproduction and decrease oxidative stress; therefore piperine could represent a novel therapeutic strategy for OLP [292]. Piperine (10 mg/day) has been used in combination with curcuminoids (1000 mg/day) to increase their bioavailability in the treatment of the metabolic syndrome [293]. Piperine (5–15 mg) per 1000 mg of curcumin was also administered in OLP for the same purpose [207], but there are no investigations that study the efficacy of piperine in OLP.

6.5 Monoclonal Antibodies

Monoclonal antibodies (MAb) are artificial antibodies identical to each other obtained by genetic engineering techniques, produced by cell lines coming from a single type of plasma cell (cell clone) and consequently directed against only one epitope of the antigen. They therefore differ from polyclonal antibodies which are instead a mixture of antibodies obtained from the immunization of an animal with an antigen: in this case different plasma cells (several cell clones) will produce genetically different antibodies capable of recognizing different epitopes of the same antigen [256].

6.5.1 Anti-TNF-α

- *Etanercept.* Competitively blocks the binding of TNF to its receptor, preventing the biological activity of the cytokine and in particular the activation of immune and inflammatory cells; etanercept is indicated in rheumatoid arthritis, ankylosing spondylitis, and severe psoriatic arthritis (25 mg twice a week or 50 mg once a week). The most common side effects are opportunistic infections and in some cases demyelination [9]. A patient with severe EOLP refractory to systemic topical agents, retinoids and azathrioprine, responsive to prednisone (but used limitedly for comorbidities such as diabetes mellitus and hypertension), was treated with etanercept 25 mg subcutaneously (twice weekly) achieving mucosal healing and pain relief starting from the fourth week; the drug was then suspended at the tenth week because it was too expensive and the disease relapsed 2 weeks after the agent was suspended [294].
- *Infliximab.* It is an antibody directed against TNF-α (preventing the binding to its receptor) indicated in rheumatoid arthritis (in association with methotrexate) and drug-resistant Crohn's disease. It is administered intravenously, and complete elimination takes several months [9]. A standard administration consists of 5 mg/kg at weeks 0, 2, and 6, followed by single infusions at intervals of 8–12 weeks. It is a relatively well-tolerated drug, but human anti-chemical antibodies (HACA) can develop during therapy and can be reduced by concomitant immunosuppressive therapy or corticosteroid premedication [22]. Possible side effects are infections with tuberculosis reactivation (all patients treated with this drug must have chest x-rays and tine tests) [9]. A single study showed a positive response from one case of severe orogenital LP to treatment with infliximab [295].
- *Adalimumab.* It is another anti-TNF monoclonal antibody approved for the treatment of rheumatoid arthritis [9]. Two cases of mucocutaneous LP with severe orogenital involvement responded positively to treatment with

adalimumab (e.g., 40 mg subcutaneously every week) [296, 297].

Some patients treated with anti-TNF-α agents (for the management of IBD) have developed oral lichenoid lesions [298] (Sect. 3.1.2). This could be due to the disruption of the delicate balance between TNF-α and IFN-α in susceptible patients [299]. Therefore, clinicians should detect possible side effects such as OLL, infections, and headaches caused by anti-TNF-α agents [300].

6.5.2 Anti-IL-2R

- *Basiliximab.* It is a monoclonal antibody directed against the alpha chain of IL-2R in T lymphocytes, blocking their clonal expansion and reducing their survival. It is administered intravenously and has a long half-life. They rarely induce the formation of neutralizing antibodies because only a small portion of the structure is of animal origin; cases of "cytokine release syndrome" have sometimes been reported [9]. Basiliximab 20 mg has been successfully infused twice in a patient with severe orogenital erosive LP; therefore this agent may be effective for short periods of treatment. However, the disorder relapsed after 4 weeks [301]; therefore the efficacy and long-term safety are not known [302].

6.5.3 Anti-CD11a

- *Efalizumab.* It is a humanized monoclonal antibody that binds to the CD11a subunit of LFA-1, a surface molecule of T lymphocytes, preventing interaction with ICAM-1 expressed on APC cells; in this way efalizumab interferes with the activation, migration, and cytotoxic function of T lymphocytes, and this block, being reversible, does not lead to a depletion of T lymphocytes, organ toxicity, opportunistic infections, or malignancy, but the platelet count is recommended [22, 303, 304]. It is administered as weekly subcutaneous injections [23]. A 54-year-old woman with EOLP resistant to application of systemic prednisone and tacrolimus ointment was treated with efalizumab (starting dose of 0.7 mg/kg per week, followed by 1.0 mg/kg per week), and an improvement in skin lesions starting from the fifth week was reported [305]. Similar results were obtained on a 29-year-old patient with generalized LP in whom, after 12 weeks of treatment with efalizumab (same dosages mentioned above), complete resolution of pruritus and lesions was observed [306]. A unicentric, open-label pilot study in four patients showed the beneficial effects of efalizumab (starting dose of 0.7 mg/kg in week 0, followed by 1.0 mg/kg through week 12) in management of the EOLP and the LP; however, two patients had severe adverse effects (urticaria, staphylococcal abscess of a hip prosthesis, and drug-induced subacute cutaneous lupus) [307]. Furthermore, close attention should be paid to the safety concerns of efalizumab mainly related to the risk of progressive multifocal leukoencephalopathy [308].

6.5.4 Anti-CD2

- *Alefacept.* It is a monoclonal antibody that binds to CD2 (blocking the interaction of LFA3 of APCs with CD2), a surface molecule of many immune cells such as DC, T, and NK lymphocytes, but mainly carries out its action on memory T cells ($CD45RO^+$) with high levels of CD2, but not naïve (CD45RA +) [9, 302]. In particular, alefacept is able to interact with two CD2 molecules, creating a bridge between two T/T, T/NK, or NK/NK cells and chaining them. In this way, being unable to carry out their biological function, they undergo apoptosis [9]. It can be administered intramuscularly or intravenously [22]. It is a well-tolerated drug with rare side effects; among them are dizziness, nausea, infections, lymphopenia, neoplasms, hypersensitivity reactions, and acute liver toxicity [9, 309]. Rarely, the drug has led to the formation of anti-alefacept antibodies [9]. The rationale for the use of alefacept in the treatment of LP ($CD4^+$ T lymphocyte-mediated disorder) is that this drug induces apoptosis of T lymphocytes through the release of granzyme by NK cells [22]. Treatment with intramuscular alefacept (15 mg per week) for 12 weeks resulted in excellent improvement in two patients with a generalized, oral form of LP resistant to other therapies. The improvement of the lesions and symptoms began from the fourth week of treatment, and after a follow-up of up to 20 weeks from the suspension of therapy, there was no relapse or worsening [310]. In a case series study by Chang et al. [311], it was observed that alefacept may induce a moderate therapeutic response in patients with EOLP, but larger, multi-center prospective studies will be needed to confirm the efficacy of this drug in the management of severe OLP.

6.5.5 Anti-CD20

- *Rituximab*. It is a monoclonal antibody that selectively binds to the CD20 antigen expressed on B lymphocytes (both mature and naïve) but not on hematopoietic stem cells, memory B lymphocytes, and plasma cells. It is believed that CD20 regulates the intracellular concentration of calcium allowing the activation of B lymphocytes [9]. This drug can be used in the desensitization of HLA-incompatible transplants; in the management of acute antibody-mediated transplant rejection; in some forms of leukemia and lymphomas; in PV, PB, GvHD (resistant to corticosteroids—see Sect. 5.5.4), and PNP caused by B lymphoma; in some forms of SLE; in rheumatoid arthritis (resistant to anti-TNF-α in association with methotrexate); in idiopathic autoimmune hemolytic anemia; and in idiopathic thrombocytopenic purpura [9, 312–316]. The most frequent adverse reaction is the infusion reaction [302]. The most serious side effects reported have been as follows: infection, pulmonary toxicity, and heart failure [9]. Some studies have reported the efficacy of rituximab (four intravenous injections [375 mg/m^2] spaced 1 week apart—lymphoma protocol) in the management of OLP with esophageal involvement (usually causing dysphagia, odynophagia, and diagnosed late); no side effects were reported, and only mild relapses were managed with local therapy after a 10-month follow-up. In particular, at the esophageal level, it was histologically observed that, before therapy, many CD4$^+$ and CD8$^+$ T lymphocytes and few CD20$^+$ B lymphocytes were present, while, after therapy, the esophageal epithelium was devoid of CD20$^+$ lymphocytes and with few lymphocytes CD8$^+$ [317, 318]. Similar results have also been reported in the management of vulvovaginal-gingival LP syndrome [319]. OLP is an immunological disorder mediated by T lymphocytes; therefore the role of rituximab remains controversial: the efficacy of this drug could suggest a direct or indirect involvement of B lymphocytes in the pathogenesis of OLP [302]. However, it has been reported that rituximab can rarely cause OLDR [320, 321].

6.5.6 Anti-VEGF

- *Bevacizumab*. It is a recombinant humanized monoclonal antibody directed against VEGF used to block the function of VEGF (see Sect. 4.4.5) in vascular endothelial cells and thus inhibit angiogenesis, on which solid tumors depend for growth and metastasis [322]. It is indicated, in combination with chemotherapy, in the treatment of advanced colorectal cancer, advanced small-cell lung cancer, renal cell carcinoma, and metastatic breast cancer [323]. Cancer cells have high metabolic rates, and this leads to a demand for oxygen and nutrients that exceeds the supply. Hypoxia is consequently determined, the primary factor that controls angiogenesis. In these conditions, the hypoxia-induced factor (HIF) favors the transcription of the VEGF gene [324]. Circulating VEGF binds to VEGFR-1 and VEGFR-2 receptors and its neuropilin co-receptors NRP-1 and NRP-2 with high binding affinity [325]. These receptors expressed on endothelial cells promote angiogenesis and stimulate their recruitment and proliferation [326]. Bevacizumab works by selectively binding circulating VEGF, thereby inhibiting binding to its receptors and leading to a reduction in microvascular growth, and thus restricts the blood supply to tumor tissues [327]. The common side effects of bevacizumab are hypertension, asymptomatic proteinuria, thromboembolic events, gastrointestinal perforation, and wound healing complications [328]. It has been shown that in the tissues of patients affected by OLP, there is an increase in the expression of pro-angiogenic factors (such as CD34, VEGF, and VEGFR-2) and a decrease in anti-angiogenic factors (such as VASH-1) compared to oral mucous membranes affected by non-specific inflammation [329]. A single clinical study has shown that patients with atrophic-erosive OLP can benefit from intralesional injections (at sites adjacent to lesions) of bevacizumab 2.5 mg/0.5 ml: this has resulted in a reduction in signs and symptoms after only 1 week of treatment and a marked reduction in the immuno-expression of VEGF and IL-8 in oral tissues; moreover, the patients did not experience the exacerbation of the lesions in the 3 months of follow-up following the suspension of therapy [330].

6.5.7 Other Monoclonal Antibodies

- *Secukinumab, Ustekinumab, and Guselkumab.* As discussed in Chap. 4, the role of the Th17 response in the pathogenesis of OLP has emerged quite recently. A single clinical study [331] showed the effects of subcutaneous treatment of secukinumab (anti-IL-17A), ustekinumab (anti-IL12/IL-23), or guselkumab (anti-IL-23) in five patients with recalcitrant forms of oral or mucocutaneous LP. Secukinumab was administered for 12/48 weeks with a dose of 300 mg in weeks 0, 1, 2, 3, and 4 followed by monthly treatment. Ustekinumab was administered for 48 weeks at a dose of 45 mg at weeks 0 and 4 and every 3 months thereafter. Guselkumab was administered for 30 weeks at a dose of 100 mg in weeks 0 and 4 and every 2 months thereafter. Treatment with secukinumab induced a rapid and prolonged clinical improvement of mucocutaneous LP and a strong reduction of Th1 and Th17/Tc17 cell and cutaneous infiltrate. Long-term treatment of a patient with recalcitrant OLP with ustekinumab resulted in the healing of the oral ulcerative lesions and a reduction in IL-17^{+} cells in peripheral blood and lesions. Finally, treatment with guselkumab resulted in marked clinical improvement in a patient with recalcitrant EOLP. The targeting of the Th17 inflammatory profile could open new therapeutic avenues in the treatment of recalcitrant forms of LP, but further studies on larger samples are needed to prove its efficacy.

6.6 Non-pharmacological Therapy

6.6.1 Psychiatric Therapy

Some authors have suggested the inclusion of psychiatric drugs in the routine therapy of OLP, given the high percentage of mental disorders found among these patients [332]. Indeed, factors such as stress and psychological problems, particularly depression and anxiety, have been cited as etiological factors in OLP (Sect. 3.2.4) because patients with such disorders report more frequent development or exacerbation of lesions during periods of increased tension [333]. However, there is still a controversy regarding the role of stress as a major or minor etiological factor in the pathogenicity of OLP [334, 335]. A study [335], but of poor quality [78], reports the effectiveness of the combination of psychiatric drug therapy and routine treatment methods.

6.6.2 Bacillus Calmette-Guerin Polysaccharide Nucleic Acid (BCG-PSN)

The introduction of biological therapies is a new challenge for the treatment of various immune-mediated disorders. Biological agents are intended by recombinant biotechnology to intercept each phase of the pathogenesis of immune-inflammatory diseases, representing a more effective and targeted approach. Structurally, biological agents include fusion receptor proteins, monoclonal antibodies, and recombinant cytokines. Functionally, however, biological agents can be distinguished into T-cell modulators or cytokines [336].

Bacillus Calmette-Guerin (BCG) is an attenuated microorganism obtained from *Mycobacterium bovis* and is used for immunization against tuberculosis and for its immunostimulating effects [9]. BCG can induce various adverse effects such as lupus vulgaris, keloid scars, hidradenitis suppurativa, and disseminated infection [337]. Bacillus Calmette-Guerin polysaccharide nucleic acid (BCG-PSN) has the immune function of the BCG vaccine without any risk of infection: it consists of a protein fraction extracted from BCG with a higher quality and fewer side effects (redness or swelling) at the injection site [338]. BCG-PSN modulates certain subsets of T cells, induces Th1 immunity, and stimulates cellular immunity [339]. It has been used in the treatment of various diseases such as idiopathic urticaria [340], alopecia areata [339], melanoma [341], warts [342], recurrent oral aphthosis [343], and vitiligo [344]. In a randomized comparative study, intralesional injections of BCG-PSN (0.5 ml every other day for 2 weeks) showed an efficacy similar to triamcinolone acetonide (intralesional injection 10 mg once a week for 2 weeks) [345]. A study by Nasr et al. [337] showed that the use of BCG-PSN injected subcutaneously (0.5 ml twice a week for 3 months) can be effective and safe in the management of cutaneous OLP and LP (the only side effect reported in less swelling at the injection site was 30% of the sample), and most patients achieved a complete response after 3 weeks of treatment.

6.6.3 Platelet-Rich Plasma (PRP)

Recently, the application of PRP, a plasma concentrate of the patient's blood containing mainly platelets, has been proposed as an adjuvant treatment for many medical conditions [346]. Platelets activated in PRP release various growth factors (epidermal growth factor or EGF, fibroblastic growth factor or FGF, transforming growth factor beta 1 or TGF-β1, and keratinocyte growth factor or KGF) that promote migration, proliferation, cell differentiation, angiogenesis, tissue debris removal, and tissue regeneration [347]. A recent case report [346] reported good results in the treatment of a case of EOLP resistant to conventional therapy through the use of autologous PRP. In particular, this was prepared according to the standardized procedure [348], and 0.5 ml of PRP was injected intralesionally per 1 cm2 of ulcerated mucosa after the application of a 2% lidocaine anesthetic solution [346, 348]. A patient with recalcitrant ulcerative OLP found benefit from the use of PRP-based oral rinses [348]. Further studies will confirm whether or not it is valid in the recalcitrant OLP. A group of researchers also treated some patients with OLP with autologous PRP in the form of a gel [349].

6.6.4 Conventional Surgery

For several years, some authors have proposed the use of conventional surgery (clearly not as a first option) in the treatment of OLP; for example, free tissue grafts were used to manage localized forms of gingival EOLP, and the complete disappearance of symptomatic OLP in the treated areas was reported up to 3.5 years of follow-up [350–352]. The excision of pathologically altered areas could be indicated in lesions of limited size, as well as in cases of histologically confirmed dysplasia. Wide excision in a diffuse form of OLP could carry the risk of postoperative scar lesions that impair function [135]. Furthermore, it should be noted that periodontal surgery has been reported to cause or worsen OLP/OLL lesions [353].

6.6.5 Cryotherapy

Cryosurgery is a therapeutic technique that exploits the effects of freezing to obtain an inflammatory and/or destructive response of the tissues. Various techniques are available, including direct contact, spray, cone nebulization, and solid contact with the probe. Liquid nitrogen is the coolant of choice for dermatological surgery because it is the coldest and most versatile. Several oral conditions have been treated with cryosurgery which may represent as an alternative to conventional surgery [354].

Cryosurgery has been used in particular in drug-resistant forms of EOLP, but lesions can develop in healing wounds and recur in scars [355].

6.6.6 Phototherapy

Phototherapy makes use of light radiation and includes various types of treatment.

1. *Laser*

The phototherapy group includes a treatment that uses various types of lasers [135]. The laser consists of an active medium struck by the energy emitted by an external source (pumping system), which absorbs photons and transfers electrons from one energy level to a higher level (population inversion). The active medium is a structure also called "optical resonator" which allows the spontaneously emitted photons to trigger the stimulation mechanism and to generate, after a threshold, the laser beam, i.e., a coherent, well-collimated, and monochromatic light beam. The emitted photons will be characterized by frequency, amplitude, and wavelength [336].

In relation to the active medium, there are several types of lasers used in oral medicine: diode lasers, excimer lasers, low-intensity laser therapy, CO2 lasers, and Er:YAG lasers [135, 336]. Depending on the type of use, laser-assisted surgery (laser ablation and laser excision) and laser biomodulation (low-intensity laser therapy (LLLT) and photodynamic laser therapy (PDLT)) can be applied in patients with OLP [135].

- *Laser-assisted surgery*. The use of laser ablation (or laser thermoablative therapy) in the treatment of OLP is based on the fact that the activating factor of immune aggression is found intraepithelially and the removal of the epithelial tunica, by means of heat, in order to eliminate the factor causal can cause the interruption of the self-sufficient immune-inflammatory process [135].

  CO2 laser. Pakfetrat et al., using CO2 laser ablation in atrophic-erosive forms of OLP, reported size reduction up to complete regression of the lesions and the transition of erosive areas to milder forms (atrophic or reticular) [356]. Van der Hem et al. [357] exposed 39 superficial OLP lesions to CO2 laser evaporation (1.5–2.0 J/mm2). During a follow-up period of 1–18 years (mean 8 years), 24 lesions no longer showed signs of oral dysfunction (pain, burning sensation), 15 lesions showed clinical relapse, and 6 of these caused pain after complete epithelialization. After CO2 laser evaporation retreatment of these six lesions, no pain complaints were observed. Complete epithelialization was observed in all patients after completion of treatment and retreatment within 3 weeks.

  Laser Er:YAG. The erbium:YAG laser (Er:YAG, 2940 nm) has been reported in two patients as being able to promote a good and fast healing process, a very low level of discomfort during and after surgery, and a rapid disappearance of symptoms [358].

  Diode laser. The diode laser is a semiconductor that uses solid-state elements (gallium, arsenide, aluminum, and indium) to transform electrical energy into light energy [359]. The light energy of the diode is greatly absorbed by the soft tissues and poorly absorbed by the teeth and bones [360]. The treatment of two patients with OLP using a diode laser (810 nm) in a defocused manner (to favor the evaporation of superficial mucosal lesions) allowed the achievement of rapid healing without scarring [359].

- *Laser biomodulation*. It could represent a promising method for treating symptomatic OLP [135].

  Low-intensity laser therapy (LLLT). Low-intensity laser therapy (LIL (low-intensity laser) or LLLT (low-level laser therapy)) includes wavelengths between 500 and 1100 nm [361]; determines local vasodilation, thus favoring the movement of immune cells in the tissue; and helps control inflammation by modulating mast cell activity [248]. LLLT promotes proliferation, maturation, and migration, as well as transformation into myofibroblasts, a reduction in the production of pro-inflammatory prostaglandins E2 and an increased production of basic growth factors [362]. Therefore the main effects are analgesic, anti-inflammatory, and regenerative ones [363]. Furthermore, LLLT implies a redox regulation that explains the clinical effects in the chronic inflammatory response (OLP) characterized by acidosis and tissue hypoxia and which has the potential for tissue healing and regeneration without systemic disturbances and undesirable effects on a healthy tissue [364, 365]. Two randomized comparative studies [362, 366] have shown some benefits on OLP; however both of these investigations have drawbacks [78]. A more recent study by Elshenawy et al. [367] showed complete remission of symptoms with no associated side effects. A series of studies have reported positive results in the treatment of cases of OLP refractory to drug therapy after the administration of ultraviolet (excimer laser, 308 nm) [368–370], KTP laser (potassium titanyl phosphate, 532 nm) [371], red (diode laser, 630 nm) [372], and infrared (diode laser, 830 [373], 904 [374], and 980 nm [375]). In particular Köllner et al. [369] employed the 308-nm excimer laser (UVB) for intraoral treatment in eight patients with OLP. During treatment, the lesions were exposed to a variable number of applications (9 to 32) and energy density per minute (75 to 175 mJ/cm2). The results showed improvement in six patients; in particular complete remission was achieved in two cases, while one patient showed recurrence of lesions after 4 weeks. In a unicentric observational study, Trehan et al. [370] evaluated the efficacy of excimer laser therapy (308 nm) (with initial energies of 100 mJ/cm2 and subsequently, once a week, 400 mJ/cm2) in the management of nine patients with conventional therapy-resistant OLP in a follow-up between 2 and 17 months. The authors conclude that low-dose treatment with the 308-nm excimer laser can be very effective in the treatment of symptomatic and recalcitrant EOLP. However Passeron et al. [368] reported unsatisfactory results in four patients presenting with EOLP. The authors evaluated the use of the 308-nm excimer laser twice weekly for 12 sessions. The lowest dose was 50 mJ/cm2, increased by 50 mJ/cm2 every two sessions up to 200 mJ/cm2: only one patient showed positive results. Cafaro et al. [374] on the other hand, using diode lasers (904 nm) with an energy density of 4 J/cm2 per minute (10 kHz, 50% duty cycle) with a distance of about 2 mm from the oral mucosa, reported a reduction in clinical signs and pain in all 13 patients analyzed. These differences show that the effectiveness of the LLLT is strongly influenced by numerous parameters such as wavelength, power, intensity, and exposure time; therefore it still remains controversial what is the number and sequence of ideal sessions [135]. Several studies conducted to compare the effects of LLLT with corticosteroid therapy have shown conflicting results [362, 376, 377]. In particular, a clinical study conducted by El Shenawy et al. [376] showed a significant improvement in signs and symptoms in patients with OLP treated with local corticosteroids compared to those treated with LLLT. Similarly it has been reported by Othman et al. [377]. On the other hand, Dillenburg et al. [378] found a statistically significant improvement with LLLT compared to topical steroid therapy in the treatment of OLP. A recent systematic review compared the data available in the literature to evaluate the efficacy of LLLT with respect to corticosteroid therapy in the treatment of OLP, but the results are conflicting. In fact, the five studies analyzed were considered at risk of partiality (four with high risk and one with moderate risk), and of these three showed a greater efficacy of topical corticosteroid therapy, one exactly the opposite, and the last showed instead of comparable results between the two therapies. Thus it remains questionable whether LLLT is more effective than corticosteroids in treating OLP, given that scientific evidence is weak [361].

Photodynamic laser therapy (PDLT (photodynamic laser therapy) or simply PDT (photodynamic therapy)). It is a form of photochemotherapy consisting in the administration of low-intensity laser radiation after local or systemic application of a photosensitizing agent [135]. In the first step, the photosensitizing agent, after administration, is accumulated in the target cells (rapidly dividing cells) to be treated [379]. This is explained by the disproportionately large number of LDL receptors on their cell membranes and by the abnormal microvasculature [380]. In the second phase, the photosensitized cells are exposed to a light source of a specific wavelength that coincides with the absorption spectrum of the photosensitizing agent [379]. The light source activates the dye and triggers a series of cytotoxic reactions, causing the generation of reactive oxygen species (ROS) that have toxic effects on target cells [381–383]. The main effects of PDLT are those immunomodulating (modulation of the activity of IL-6 and IL-10, but not TNF-α) [379] and induction of apoptosis of hyper-proliferating inflammatory cells [384, 385]. Photosensitizing agents do not accumulate in the nucleus; therefore they have low DNA mutagenic or carcinogenic potential [386]. Several studies have shown a consistent improvement in the clinical presentation of OLP lesions with no adverse effects regardless of the type of photosensitizing agent used: methylene blue [384], Photolon [387], or porphyrin [379]. Methylene blue is an optimal photosensitizer for PDT, has strong absorption at wavelengths above 620 nm, and may be a preferred choice for superficial lesions of the skin and oral cavity [336]. In particular Aghahosseini et al. [388] used the diode laser (632 nm, 120 J/cm2) for 2 min after instructing patients to gargle for 5 min with an aqueous solution of 5% methylene blue (0.05 gr per 100 cc) 10 min before treatment. The data analyzed showed a significant reduction in the size of lesions resistant to conventional therapies and a decrease in pain in 16 of the 26 lesions. To date, however, there is no photosensitizing agent capable of meeting all clinical needs [379]. Most of them have disadvantages such as prolonged skin photosensitivity, limited capacity of cell selectivity, and unpredictable efficacy [389].

2. *Psoralen and UVA treatment (PUVA)*

In addition to laser treatment, phototherapy includes other types of treatment including PUVA therapy, another form of photochemotherapy. It consists of exposure to UVA rays (wavelengths between 320 and 400 nm) after the injection of a psoralen (8-methoxypsoralen) [119]. Psoralens are compounds found in many plants, which make the skin and mucous membranes temporarily sensitive to UV radiation. Methoxypsoralen is administered orally, followed by a 2-h exposure of UV radiation intraorally in the affected sites [23].

The possible positive effect of PUVA therapy in cases of severe OLP lesions refractory to conventional therapies has been observed for some time. In particular Lundquist et al. [390] found side effects, even severe ones, in 14 out of 16 patients who were injected in 12 sessions at a distance of 2–3 days from each other, before UV radiation of 16.5 J/cm2, 0.6 mg/kg of methoxypsoralen (Puvamet) per visit. Nine of these patients showed marked improvement, but the authors suggested using topical psoralens to avoid side effects seen with systemic administration. PUVA therapy includes adverse effects including nausea and dizziness due to psoralen and a photosensitivity for 24 h when the drug is taken orally. Dosimetry can be difficult to establish within the complex geometry of the mouth, as PUVA is generally administered to the skin over large open surfaces [23]. Furthermore, because of its oncogenic potential, PUVA therapy has been replaced by other safer types of phototherapy [3, 385].

PUVA is also not recommended for OLL-GvHD due to its oncogenic potential [3].

3. *Narrowband UVB (NB-UVB) therapy*

Narrowband UVB therapy (NB-UVB, 311–313 nm) is efficient and probably with a lower malignant potential than PUVA [391]. Kassem et al. [392] achieved positive effects on the clinical presentation of EOLP lesions using UVB therapy.

4. *Photopheresis or extracorporeal photochemotherapy (ECP)*

Extracorporeal photopheresis or photochemotherapy (ECP), a type of PDT, is an emerging treatment in which a centrifugal apheresis machine is used to separate the patient's blood cells. The removed cells are treated with a photosensitizing compound (8-methoxypsoralen), which has been intercalated into the DNA of the treated cells making them more sensitive to apoptosis when exposed to UVA light and then reinfused into the patient [336]. Kunte et al. [393] reported an improvement in EOLP symptoms and lesions in all four subjects after seven to nine courses of therapy. Therapy was performed for two consecutive days (therapeutic cycle) every 2 weeks. After clinical improvement, the therapy intervals were prolonged. In a study conducted by Guyot et al. [394], 12 patients affected by refractory EOLP underwent the standardized protocol of ECP: performed twice a week for 3 weeks while the following sessions were planned according to clinical improvement. Researchers monitored $CD4^+$ and $CD8^+$ peripheral blood T-cell counts every 3 months and observed clinical improvements in all treated patients. Another group of researchers also successfully treated two patients with EOLP lesions resistant to corticosteroid therapy [395].

6.6.7 Final Considerations

Although the LP has been known for over 150 years, to date there is no treatment capable of bringing the patient to complete recovery. This could be due to the various immune responses and conditions of the individual patient or to the fact that the etiopathogenesis is not fully understood [248]. Thanks to the use of topical corticosteroids such as super-potent halogenates and calcineurin inhibitors, it is possible to obtain a safe and satisfactory control of the symptoms caused by OLP lesions in most cases [2]. As reported in the new textbook "Patologia e Medicina Orale" [396] written by the Italian Society of Oral Pathology and Medicine (SIPMO) it is hypothesized that the long-lasting inflammatory stimulus, typical of OLP, could be one of the mechanisms underlying the malignant potential. For this reason it is possible that the drugs administered to control the symptoms (particularly corticosteroids) during the acute phase may have a protective effect on the onset of the cancer itself. But these same drugs, due to their immunosuppressive effects, could themselves be promoters of the onset of oral cancer. Some new treatment modalities are potentially interesting for cases refractory to conventional therapies, such as the oxygen-ozone mixture injections [397], but the positive preliminary results need confirmation [78]. In this regard, it is worth mentioning the recent use of psychotropic agents (topical clonazepam and systemic benzodiazepine and antidepressant drugs) which have proved effective in the management of burning mouth syndrome-like oral symptoms in symptomatic reticular OLP patients refractory to conventional immunosuppressive therapy, although in a long-term period [398].

References

1. Spadari F, Pallotti F, Bombeccari GP, di Patologia A, Oss D. Lichen planus orale: revisione della letteratura.
2. Carrozzo M. Lichen planus orale: quale approccio? Stomatologia dermatologica. 2014:30–5.
3. Al-Hashimi I, Schifter M, Lockhart PB, Wray D, Brennan M, Migliorati CA, et al. Oral lichen planus and oral lichenoid lesions: diagnostic and therapeutic considerations. Oral Surg Oral Med Oral Pathol Oral Radiol Endodontol. 2007;103:S25. e1–S. e12.
4. Córdova P, Rubio A, Echeverría P. Oral lichen planus: a look from diagnosis to treatment. J Oral Res. 2014;3(1):62–7.
5. Motta ACF, Komesu MC, Grisi MFM, Souza CS, Roselino AMF, Migliari DA. Topical occlusive cor-

ticosteroid for the treatment of gingival manifestations of vesicobullous autoimmune diseases. An Bras Dermatol. 2006;81:283–5.
6. Thongprasom K, Carrozzo M, Furness S, Lodi G. Interventions for treating oral lichen planus. Cochrane Database Syst Rev. 2011;7
7. Scully C, Eisen D, Carrozzo M. Management of oral lichen planus. Am J Clin Dermatol. 2000;1(5):287–306.
8. Amico-Roxas MCA, Del Tacca M. Farmacologia in odontoiatria. Florence: Utet; 2006.
9. Annunziato L, Di Renzo G, Abbracchio MP. Trattato di farmacologia. Idelson-Gnocchi; 2021.
10. Carbone M, Goss E, Carrozzo M, Castellano S, Conrotto D, Broccoletti R, et al. Systemic and topical corticosteroid treatment of oral lichen planus: a comparative study with long-term follow-up. J Oral Pathol Med. 2003;32(6):323–9.
11. Kuo R-C, Lin H-P, Sun A, Wang Y-P. Prompt healing of erosive oral lichen planus lesion after combined corticosteroid treatment with locally injected triamcinolone acetonide plus oral prednisolone. J Formos Med Assoc. 2013;112(4):216–20.
12. Savage N, McCullough M. Topical corticosteroids in dental practice. Aust Dent J. 2005;50:S40–S4.
13. Cheng Y-SL, Gould A, Kurago Z, Fantasia J, Muller S. Diagnosis of oral lichen planus: a position paper of the American Academy of Oral and maxillofacial pathology. Oral Surg Oral Med Oral Pathol Oral Radiol. 2016;122(3):332–54.
14. Silverman S Jr, Gorsky M, Lozada-Nur F, Giannotti K. A prospective study of findings and management in 214 patients with oral lichen planus. Oral Surg Oral Med Oral Pathol. 1991;72(6):665–70.
15. Carrozzo M, Porter S, Mercadante V, Fedele S. Oral lichen planus: a disease or a spectrum of tissue reactions? Types, causes, diagnostic algorhythms, prognosis, management strategies. Periodontology 2000. 2019;80(1):105–25.
16. Lozada F, Silverman S Jr, Migliorati C. Adverse side effects associated with prednisone in the treatment of patients with oral inflammatory ulcerative diseases. J Am Dent Assoc. 1984;109(2):269–70.
17. Carbone M, Conrotto D, Carrozzo M, Broccoletti R, Gandolfo S, Scully C. Topical corticosteroids in association with miconazole and chlorhexidine in the long-term management of atrophic-erosive oral lichen planus: a placebo-controlled and comparative study between clobetasol and fluocinonide. Oral Dis. 1999;5(1):44–9.
18. Thongprasom K, Luengvisut P, Wongwatanakij A, Boonjatturus C. Clinical evaluation in treatment of oral lichen planus with topical fluocinolone acetonide: a 2-year follow-up. J Oral Pathol Med. 2003;32(6):315–22.
19. Bagan J-V, Eisen D, Scully C. The diagnosis and management of oral lichen planus: a consensus approach. Oral Biosci Med. 2004;1:21–7.
20. Vincent S, Fotos P, Baker K, Williams T. Oral lichen planus: the clinical, historical, and therapeutic features of 100 cases. Oral Surg Oral Med Oral Pathol. 1990;70(2):165–71.
21. Mansourian A, Saheb-Jamee M, Momen-Beitollahi J, Momen-Heravi F, Esfehani M, Khalilzadeh O. Comparison of aloe vera mouthwash with triamcinolone acetonide 0.1% on oral lichen planus: a randomized double-blinded clinical trial. Am J Med Sci. 2011;342(6):447–51.
22. Crincoli V, Di Bisceglie MB, Scivetti M, Lucchese A, Tecco S, Festa F. Oral lichen planus: update on etiopathogenesis, diagnosis and treatment. Immunopharmacol Immunotoxicol. 2011;33(1):11–20.
23. Lavanya N, Jayanthi P, Rao UK, Ranganathan K. Oral lichen planus: an update on pathogenesis and treatment. J Oral Maxillofacial Pathol: JOMFP. 2011;15(2):127.
24. Scully C, Carrozzo M. Oral mucosal disease: lichen planus. Br J Oral Maxillofac Surg. 2008;46(1):15–21. https://doi.org/10.1016/j.bjoms.2007.07.199.
25. Rhodus N, Cheng B, Bowles W, Myers S, Miller L, Ondrey F. Proinflammatory cytokine levels in saliva before and after treatment of (erosive) oral lichen planus with dexamethasone. Oral Dis. 2006;12(2):112–6.
26. Fu J, Zhu X, Dan H, Zhou Y, Liu C, Wang F, et al. Amlexanox is as effective as dexamethasone in topical treatment of erosive oral lichen planus: a short-term pilot study. Oral Surg Oral Med Oral Pathol Oral Radiol. 2012;113(5):638–43.
27. Jaffe GJ, Yang CH, Guo H, Denny JP, Lima C, Ashton P. Safety and pharmacokinetics of an intraocular fluocinolone acetonide sustained delivery device. Invest Ophthalmol Vis Sci. 2000;41(11):3569–75.
28. Buajeeb W, Pobrurksa C, Kraivaphan P. Efficacy of fluocinolone acetonide gel in the treatment of oral lichen planus. Oral Surg Oral Med Oral Pathol Oral Radiol Endodontol. 2000;89(1):42–5.
29. Buajeeb W, Kraivaphan P, Pobrurksa C. Efficacy of topical retinoic acid compared with topical fluocinolone acetonide in the treatment of oral lichen planus. Oral Surg Oral Med Oral Pathol Oral Radiol Endodontol. 1997;83(1):21–5.
30. Thongprasom K, Luangjarmekorn L, Sererat T, Taweesap W. Relative efficacy of fluocinolone acetonide compared with triamcinolone acetonide in treatment of oral lichen planus. J Oral Pathol Med. 1992;21(10):456–8.
31. Thongprasom K, Dhanuthai K, Sarideechaigul W, Chaiyarit P, Chaimusig M. Expression of TNF-α in oral lichen planus treated with fluocinolone acetonide 0.1%. J Oral Pathol Med. 2006;35(3):161–6.
32. Stoughton R. Perspectives in topical glucocorticosteroid therapy. Prog Dermatol. 1975;9:7–11.
33. Voûte AB, Schulten EA, Langendijk PN, Kostense PJ, van der Waal I. Fluocinonide in an adhesive base for treatment of oral lichen planus: a double-blind, placebo-controlled clinical study. Oral Surg Oral Med Oral Pathol. 1993;75(2):181–5.
34. Lozada-Nur F, Miranda C, Maliksi R. Double-blind clinical trial of 0.05% clobetasol proprionate ointment in orabase and 0.05% fluocinonide ointment in orabase in the treatment of patients with oral vesiculoerosive diseases. Oral Surg Oral Med Oral Pathol. 1994;77(6):598–604.

35. Lozada-Nur F, Huang MZ. Open preliminary clinical trial of clobetasol propionate ointment in adhesive paste for treatment of chronic oral vesiculoerosive diseases. Oral Surg Oral Med Oral Pathol. 1991;71(3):283–7.
36. Sarfaraz S, Javed A, Khan F, Raees H, Nasir I, Shahid J. Treatment of lichen planus-a review. 2019.
37. Rödström P, Hakeberg M, Jontell M, Nordin P. Erosive oral lichen planus treated with clobetasol propionate and triamcinolone acetonide in Orabase: a double-blind clinical trial. J Dermatol Treat. 1994;5(1):7–10.
38. Lodi G, Manfredi M, Mercadante V, Murphy R, Carrozzo M. Interventions for treating oral lichen planus: corticosteroid therapies. Cochrane Database Syst Rev. 2020;2 https://doi.org/10.1002/14651858.CD001168.pub3.
39. Carbone M, Arduino PG, Carrozzo M, Caiazzo G, Broccoletti R, Conrotto D, et al. Topical clobetasol in the treatment of atrophic-erosive oral lichen planus: a randomized controlled trial to compare two preparations with different concentrations. J Oral Pathol Med. 2009;38(2):227–33.
40. Chamani G, Rad M, Zarei MR, Lotfi S, Sadeghi M, Ahmadi Z. Efficacy of tacrolimus and clobetasol in the treatment of oral lichen planus: a systematic review and meta-analysis. Int J Dermatol. 2015;54(9):996–1004.
41. Conrotto D, Carbone M, Carrozzo M, Arduino P, Broccoletti R, Pentenero M, et al. Ciclosporin vs. clobetasol in the topical management of atrophic and erosive oral lichen planus: a double-blind, randomized controlled trial. Br J Dermatol. 2006;154(1):139–45.
42. Muzio LL, Della Valle A, Mignogna MD, Pannone G, Bucci P, Bucci E, et al. The treatment of oral aphthous ulceration or erosive lichen planus with topical clobetasol propionate in three preparations: a clinical and pilot study on 54 patients. J Oral Pathol Med. 2001;30(10):611–7.
43. Campisi G, Giandalia G, De Caro V, Di Liberto C, Arico P, Giannola L. A new delivery system of clobetasol-17-propionate (lipid-loaded microspheres 0· 025%) compared with a conventional formulation (lipophilic ointment in a hydrophilic phase 0· 025%) in topical treatment of atrophic/erosive oral lichen planus. A phase IV, randomized, observer-blinded, parallel group clinical trial. Br J Dermatol. 2004;150(5):984–90.
44. Gonzalez-Moles MA, Ruiz-Avila I, Rodriguez-Archilla A, Morales-Garcia P, Mesa-Aguado F, Bascones-Martinez A, et al. Treatment of severe erosive gingival lesions by topical application of clobetasol propionate in custom trays. Oral Surg Oral Med Oral Pathol Oral Radiol Endodontol. 2003;95(6):688–92.
45. Gonzalez-Moles MA, Morales P, Rodriguez-Archilla A, Isabel IR-A, Gonzalez-Moles S. Treatment of severe chronic oral erosive lesions with clobetasol propionate in aqueous solution. Oral Surg Oral Med Oral Pathol Oral Radiol Endodontol. 2002;93(3):264–70.
46. Sugerman PB, Savage NW, Zhou X, Walsh LJ, Bigby M. Oral lichen planus. Clin Dermatol. 2000;18(5):533–9.
47. Yang H, Wu Y, Ma H, Jiang L, Zeng X, Dan H, et al. Possible alternative therapies for oral lichen planus cases refractory to steroid therapies. Oral Surg Oral Med Oral Pathol Oral Radiol. 2016;121(5):496–509.
48. Thongprasom K, Dhanuthai K. Steriods in the treatment of lichen planus: a review. J Oral Sci. 2008;50(4):377–85.
49. Lodi G, Tarozzi M, Sardella A, Demarosi F, Canegallo L, Di Benedetto D, et al. Miconazole as adjuvant therapy for oral lichen planus: a double-blind randomized controlled trial. Br J Dermatol. 2007;156(6):1336–41.
50. Hettiarachchi PVKS, Hettiarachchi RM, Jayasinghe RD, Sitheeque M. Comparison of topical tacrolimus and clobetasol in the management of symptomatic oral lichen planus: a double-blinded, randomized clinical trial in Sri Lanka. J Investig Clin Dent. 2017;8(4):e12237.
51. Arunkumar S, Kalappanavar AN, Annigeri RG, Kalappa SG. Relative efficacy of pimecrolimus cream and triamcinolone acetonide paste in the treatment of symptomatic oral lichen planus. Ind J Dent. 2015;6(1):14.
52. Sieg P, Von Domarus H, Von Zitzewitz V, Iven H, Färber L. Topical cyclosporin in oral lichen planus: a controlled, randomized, prospective trial. Br J Dermatol. 1995;132(5):790–4.
53. Thongprasom K, Chaimusig M, Korkij W, Sererat T, Luangjarmekorn L, Rojwattanasirivej S. A randomized-controlled trial to compare topical cyclosporin with triamcinolone acetonide for the treatment of oral lichen planus. J Oral Pathol Med. 2007;36(3):142–6.
54. Eisen D, Ellis CN, Duell EA, Griffiths CE, Voorhees JJ. Effect of topical cyclosporine rinse on oral lichen planus: a double-blind analysis. N Engl J Med. 1990;323(5):290–4.
55. Levell N, Munro C, Marks JM. Severe lichen planus clears with very low-dose cyclosporin. Br J Dermatol. 1992;127(1):66–7.
56. Bécherel P-A, Chosidow O, Boisnic S, Moyal-Barraco M, Pelisse M, Reigneau O, et al. Topical cyclosporine in the treatment of oral and vulvar erosive lichen planus: a blood level monitoring study. Arch Dermatol. 1995;131(4):495–6.
57. Oberti L, Alberta L, Massimo P, Francesco C, Dorina L. Clinical Management of Oral Lichen Planus: a systematic review. Mini Rev Med Chem. 2019;19(13):1049–59. https://doi.org/10.2174/1389557519666190301144157.
58. Eisen D, Carrozzo M, Bagan Sebastian JV, Thongprasom K. Number V Oral lichen planus: clinical features and management. Oral Dis. 2005;11(6):338–49.
59. Ruzicka T, Assmann T, Homey B. Tacrolimus: the drug for the turn of the millennium? Arch Dermatol. 1999;135(5):574–80.
60. Washio K, Nakamura A, Fukuda S, Hashimoto T, Horikawa T. A case of lichen planus pemphigoides

successfully treated with a combination of cyclosporine a and prednisolone. Case Rep Dermatol. 2013;5(1):84–7.
61. Sun SL, Liu JJ, Zhong B, Wang JK, Jin X, Xu H, et al. Topical calcineurin inhibitors in the treatment of oral lichen planus: a systematic review and meta-analysis. Br J Dermatol. 2019;181(6):1166–76.
62. Kaliakatsou F, Hodgson T, Lewsey J, Hegarty A, Murphy A, Porter S. Management of recalcitrant ulcerative oral lichen planus with topical tacrolimus. J Am Acad Dermatol. 2002;46(1):35–41.
63. Conrotto D, Carrozzo M, Ubertalli AV, Gandolfo S, Giaccone L, Boccadoro M, et al. Dramatic increase of tacrolimus plasma concentration during topical treatment for oral graft-versus-host disease. Transplantation. 2006;82(8):1113–5.
64. Hodgson TA, Sahni N, Kaliakatsou F, Buchanan JA, Porter SR. Long-term efficacy and safety of topical tacrolimus in the management of ulcerative\erosive oral lichen planus. Eur J Dermatol. 2003;13(5):466–70.
65. Lener EV, Brieva J, Schachter M, West LE, West DP, El-Azhary RA. Successful treatment of erosive lichen planus with topical tacrolimus. Arch Dermatol. 2001;137(4):419–22.
66. Morrison L, Kratochvil FJ III, Gorman A. An open trial of topical tacrolimus for erosive oral lichen planus. J Am Acad Dermatol. 2002;47(4):617–20.
67. Olivier V, Lacour J-P, Mousnier A, Garraffo R, Monteil RA, Ortonne J-P. Treatment of chronic erosive oral lichen planus with low concentrations of topical tacrolimus: an open prospective study. Arch Dermatol. 2002;138(10):1335–8.
68. Rozycki TW, Rogers RS III, Pittelkow MR, McEvoy MT, El-Azhary RA, Bruce AJ, et al. Topical tacrolimus in the treatment of symptomatic oral lichen planus: a series of 13 patients. J Am Acad Dermatol. 2002;46(1):27–34.
69. Samycia M, Lin AN. Efficacy of topical calcineurin inhibitors in lichen planus. J Cutan Med Surg. 2012;16(4):221–9.
70. Arash A, Shirin L. The comparison of efficacy of adcortyl ointment and topical tacrolimus in treatment of erosive oral lichen planus. 2007.
71. Singh A, Rai A, Aftab M, Jain S, Singh M. Efficacy of steroidal vs non-steroidal agents in oral lichen planus: a randomised, open-label study. J Laryngol Otol. 2017;131(1):69–76.
72. Polizzi A, Santonocito S, Lo Giudice A, Alibrandi A, De Pasquale R, Isola G. Analysis of the response to two pharmacological protocols in patients with oral lichen planus: a randomized clinical trial. Oral Dis. 2021;
73. Ribero S, Stieger M, Quaglino P, Hongang T, Bornstein M, Naldi L, et al. Efficacy of topical tacrolimus for oral lichen planus: real-life experience in a retrospective cohort of patients with a review of the literature. J Eur Acad Dermatol Venereol. 2015;29(6):1107–13.
74. Arduino PG, Carbone M, Della Ferrera F, Elia A, Conrotto D, Gambino A, et al. Pimecrolimus vs. tacrolimus for the topical treatment of unresponsive oral erosive lichen planus: a 8 week randomized double-blind controlled study. J Eur Acad Dermatol Venereol. 2014;28(4):475–82.
75. Becker JC, Houben R, Vetter CS, Bröcker EB. The carcinogenic potential of tacrolimus ointment beyond immune suppression: a hypothesis creating case report. BMC Cancer. 2006;6(1):1–6.
76. Mattsson U, Magnusson B, Jontell M. Squamous cell carcinoma in a patient with oral lichen planus treated with topical application of tacrolimus. Oral Surg Oral Med Oral Pathol Oral Radiol Endodontol. 2010;110(1):e19–25.
77. Goel S, Marwah A, Kaushik S, Garg VK, Gupta S. Role of serum interleukin-6 in deciding therapy for multidrug resistant oral lichen planus. J Clin Exp Dent. 2015;7(4):e477.
78. Thongprasom K, Prapinjumrune C, Carrozzo M. Novel therapies for oral lichen planus. J Oral Pathol Med. 2013;42(10):721–7.
79. Ibrahim SS, Hazzaa HH. Topical pimecrolimus effect on Fas inducing apoptosis in oral lichen planus: a clinical immunohistochemical study. J Oral Pathol Med. 2012;41(4):315–21.
80. Gorouhi F, Solhpour A, Beitollahi JM, Afshar S, Davari P, Hashemi P, et al. Randomized trial of pimecrolimus cream versus triamcinolone acetonide paste in the treatment of oral lichen planus. J Am Acad Dermatol. 2007;57(5):806–13.
81. McCaughey C, Machan M, Bennett R, Zone J, Hull C. Pimecrolimus 1% cream for oral erosive lichen planus: a 6-week randomized, double-blind, vehicle-controlled study with a 6-week open-label extension to assess efficacy and safety. J Eur Acad Dermatol Venereol. 2011;25(9):1061–7.
82. Passeron T, Lacour J-P, Fontas E, Ortonne J-P. Treatment of oral erosive lichen planus with 1% pimecrolimus cream: a double-blind, randomized, prospective trial with measurement of pimecrolimus levels in the blood. Arch Dermatol. 2007;143(4):472–6.
83. Swift JC, Rees TD, Plemons JM, Hallmon WW, Wright JC. The effectiveness of 1% pimecrolimus cream in the treatment of oral erosive lichen planus. J Periodontol. 2005;76(4):627–35.
84. Volz T, Caroli U, Lüdtke H, Bräutigam M, Kohler-Späth H, Röcken M, et al. Pimecrolimus cream 1% in erosive oral lichen planus—a prospective randomized double-blind vehicle-controlled study. Br J Dermatol. 2008;159(4):936–41.
85. Siegfried EC, Jaworski JC, Hebert AA. Topical calcineurin inhibitors and lymphoma risk: evidence update with implications for daily practice. Am J Clin Dermatol. 2013;14(3):163–78.
86. Tennis P, Gelfand J, Rothman K. Evaluation of cancer risk related to atopic dermatitis and use of topical calcineurin inhibitors. Br J Dermatol. 2011;165(3):465–73.
87. Dalmau J, Puig L, Roé E, Peramiquel L, Campos M, Alomar A. Successful treatment of oral erosive lichen planus with mycophenolate mofetil. J Eur Acad Dermatol Venereol. 2007;21(2):259–60.
88. Wee J, Shirlaw P, Challacombe S, Setterfield J. Efficacy of mycophenolate mofetil in severe

mucocutaneous lichen planus: a retrospective review of 10 patients. Br J Dermatol. 2012;167(1):36–43.
89. Frieling U, Bonsmann G, Schwarz T, Luger TA, Beissert S. Treatment of severe lichen planus with mycophenolate mofetil. J Am Acad Dermatol. 2003;49(6):1063–6.
90. Nousari HC, Goyal S, Anhalt GJ. Successful treatment of resistant hypertrophic and bullous lichen planus with mycophenolate mofetil. Arch Dermatol. 1999;135(11):1420–1.
91. Liu V, Mackool B. Mycophenolate in dermatology. J Dermatol Treat. 2003;14(4):203–11.
92. Eisen D. The clinical manifestations and treatment of oral lichen planus. Dermatol Clin. 2003;21(1):79–89. https://doi.org/10.1016/s0733-8635(02)00067-0.
93. Zenuz AT, Mehdipour M, Shokri J, Samiei N, Aghazadeh M. Effect of mucoadhesive form of mycophenolate mofetil on oral erosive lichen planus lesions. Oral Surg Oral Med Oral Pathol Oral Radiol. 2015;119(3):e167.
94. Lear J, English J. Erosive and generalized lichen planus responsive to azathioprine. Clin Exp Dermatol. 1996;21(1):56–7.
95. Klein L, Callen J. Azathioprine: effective steroid-sparing therapy for generalized lichen planus. South Med J. 1992;85(2):198–201.
96. Verma K, Sirka C, Khaitan B. Generalized severe lichen planus treated with azathioprine. Acta Derm Venereol. 1999;79(6):493.
97. Lozada F. Prednisone and azathioprine in the treatment of oral inflammatory mucocutaneous diseases. Oral Surg Oral Med Oral Pathol. 1981;52: 257–60.
98. Epstein J, Nantel S, Sheoltch S. Topical azathioprine in the combined treatment of chronic oral graft-versus-host disease. Bone Marrow Transplant. 2000;25(6):683–7.
99. Epstein J, Gorsky M, Epstein M, Nantel S. Topical azathioprine in the treatment of immune-mediated chronic oral inflammatory conditions: a series of cases. Oral Surg Oral Med Oral Pathol Oral Radiol Endodontol. 2001;91(1):56–61.
100. Lajevardi V, Ghodsi SZ, Hallaji Z, Shafiei Z, Aghazadeh N, Akbari Z. Treatment of erosive oral lichen planus with methotrexate. JDDG. J Dtsch Dermatol Ges. 2016;14(3):286–93.
101. Torti DC, Jorizzo JL, McCarty MA. Oral lichen planus: a case series with emphasis on therapy. Arch Dermatol. 2007;143(4):511–5.
102. Lundqvist EN, Wahlin YB, Hofer P-A. Methotrexate supplemented with steroid ointments for the treatment of severe erosive lichen ruber. Acta Derm Venereol. 2002;82(1):63–4.
103. Soria A, Agbo-Godeau S, Taïeb A, Francès C. Treatment of refractory oral erosive lichen planus with topical rapamycin: 7 cases. Dermatology. 2009;218(1):22–5.
104. Franks ME, Macpherson GR, Figg WD. Thalidomide. Lancet. 2004;363(9423):1802–11.
105. Matthews SJ, McCoy C. Thalidomide: a review of approved and investigational uses. Clin Ther. 2003;25(2):342–95.
106. Camisa C, Popovsky JL. Effective treatment of oral erosive lichen planus with thalidomide. Arch Dermatol. 2000;136(12):1442–3.
107. Macario-Barrel A, Balguerie X, Joly P. Treatment of erosive oral lichen planus with thalidomide. Ann Dermatol Venereol. 2003;130:1109–12.
108. Wu Y, Zhou G, Zeng H, Xiong C-r, Lin M, Zhou H-m. A randomized double-blind, positive-control trial of topical thalidomide in erosive oral lichen planus. Oral Surg Oral Med, Oral Pathol, Oral Radiol, Endodontol. 2010;110(2):188–95.
109. Bell J. Amlexanox for the treatment of recurrent aphthous ulcers. Clin Drug Investig. 2005;25(9):555–66.
110. Zhang Y, Guan H, Li J, Fang Z, Chen W, Li F. Amlexanox suppresses osteoclastogenesis and prevents ovariectomy-induced bone loss. Sci Rep. 2015;5(1):1–13.
111. Saijo T, Kuriki H, Ashida Y, Makino H, Maki Y. Mechanism of the action of amoxanox (AA-673), an orally active antiallergic agent. Int Arch Allergy Appl Immunol. 1985;78(1):43–50. https://doi.org/10.1159/000233861.
112. Patil K, Joshy A, Doggalli N, Shankar J, Gowda CJ, Deshpande P. Recent advancements in Oral lichen planus management: an overview. World J Dent. 2018;9(3):249–51.
113. Beck H, Brandrup F. Treatment of erosive lichen planus with dapsone. Acta Derm Venereol. 1986;66(4):366–7.
114. Begon E, Chosidow O, Wolkenstein P. Disulone. Annales de dermatologie et de vénéréologie: Elsevier; 2004. p. 1062–73.
115. Sugerman PB, Sabage N. Oral lichen planus: causes, diagnosis and management. Aust Dent J. 2002;47(4):290–7.
116. Graham WR Jr. Adverse effects of dapsone. Int J Dermatol. 1975;14(7):494–500.
117. Lundström IM, Anneroth GB, Holmberg K. Candida in patients with oral lichen planus. Int J Oral Surg. 1984;13(3):226–38.
118. Barrett A, Kingsmill V, Speight P. The frequency of fungal infection in biopsies of oral mucosal lesions. Oral Dis. 1998;4(1):26–31.
119. Gupta S, Jawanda MK. Oral lichen planus: an update on etiology, pathogenesis, clinical presentation, diagnosis and management. Indian J Dermatol. 2015;60(3):222.
120. Sehgal V, Abraham G, MALIK GB. Griseofulvin therapy in lichen planus: a double-blind controlled trial. Br J Dermatol. 1972;87(4):383–5.
121. Massa M, Rogers R 3rd. Griseofulvin therapy of lichen planus. Acta Derm Venereol. 1981;61(6):547–50.
122. Aufdemorte TB, De Villez RL, Gieseker DR. Griseofulvin in the treatment of three cases of oral erosive lichen planus. Oral Surg Oral Med Oral Pathol. 1983;55(5):459–62.
123. Parmar D, Thacker K, Shah J. Assessment of griseofulvin in the management of lichen planus. Int J Res. 2017;3(4):523.
124. Lamey P, Boyle M, Simpson N, Ferguson M. A pilot study of griseofulvin therapy in erosive oral lichen planus. J Oral Med. 1987;42(233):59.

125. Matthews R, Scully C. Griseofulvin in the treatment of oral lichen planus: adverse drug reactions, but little beneficial effect. Ann Dent. 1992;51(2):10–1.
126. Naylor GD. Treating erosive lichen planus with griseofulvin: a report of four cases. Quintessence Int. 1990;21(12):943–7.
127. Büyük AY, Kavala M. Oral metronidazole treatment of lichen planus. J Am Acad Dermatol. 2000;43(2):260–2.
128. Rasi A, Behzadi AH, Davoudi S, Rafizadeh P, Honarbakhsh Y, Mehran M, et al. Efficacy of oral metronidazole in treatment of cutaneous and mucosal lichen planus. J Drug Dermatol: JDD. 2010;9(10):1186–90.
129. Ohkuma S, Poole B. Fluorescence probe measurement of the intralysosomal pH in living cells and the perturbation of pH by various agents. Proc Natl Acad Sci. 1978;75(7):3327–31.
130. Ohkuma S, Chudzik J, Poole B. The effects of basic substances and acidic ionophores on the digestion of exogenous and endogenous proteins in mouse peritoneal macrophages. J Cell Biol. 1986;102(3):959–66.
131. Oda K, Koriyama Y, Yamada E, Ikehara Y. Effects of weakly basic amines on proteolytic processing and terminal glycosylation of secretory proteins in cultured rat hepatocytes. Biochem J. 1986;240(3):739–45.
132. Hurst N, French J, Gorjatschko L, Betts W. Chloroquine and hydroxychloroquine inhibit multiple sites in metabolic pathways leading to neutrophil superoxide release. J Rheumatol. 1988;15(1):23–7.
133. Jessop S, Whitelaw DA, Grainge MJ, Jayasekera P. Drugs for discoid lupus erythematosus. Cochrane Database Syst Rev. 2017;5
134. Chew CY, Mar A, Nikpour M, Saracino AM. Hydroxychloroquine in dermatology: new perspectives on an old drug. Australas J Dermatol. 2020;61(2):e150–e7.
135. Mutafchieva MZ, Draganova-Filipova MN, Zagorchev PI, Tomov GT. Oral lichen planus–known and unknown: a review. Folia Med (Plovdiv). 2018;60(4):528–35.
136. Bhuiyan I, Wahab M, Ali A, Sultana A, Siddique RU, Hawlader AR, et al. Comparative efficacy of hydroxychloroquine and griseofulvin in the treatment of lichen planus. J Pak Assoc Dermatol. 2010;20(2):79–83.
137. Eisen D. Hydroxychloroquine sulfate (Plaquenil) improves oral lichen planus: an open trial. J Am Acad Dermatol. 1993;28(4):609–12.
138. Yeshurun A, Bergman R, Bathish N, Khamaysi Z. Hydroxychloroquine sulphate therapy of erosive oral lichen planus. Australas J Dermatol. 2019;60(2):e109–e12.
139. Hussein H, Brown R. Hydroxychloroquine and the treatment of Sjogren syndrome, chronic ulcerative stomatitis, and oral lichen planus in the age of COVID-19. Oral Surg Oral Med Oral Pathol Oral Radiol. 2021;131(1):e9–e13.
140. Bendas ER, Abdullah H, El-Komy MH, Kassem MA. Hydroxychloroquine niosomes: a new trend in topical management of oral lichen planus. Int J Pharm. 2013;458(2):287–95. https://doi.org/10.1016/j.ijpharm.2013.10.042.
141. Lu S-Y, Chen W-J, Eng H-L. Dramatic response to levamisole and low-dose prednisolone in 23 patients with oral lichen planus: a 6-year prospective follow-up study. Oral Surg Oral Med Oral Pathol Oral Radiol Endodontol. 1995;80(6):705–9.
142. Kirby JD, Black M, McGibbon D. Levamisole-induced lichenoid eruptions. J R Soc Med. 1980;73(3):208–11.
143. Sardella A, Demarosi F, Oltolina A, Rimondini L, Carrassi A. Efficacy of topical mesalazine compared with clobetasol propionate in treatment of symptomatic oral lichen planus. Oral Dis. 1998;4(4):255–9.
144. Alstead E, Wilson A, Farthing M. Lichen planus and mesalazine. J Clin Gastroenterol. 1991;13(3):335–7.
145. Hodak E, Yosipovitch G, David M, Ingber A, Chorev L, Lider O, et al. Low-dose low-molecular-weight heparin (enoxaparin) is beneficial in lichen planus: a preliminary report. J Am Acad Dermatol. 1998;38(4):564–8.
146. Stefanidou M, Ioannidou D, Panayiotides J, Tosca A. Low molecular weight heparin; a novel alternative therapeutic approach for lichen planus. Br J Dermatol. 1999;141(6):1040–5.
147. Iraji F, Asilian A, Saeidi A, Siadat AH, Saeidi AR, Hassanzadeh A. Comparison of therapeutic effect of low-dose low-molecular-weight heparin (enoxaparin) vs. oral prednisone in treatment of patients with lichen planus; a clinical trial. Advanced. Biomed Res. 2013:2.
148. Kövesi G. Evaluation of clinical data and immunomodulating treatment of patients with oral lichen planus. Fogorv Sz. 2001;94(1):9–14.
149. Sato M, Yoshida H, Yanagawa T, Yura Y, Urata M, Nitta T, et al. Therapeutic effect of human fibroblast interferon on premalignant lesions arising in oral mucosa: a pilot study. Int J Oral Surg. 1985;14(2):184–94.
150. Pedersen A. IFN-a cream in the treatment of oral lichen planus. Oral Dis. 1998;4(2):155–6.
151. Doutre M, Beylot C, Couzigou P, Long P, Royer P, Beylot J. Lichen planus and virus C hepatitis: disappearance of the lichen under interferon alfa therapy. Dermatology. 1992;184(3):229.
152. Hildebrand A, Kolde G, Luger TA, Schwarz T. Successful treatment of generalized lichen planus with recombinant interferon alfa-2b. J Am Acad Dermatol. 1995;33(5):880–3.
153. Nagao Y, Sata M, Suzuki H, Kameyama T, Ueno T. Histological improvement of oral lichen planus in patients with chronic hepatitis C treated with interferon. Gastroenterology. 1999;117(1):283–4.
154. Nagao Y, Sata M, Ide T, Suzuki H, Tanikawa K, Itoh K, et al. Development and exacerbation of oral lichen planus during and after interferon therapy for hepatitis C. Eur J Clin Investig. 1996;26(12):1171–4.
155. Schlesinger TE, Camisa C, Gay JD, Bergfeld WF. Oral erosive lichen planus with epidermolytic hyperkeratosis during interferon alfa-2b therapy for chronic hepatitis C virus infection. J Am Acad Dermatol. 1997;36(6):1023–5.

156. Kütting B, Bühm M, Luger T, Bonsmann G. Ornpharyngeal lichen planus associated with interferon-α treatment for mycosis fungoides: a rare side-effect in the therapy of cutaneous lymphomas. Br J Dermatol. 1997;137(5):836–7.
157. Shiohara T, Nickoloff BJ, Moriya N, Gotoh C, Nagashima M. In vivo effects of interferon-γ and anti-interferon-γ antibody on the experimentally induced lichenoid tissue reaction. Br J Dermatol. 1988;119(2):199–206.
158. Nagao Y, Kimura K, Kawahigashi Y, Sata M. Successful treatment of hepatitis C virus-associated oral lichen planus by interferon-free therapy with direct-acting antivirals. Clin Transl Gastroenterol. 2016;7(7):e179.
159. Misaka K, Kishimoto T, Kawahigashi Y, Sata M, Nagao Y. Use of direct-acting antivirals for the treatment of hepatitis C virus-associated oral lichen planus: a case report. Case Rep Gastroenterol. 2016;10(3):617–22.
160. Nagao Y, Kawaguchi T, Ide T, Kumashiro R, Sata M. Exacerbation of oral erosive lichen planus by combination of interferon and ribavirin therapy for chronic hepatitis C. Int J Mol Med. 2005;15(2):237–41.
161. Grossmann SMC, Teixeira R, de Aguiar MCF, do Carmo MAV. Exacerbation of oral lichen planus lesions during treatment of chronic hepatitis C with pegylated interferon and ribavirin. Eur J Gastroenterol Hepatol. 2008;20(7):702–6.
162. Javadzadeh A, Vatanpour H, Delavarian Z, Momajed A, Esmaeili HE, Vatanpour M, et al. Efficacy of clobetasol, ketoconazole and amitryptiline mouthwash on Oral lichen planus. 2008.
163. Costantini AM, Cannella C, Tomassi G. Fondamenti di nutrizione umana. Il pensiero scientifico; 1999.
164. Nosratzehi T. Oral lichen planus: an overview of potential risk factors, biomarkers and treatments. Asian Pac J Cancer Prev: APJCP. 2018;19(5):1161.
165. Sloberg K, Hersle K, Mobacken H, Thilander H. Topical tretinoin therapy and oral lichen planus. Arch Dermatol. 1979;115(6):716–8.
166. Giustina TA, Stewart JC, Ellis CN, Regezi JA, Annesley T, Woo TY, et al. Topical application of isotretinoin gel improves oral lichen planus: a double-blind study. Arch Dermatol. 1986;122(5):534–6.
167. Scardina G, Messina P, Carini F, Maresi E. A randomized trial assessing the effectiveness of different concentrations of isotretinoin in the management of lichen planus. Int J Oral Maxillofac Surg. 2006;35(1):67–71.
168. Boisnic S, Branchet M, Pascal F, Benslama L, Rostin M, Szpirglas H. Topical tretinoin for treatment of oral lichen-planus and oral leukoplakia-clinical-study. Annales de dermatologie et de venereologie: masson editeur 120 BLVD SAINT-GERMAIN, 75280 PARIS 06, FRANCE; 1994. p. 459–463.
169. Boisnic S, Licu D, Slama B, Branchet-Gumila M, Szpirglas H, Dupuy P. Topical retinaldehyde treatment in oral lichen planus and leukoplakia. Int J Tissue React. 2002;24(4):123–30.
170. Regezi JA, Ellis CN, Stewart JC, Giustina TA. Histologic changes associated with the topical use of isotretinoin on oral lichen planus. Oral Surg Oral Med Oral Pathol. 1986;61(5):479–84.
171. Levy J, Sharoni Y. Functions of tomato lycopene and its role in human health. HerbalGram. 2004;62:49–56.
172. Stahl W, Sies H. Lycopene: a biologically important carotenoid for humans? Arch Biochem Biophys. 1996;336(1):1–9.
173. Salehi B, Jornet PL, López EP-F, Calina D, Sharifi-Rad M, Ramírez-Alarcón K, et al. Plant-derived bioactives in oral mucosal lesions: a key emphasis to curcumin, lycopene, chamomile, aloe vera, green tea and coffee properties. Biomol Ther. 2019;9(3):106.
174. Nagao T, Ikeda N, Warnakulasuriya S, Fukano H, Yuasa H, Yano M, et al. Serum antioxidant micronutrients and the risk of oral leukoplakia among Japanese. Oral Oncol. 2000;36(5):466–70.
175. Nagao T, Warnakulasuriya S, Ikeda N, Fukano H, Yamamoto S, Yano M, et al. Serum antioxidant micronutrient levels in oral lichen planus. J Oral Pathol Med. 2001;30(5):264–7.
176. Saawarn N, Shashikanth M, Saawarn S, Jirge V, Chaitanya NC, Pinakapani R. Lycopene in the management of oral lichen planus: a placebo-controlled study. Indian J Dent Res. 2011;22(5):639.
177. Miyachi M, Matsuno T, Asano K, Mataga I. Anti-inflammatory effects of astaxanthin in the human gingival keratinocyte line NDUSD-1. J Clin Biochem Nutr. 2015;56:14–109.
178. Tradati N, Chiesa F, Rossi N, Grigolato R, Formelli F, Costa A, et al. Successful topical treatment of oral lichen planus and leukoplakias with fenretinide (4-HPR). Cancer Lett. 1994;76(2–3):109–11.
179. Hersle K, Mobacken H, Sloberg K, Thilander H. Severe oral lichen planus: treatment with an aromatic retinoid (etretinate). Br J Dermatol. 1982;106(1):77–80.
180. Laurberg G, Geiger J-M, Hjorth N, Holm P, Hou-Jensen K, Jacobsen KU, et al. Treatment of lichen planus with acitretin: a double-blind, placebo-controlled study in 65 patients. J Am Acad Dermatol. 1991;24(3):434–7.
181. Deshpande A. Successful use of oral acitretin in oral lichen planus. Ind J Drug Dermatol. 2017;3(1):24.
182. Petruzzi M, De Benedittis M, Grassi R, Cassano N, Vena G, Serpico R. Oral lichen planus: a preliminary clinical study on treatment with tazarotene. Oral Dis. 2002;8(6):291–5.
183. Bollag W, Ott F. Treatment of lichen planus with temarotene. Lancet. 1989;334(8669):974.
184. Challacombe S. Haematological abnormalities in oral lichen planus, candidiasis, leukoplakia and nonspecific stomatitis. Int J Oral Maxillofac Surg. 1986;15(1):72–80.
185. Chen H-M, Wang Y-P, Chang JY-F, Wu Y-C, Cheng S-J, Sun A. Significant association of deficiencies of hemoglobin, iron, folic acid, and vitamin B12 and high homocysteine level with oral lichen planus. J Formos Med Assoc. 2015;114(2):124–9.

186. Lin HP, Wang YP, Chia JS, Chiang CP, Sun A. Modulation of serum gastric parietal cell antibody level by levamisole and vitamin B12 in oral lichen planus. Oral Dis. 2011;17(1):95–101.
187. Sun A, Wang J, Chia J, Chiang C. Serum interleukin-8 level is a more sensitive marker than serum interleukin-6 level in monitoring the disease activity of oral lichen planus. Br J Dermatol. 2005;152(6):1187–92.
188. Sun A, Chia J, Wang J-T, Chiang C. Levamisole can reduce the high serum tumour necrosis factor-α level to a normal level in patients with erosive oral lichen planus. Clin Exp Dermatol: Exp Dermatol. 2007;32(3):308–10.
189. Chang JYF, Chiang CP, Hsiao CK, Sun A. Significantly higher frequencies of presence of serum autoantibodies in Chinese patients with oral lichen planus. J Oral Pathol Med. 2009;38(1):48–54.
190. Ahmed SA. The role of serum vitamin D Deficency in oral lichen planus case control study. Diyala J Med. 2019;17(2):189–98.
191. Gupta J, Aggarwal A, Asadullah M, Khan MH, Agrawal N, Khwaja KJ. Vitamin D in the treatment of oral lichen planus: a pilot clinical study. J Ind Acad Oral Med Radiol. 2019;31(3):222.
192. Rai B, Kaur J, Jacobs R, Singh J. Possible action mechanism for curcumin in pre-cancerous lesions based on serum and salivary markers of oxidative stress. J Oral Sci. 2010;52(2):251–6.
193. Azizi A, Farshchi F. Comparison of salivary and plasma antioxidant levels in lichen planus patients and healthy subjects. J Oral Pathol Med. 2012;41(7):524–6.
194. Yang L-L, Liu X-Q, Liu W, Cheng B, Li M-T. Comparative analysis of whole saliva proteomes for the screening of biomarkers for oral lichen planus. Inflamm Res. 2006;55(10):405–7.
195. Keller KL, Fenske NA. Uses of vitamins a, C, and E and related compounds in dermatology: a review. J Am Acad Dermatol. 1998;39(4):611–25.
196. Bacci C, Vanzo V, Frigo A, Stellini E, Sbricoli L, Valente M. Topical tocopherol for treatment of reticular oral lichen planus: a randomized, double-blind, crossover study. Oral Dis. 2017;23(1):62–8.
197. Heim KE, Tagliaferro AR, Bobilya DJ. Flavonoid antioxidants: chemistry, metabolism and structure-activity relationships. J Nutr Biochem. 2002;13(10):572–84.
198. de Gutierrez ER, Di Fabio A, Salomón S, Lanfranchi H. Topical treatment of oral lichen planus with anthocyanins. Med Oral Patol Oral Cir Bucal. 2014;19(5):e459.
199. Wildman RE. Nutraceuticals: a brief review of historical and teleological aspects. In: Handbook of nutraceuticals and functional foods; 2001. p. 2–12.
200. Aggarwal BB, Kumar A, Bharti AC. Anticancer potential of curcumin: preclinical and clinical studies. Anticancer Res. 2003;23(1/A):363–98.
201. Singh V, Pal M, Gupta S, Tiwari S, Malkunje L, Das S. Turmeric-a new treatment option for lichen planus: a pilot study. Natl J Maxillofac Surg. 2013;4(2):198.
202. Atsumi T, Fujisawa S, Tonosaki K. Relationship between intracellular ROS production and membrane mobility in curcumin-and tetrahydrocurcumin-treated human gingival fibroblasts and human submandibular gland carcinoma cells. Oral Dis. 2005;11(4):236–42.
203. Krishnaswamy K, Prasad M, Krishna T, Annapurna V, Reddy GA. A case study of nutrient intervention of oral precancerous lesions in India. Eur J Cancer B Oral Oncol. 1995;31(1):41–8.
204. Chainani-Wu N, Silverman S Jr, Reingold A, Bostrom A, Mc Culloch C, Lozada-Nur F, et al. A randomized, placebo-controlled, double-blind clinical trial of curcuminoids in oral lichen planus. Phytomedicine. 2007;14(7–8):437–46.
205. Amirchaghmaghi M, Pakfetrat A, Delavarian Z, Ghalavani H, Ghazi A. Evaluation of the efficacy of curcumin in the treatment of oral lichen planus: a randomized controlled trial. J Clin Diagn Res. 2016;10(5):ZC134.
206. Chainani-Wu N, Madden E, Lozada-Nur F, Silverman S Jr. High-dose curcuminoids are efficacious in the reduction in symptoms and signs of oral lichen planus. J Am Acad Dermatol. 2012;66(5):752–60.
207. Chainani-Wu N, Collins K, Silverman S Jr. Use of curcuminoids in a cohort of patients with oral lichen planus, an autoimmune disease. Phytomedicine. 2012;19(5):418–23.
208. Kia SJ, Shirazian S, Mansourian A, Fard LK, Ashnagar S. Comparative efficacy of topical curcumin and triamcinolone for oral lichen planus: a randomized, controlled clinical trial. J Dent (Tehran, Iran). 2015;12(11):789.
209. Nosratzehi T, Arbabi-Kalati F, Hamishehkar H, Bagheri S. Comparison of the effects of curcumin mucoadhesive paste and local corticosteroid on the treatment of erosive oral lichen planus lesions. J Natl Med Assoc. 2018;110(1):92–7.
210. Thomas AE, Varma B, Kurup S, Jose R, Chandy ML, Kumar SP, et al. Evaluation of efficacy of 1% curcuminoids as local application in management of oral lichen planus–interventional study. J Clin Diagn Res. 2017;11(4):ZC89.
211. White CM, Chamberlin K, Eisenberg E. Curcumin, a turmeric extract, for oral lichen planus: a systematic review. Oral Dis. 2019;25(3):720–5.
212. Lv K-J, Chen T-C, Wang G-H, Yao Y-N, Yao H. Clinical safety and efficacy of curcumin use for oral lichen planus: a systematic review. J Dermatol Treat. 2018;30(6):605–11.
213. Yagi A, Kabash A, Okamura N, Haraguchi H, Moustafa S, Khalifa T. Antioxidant, free radical scavenging and anti-inflammatory effects of aloesin derivatives in Aloe vera. Planta Med. 2002;68(11):957–60.
214. Shelton RM. Aloe vera: its chemical and therapeutic properties. Int J Dermatol. 1991;30(10):679–83.
215. Vogler B, Ernst E. Aloe vera: a systematic review of its clinical effectiveness. Br J Gen Pract. 1999;49(447):823–8.
216. Choi SW, Son BW, Son YS, Park YI, Lee SK, Chung MH. The wound-healing effect of a glycoprotein

fraction isolated from aloe vera. Br J Dermatol. 2001;145(4):535–45.
217. Klein AD, Penneys NS. Aloe vera. J Am Acad Dermatol. 1988;18(4):714–20.
218. Williams MS, Burk M, Loprinzi CL, Hill M, Schomberg PJ, Nearhood K, et al. Phase III double-blind evaluation of an aloe vera gel as a prophylactic agent for radiation-induced skin toxicity. Int J Radiat Oncol Biol Phys. 1996;36(2):345–9.
219. Nair GR, Naidu GS, Jain S, Nagi R, Makkad RS, Jha A. Clinical effectiveness of aloe vera in the management of oral mucosal diseases-a systematic review. J Clin Diagn Res. 2016;10(8):ZE01.
220. Hayes S. Lichen planus–report of successful treatment with aloe vera. Gen Dent. 1999;47(3):268–72.
221. Choonhakarn C, Busaracome P, Sripanidkulchai B, Sarakarn P. The efficacy of aloe vera gel in the treatment of oral lichen planus: a randomized controlled trial. Br J Dermatol. 2008;158(3):573–7.
222. Salazar-Sánchez N, López-Jornet P, Camacho-Alonso F, Sánchez-Siles M. Efficacy of topical Aloe vera in patients with oral lichen planus: a randomized double-blind study. J Oral Pathol Med. 2010;39(10):735–40.
223. Reddy RL, Reddy RS, Ramesh T, Singh TR, Swapna LA, Laxmi NV. Randomized trial of aloe vera gel vs triamcinolone acetonide ointment in the treatment of oral lichen planus. Quintessence Int. 2012;43(9):793–800.
224. Ialenti A, Di Rosa M. Hyaluronic acid modulates acute and chronic inflammation. Agents Actions. 1994;43(1):44–7.
225. Radwan-Oczko M. Topical application of drugs used in treatment of oral lichen planus lesions. Adv Clin Exp Med. 2013;22(6):893–8.
226. Nolan A, Badminton J, Maguire J, Seymour R. The efficacy of topical hyaluronic acid in the management of oral lichen planus. J Oral Pathol Med. 2009;38(3):299–303.
227. Hashem AS, Issrani R, Elsayed TE, Prabhu N. Topical hyaluronic acid in the management of oral lichen planus: a comparative study. J Investig Clin Dent. 2019;10(2):e12385.
228. Shetty RR, Burde KN, Guttal KS. The efficacy of topical hyaluronic acid 0.2% in the management of symptomatic oral lichen planus. J Clin Diagn Res. 2016;10(1):ZC46.
229. Khan N, Mukhtar H. Tea and health: studies in humans. Curr Pharm Des. 2013;19(34):6141–7.
230. Cabrera C, Artacho R, Giménez R. Beneficial effects of green tea—a review. J Am Coll Nutr. 2006;25(2):79–99.
231. Basu A, Masek E, Ebersole JL. Dietary polyphenols and periodontitis—a mini-review of literature. Molecules. 2018;23(7):1786.
232. Hirasawa M, Takada K, Makimura M, Otake S. Improvement of periodontal status by green tea catechin using a local delivery system: a clinical pilot study. J Periodontal Res. 2002;37(6):433–8.
233. Welsh EJ, Bara A, Barley E, Cates CJ. Caffeine for asthma. Cochrane Database Syst Rev. 2010;1:CD001112.
234. Furtado KS, Prado MG, Aguiar e Silva MA, Dias MC, Rivelli DP, Rodrigues MA, et al. Coffee and caffeine protect against liver injury induced by thioacetamide in male Wistar rats. Basic Clin Pharmacol Toxicol. 2012;111(5):339–47.
235. Yoneyama S, Kawai K, Tsuno NH, Okaji Y, Asakage M, Tsuchiya T, et al. Epigallocatechin gallate affects human dendritic cell differentiation and maturation. J Allergy Clin Immunol. 2008;121(1):209–14.
236. Kawai K, Tsuno NH, Kitayama J, Okaji Y, Yazawa K, Asakage M, et al. Epigallocatechin gallate induces apoptosis of monocytes. J Allergy Clin Immunol. 2005;115(1):186–91.
237. Zhang J, Zhou G. Green tea consumption: an alternative approach to managing oral lichen planus. Inflamm Res. 2012;61(6):535–9.
238. Contessi A, Celli G. Le api: biologia, allevamento, prodotti. Edagricole Bologna; 1983.
239. Grange J, Davey R. Antibacterial properties of propolis (bee glue). J R Soc Med. 1990;83(3):159–60.
240. Ansorge S, Reinhold D, Lendeckel U. Propolis and some of its constituents down-regulate DNA synthesis and inflammatory cytokine production but induce TGF-β1 production of human immune cells. Zeitschrift für Naturforschung C. 2003;58(7–8):580–9.
241. Bankova V. Recent trends and important developments in propolis research. Evid Based Complement Alternat Med. 2005;2(1):29–32.
242. Cowan MM. Plant products as antimicrobial agents. Clin Microbiol Rev. 1999;12(4):564–82.
243. Paintz M, Metzner J. On the local anaesthetic action of propolis and some of its constituents. Pharmazie. 1979;34(12):839–41.
244. Lotfy M, Badra G, Burham W, Alenzi F. Combined use of honey, bee propolis and myrrh in healing a deep, infected wound in a patient with diabetes mellitus. Br J Biomed Sci. 2006;63(4):171–3.
245. Murray TJ, Yang X, Sherr DH. Growth of a human mammary tumor cell line is blocked by galangin, a naturally occurring bioflavonoid, and is accompanied by down-regulation of cyclins D3, E, and a. Breast Cancer Res. 2006;8(2):1–12.
246. Zenouz AT, Mehdipour M, Abadi RTA, Shokri J, Rajaee M, Aghazadeh M, et al. Effect of use of propolis on serum levels of il-17 and clinical symptoms and signs in patients with ulcerative oral lichen planus. Oral Surg Oral Med Oral Pathol Oral Radiol. 2015;119(3):e166–e7.
247. Zyada M, El-Said Elewa M, El-Meadawy S, El-Sharkawy H. Effectiveness of topical mucoadhesive gel containing propolis in management of patients with atrophic and erosive oral lichen planus: clinical and immunohistochemical study. Egypt Dent Assoc. 2012;58:1–3.
248. Joshy A, Doggalli N, Patil K, Kulkarni P. To evaluate the efficacy of topical propolis in the management of symptomatic oral lichen planus: a randomized controlled trial. Contemp Clin Dent. 2018;9(1):65.
249. Srivastava JK, Shankar E, Gupta S. Chamomile: a herbal medicine of the past with a bright future. Mol Med Rep. 2010;3(6):895–901.

250. McKay DL, Blumberg JB. A review of the bioactivity and potential health benefits of chamomile tea (Matricaria recutita L.). Phytother Res. 2006;20(7):519–30.
251. Avallone R, Zanoli P, Puia G, Kleinschnitz M, Schreier P, Baraldi M. Pharmacological profile of apigenin, a flavonoid isolated from Matricaria chamomilla. Biochem Pharmacol. 2000;59(11):1387–94.
252. Pino JA, Bayat F, Marbot R, Aguero J. Essential oil of chamomile Chamomilla recutita (L.) Rausch from Iran. J Essent Oil Res. 2002;14(6):407–8.
253. Pirzad A, Alyari H, Shakiba M, Zehtab-Salmasi S, Mohammadi A. Essential oil content and composition of German chamomile (Matricaria chamomilla L.) at different irrigation regimes. J Agron. 2006;5(3):451–5.
254. Zhany Y, Kang Y, Ding X. Clinical effect of compound chamomile and lidocaine hydrochloride gell and dexamethasone in the treatment of oral lichen planus. Chinese J Clin Pharmacol. 2008;24(2):107.
255. Lopez Jornet P, Aznar-Cayuela C. Efficacy of topical chamomile management vs. placebo in patients with oral lichen planus: a randomized double-blind study. J Eur Acad Dermatol Venereol. 2016;30(10):1783–6.
256. Britannica T. Editors of encyclopaedia. Argon Encyclopedia Britannica; 2020.
257. Abe N, Ebina T, Ishida N. Interferon induction by glycyrrhizin and glycyrrhetinic acid in mice. Microbiol Immunol. 1982;26(6):535–9.
258. Arbabi KF, Nosratzehi T, Hamishehkar H, Delazar A. Comparison of effectiveness of the bioadhesive pastes containing licorice 5% and topical corticosteroid for the treatment of oral lichen planus: a pilot study. 2014.
259. Nagao Y. A case of oral lichen planus with chronic hepatitis C successfully treated by glycyrrhizin. Kansenshogaku Zasshi. 1995;69:940–3.
260. Nagao Y, Sata M, Suzuki H, Tanikawa K, Itoh K, Kameyama T. Effectiveness of glycyrrhizin for oral lichen planus in patients with chronic HCV infection. J Gastroenterol. 1996;31(5):691–5.
261. Nagao Y, Nakasone K, Maeshiro T, Nishida N, Kimura K, Kawahigashi Y, et al. Successful treatment of oral lichen planus with direct-acting antiviral agents after liver transplantation for hepatitis C virus-associated hepatocellular carcinoma. Case Rep Gastroenterol. 2017;11(3):701–10.
262. Sorokin E, Smoliakova G, Bachaldin I. Clinical efficacy of eiconol in patients with diabetic retinopathy. Vestn oftalmol. 1997;113(4):37–9.
263. Isaev V, Kaplan AI, Kochetova A, Platonova R, Ashmarin I. Eiconol, a complex of unsaturated fatty acids, optimizes human cognitive activities. Fiziol Cheloveka. 2000;26(2):99–104.
264. Barer G, Polovets M. The use of eiconol in the combined treatment of lichen ruber planus of the oral mucosa. Stomatologiia. 1995;74(1):22–5.
265. Rayman MP. The use of high-selenium yeast to raise selenium status: how does it measure up? Br J Nutr. 2004;92(4):557–73.
266. Selenium. Monograph. Altern Med Rev. 2003;8(1):63–71.
267. Canter P, Wider B, Ernst E. The antioxidant vitamins a, C, E and selenium in the treatment of arthritis: a systematic review of randomized clinical trials. Rheumatology. 2007;46(8):1223–33.
268. Matloob NA. Selenium level in lichen planus and in psoriasis and its relation to chronicity and severity of both diseases. Iraqi. J Med Sci. 2011;9(1)
269. Belal MH. Management of symptomatic erosive-ulcerative lesions of oral lichen planus in an adult Egyptian population using Selenium-ACE combined with topical corticosteroids plus antifungal agent. Contemp Clin Dent. 2015;6(4):454.
270. Qataya PO, Elsayed NM, Elguindy NM, Ahmed Hafiz M, Samy WM. Selenium: a sole treatment for erosive oral lichen planus (randomized controlled clinical trial). Oral Dis. 2020;26(4):789–804.
271. Marzotto M, Conforti A, Magnani P, Zanolin ME, Bellavite P. Effects of Ignatia Amara in mouse behavioural models. Homeopathy. 2012;101(01):57–67.
272. Mousavi F, Sherafati S, Mojaver YN. Ignatia in the treatment of oral lichen planus. Homeopathy. 2009;98(01):40–4.
273. Movahedian A, Ghannadi A, Vashirnia M. Hypocholesterolemic effects of purslane extract on serum lipids in rabbits fed with high cholesterol levels. Int J Pharmacol. 2007;3(3):285–9.
274. Agha-Hosseini F, Borhan-Mojabi K, Monsef-Esfahani HR, Mirzaii-Dizgah I, Etemad-Moghadam S, Karagah A. Efficacy of purslane in the treatment of oral lichen planus. Phytother Res. 2010;24(2):240–4.
275. Wu C. A review on the pharmacology of Paeonia lactiflora and its chemical components. Zhong yao Tong bao (Beijing, China: 1981). 1985;10(6):43–5.
276. Li J, Chen CX, Shen YH. Effects of total glucosides from paeony (Paeonia lactiflora pall) roots on experimental atherosclerosis in rats. J Ethnopharmacol. 2011;135(2):469–75.
277. Xiang N, Li X-M, Zhang M-J, Zhao D-B, Zhu P, Zuo X-X, et al. Total glucosides of paeony can reduce the hepatotoxicity caused by methotrexate and Leflunomide combination treatment of active rheumatoid arthritis. Int Immunopharmacol. 2015;28(1):802–7.
278. Li CL, He J, Li ZG, Zheng LW, Hua H. Effects of total glucosides of paeony for delaying onset of Sjogren's syndrome: an animal study. J Cranio-Maxillofac Surg. 2013;41(7):610–5.
279. Chen Z, Li X-P, Li Z-J, Xu L, Li X-M. Reduced hepatotoxicity by total glucosides of paeony in combination treatment with leflunomide and methotrexate for patients with active rheumatoid arthritis. Int Immunopharmacol. 2013;15(3):474–7.
280. Long J-w, Wang Y-y, Pi X-m, Tu Y-t. Clinical observation on the treatment of chronic urticaria with total glucosides of paeony capsule combined with citirizine. Chin J Integr Med. 2010;16(4):353–6.
281. Zhao M, Liang G-p, Tang M-n, Luo S-y, Zhang J, Cheng W-j, et al. Total glucosides of paeony induces

regulatory CD4+ CD25+ T cells by increasing Foxp3 demethylation in lupus CD4+ T cells. Clin Immunol. 2012;143(2):180–7.
282. Lin J, Xiao L, Ouyang G, Shen Y, Huo R, Zhou Z, et al. Total glucosides of paeony inhibits Th1/Th17 cells via decreasing dendritic cells activation in rheumatoid arthritis. Cell Immunol. 2012;280(2):156–63.
283. Wang Y, Zhang H, Du G, Wang Y, Cao T, Luo Q, et al. Total glucosides of paeony (TGP) inhibits the production of inflammatory cytokines in oral lichen planus by suppressing the NF-κB signaling pathway. Int Immunopharmacol. 2016;36:67–72.
284. Zhao Z, Han Y, Zhang Z, Li W, Ji X, Liu X, et al. Total glucosides of paeony improves the immunomodulatory capacity of MSCs partially via the miR-124/STAT3 pathway in oral lichen planus. Biomed Pharmacother. 2018;105:151–8.
285. Zhou L, Cao T, Wang Y, Yao H, Du G, Tian Z, et al. Clinical observation on the treatment of oral lichen planus with total glucosides of paeony capsule combined with corticosteroids. Int Immunopharmacol. 2016;36:106–10.
286. Ai-ping H. Clinical effect of Nd: YAG laser combined with total glucosides of paeony for the treatment of erosive oral lichen planus. Shanghai Kou Qiang Yi Xue. 2016;25(4):481.
287. Srinivasan K. Black pepper and its pungent principle-piperine: a review of diverse physiological effects. Crit Rev Food Sci Nutr. 2007;47(8):735–48.
288. Bae G-S, Kim M-S, Jung W-S, Seo S-W, Yun S-W, Kim SG, et al. Inhibition of lipopolysaccharide-induced inflammatory responses by piperine. Eur J Pharmacol. 2010;642(1–3):154–62.
289. Butt MS, Pasha I, Sultan MT, Randhawa MA, Saeed F, Ahmed W. Black pepper and health claims: a comprehensive treatise. Crit Rev Food Sci Nutr. 2013;53(9):875–86.
290. Derosa G, Maffioli P, Sahebkar A. Piperine and its role in chronic diseases. Adv Exp Med Biol. 2016;928:173–84.
291. Meghwal M, Goswami T. Piper nigrum and piperine: an update. Phytother Res. 2013;27(8):1121–30.
292. Yang J-Y, Zhang J, Zhou G. Black pepper and its bioactive constituent piperine: promising therapeutic strategies for oral lichen planus. Inflammopharmacology. 2019;27(1):5–13.
293. Panahi Y, Hosseini MS, Khalili N, Naimi E, Majeed M, Sahebkar A. Antioxidant and anti-inflammatory effects of curcuminoid-piperine combination in subjects with metabolic syndrome: a randomized controlled trial and an updated meta-analysis. Clin Nutr. 2015;34(6):1101–8.
294. Yarom N. Etanercept for the management of oral lichen planus. Am J Clin Dermatol. 2007;8(2):121.
295. Muller S, McCreary C, Murphy M. Vulvovaginal-gingival lichen planus with initial response to infliximab. Irish Association of Dermatologists Spring Meeting 2008.
296. Chao TJ. Adalimumab in the management of cutaneous and oral lichen planus. Cutis. 2009;84(6):325–8.
297. Ho JK, Hantash BM. Treatment of recalcitrant vulvovaginal gingival syndrome with adalimumab. J Am Acad Dermatol. 2011;65(2):e55–e7.
298. Andrade P, Lopes S, Albuquerque A, Osório F, Pardal J, Macedo G. Oral lichen planus in ibd patients: a paradoxical adverse effect of anti-TNF-α therapy. Dig Dis Sci. 2015;60(9):2746–9.
299. Asarch A, Gottlieb AB, Lee J, Masterpol KS, Scheinman PL, Stadecker MJ, et al. Lichen planus–like eruptions: an emerging side effect of tumor necrosis factor-α antagonists. J Am Acad Dermatol. 2009;61(1):104–11.
300. Sivamani RK, Correa G, Ono Y, Bowen MP, Raychaudhuri SP, Maverakis E. Biological therapy of psoriasis. Indian J Dermatol. 2010;55(2):161.
301. Rebora A, Parodi A, Murialdo G. Basiliximab is effective for erosive lichen planus. Arch Dermatol. 2002;138(8):1100–1.
302. Zhang J, Zhou G, Du GF, Xu XY, Zhou HM. Biologics, an alternative therapeutic approach for oral lichen planus. J Oral Pathol Med. 2011;40(7):521–4.
303. Gisondi P, Girolomoni G. Biologic therapies in psoriasis: a new therapeutic approach. Autoimmun Rev. 2007;6(8):515–9.
304. Gottlieb AB, Gordon KB, Hamilton TK, Caro I, Kwon P, Compton P. Maintenance of efficacy and safety with continuous efalizumab therapy in patients with moderate to severe chronic plaque psoriasis: final phase IIIb study results. 63rd Annual Meeting of the American Academy of Dermatology 2005. pp. 18–22.
305. Cheng A, Mann C. Oral erosive lichen planus treated with efalizumab. Arch Dermatol. 2006;142(6):680–2.
306. Böhm M, Luger TA. Lichen planus responding to efalizumab. J Am Acad Dermatol. 2007;56(5):S92–S3.
307. Heffernan MP, Smith DI, Bentley D, Tabacchi M, Graves JE. A single-center, open-label, prospective pilot study of subcutaneous efalizumab for oral erosive lichen planus. J Drug Dermatol. 2007;6(3):310–4.
308. Korman BD, Tyler KL, Korman NJ. Progressive multifocal leukoencephalopathy, efalizumab, and immunosuppression: a cautionary tale for dermatologists. Arch Dermatol. 2009;145(8):937–42.
309. Ellis CN, Krueger GG. Treatment of chronic plaque psoriasis by selective targeting of memory effector T lymphocytes. N Engl J Med. 2001;345(4):248–55.
310. Fivenson DP, Mathes B. Treatment of generalized lichen planus with alefacept. Arch Dermatol. 2006;142(2):151–2.
311. Chang A, Badger J, Rehmus W, Kimball AB. Alefacept for erosive lichen planus: a case series. J Drug Dermatol. 2008;7(4):379–83.
312. Colliou N, Picard D, Caillot F, Calbo S, Le Corre S, Lim A, et al. Long-term remissions of severe pemphigus after rituximab therapy are associated with prolonged failure of desmoglein B cell response. Sci Transl Med. 2013;5(175):175ra30-ra30.

313. Kenneth KY, Crew AB, Messingham KA, Fairley JA, Woodley DT. Omalizumab therapy for bullous pemphigoid. J Am Acad Dermatol. 2014;71(3):468–74.
314. Hainsworth JD, Burris HA III, Morrissey LH, Litchy S, Scullin DC Jr, Bearden JD III, et al. Rituximab monoclonal antibody as initial systemic therapy for patients with low-grade non-Hodgkin lymphoma. Blood. 2000;95(10):3052–6.
315. Chong BF, Werth VP. Management of cutaneous lupus erythematosus. Dubois' Lupus Erythematosus and related syndromes. Elsevier; 2019. pp. 719–726.
316. Cutler C, Miklos D, Kim HT, Treister N, Woo S-B, Bienfang D, et al. Rituximab for steroid-refractory chronic graft-versus-host disease. Blood. 2006;108(2):756–62.
317. Parmentier L, Bron B-A, Prins C, Samson J, Masouyé I, Borradori L. Mucocutaneous lichen planus with esophageal involvement: successful treatment with an anti-CD20 monoclonal antibody. Arch Dermatol. 2008;144(11):1427–30.
318. Esarte SG, Letamendía AA, Costas JJV, Pérez FJJ. Rituximab as rescue therapy in refractory esophageal lichen planus. Gastroenterol Hepatol. 2012;36(4):264–7.
319. Heelan K, McAleer M, Roche L, McCreary C, Murphy M. Intractable erosive lichen planus treated successfully with rituximab. Br J Dermatol. 2015;172(2):538–40.
320. Giudice A, Liborio F, Averta F, Barone S, Fortunato L. Oral lichenoid reaction: an uncommon side effect of rituximab. Case reports in Dentistry 2019;2019.
321. Kuten-Shorrer M, Hochberg EP, Woo S-B. Lichenoid mucosal reaction to rituximab. Oncologist. 2014;19(10):e12–e3.
322. McCormack PL, Keam SJ. Bevacizumab. Drugs. 2008;68(4):487–506.
323. Food U, Administration D. Center for Drug Evaluation and Research. Final Labeling Text, BL125085 Supplement. 2008.
324. Tanimoto K, Yoshiga K, Eguchi H, Kaneyasu M, Ukon K, Kumazaki T, et al. Hypoxia-inducible factor-1α polymorphisms associated with enhanced transactivation capacity, implying clinical significance. Carcinogenesis. 2003;24(11):1779–83.
325. Muller YA, Chen Y, Christinger HW, Li B, Cunningham BC, Lowman HB, et al. VEGF and the fab fragment of a humanized neutralizing antibody: crystal structure of the complex at 2.4 Å resolution and mutational analysis of the interface. Structure. 1998;6(9):1153–67.
326. Mancuso MR, Davis R, Norberg SM, O'Brien S, Sennino B, Nakahara T, et al. Rapid vascular regrowth in tumors after reversal of VEGF inhibition. J Clin Invest. 2006;116(10):2610–21.
327. Shih T, Lindley C. Bevacizumab: an angiogenesis inhibitor for the treatment of solid malignancies. Clin Ther. 2006;28(11):1779–802.
328. Kazazi-Hyseni F, Beijnen JH, Schellens JH. Bevacizumab. Oncologist. 2010;15(8):819.
329. Al-Hassiny A, Friedlander L, Parachuru V, Seo B, Hussaini H, Rich A. Upregulation of angiogenesis in oral lichen planus. J Oral Pathol Med. 2018;47(2):173–8.
330. Mahmoud MM, Afifi MM. Anti-angiogenic therapy (bevacizumab) in the management of oral lichen planus. Eur J Oral Sci. 2016;124(2):119–26.
331. Solimani F, Pollmann R, Schmidt T, Schmidt A, Zheng X, Savai R, et al. Therapeutic targeting of Th17/Tc17 cells leads to clinical improvement of lichen planus. Front Immunol. 2019;10:1808.
332. Dalirsani Z, Delavarian Z, Javadzade-Bolouri A, Hashemian P. Psychiatric comorbidity and pharmacotherapy in patients with oral lichen planus. Psychiatric Disorders–Worldwide Advances 2011;223.
333. Vallejo MG-P, Huerta G, Cerero R, Seoane J. Anxiety and depression as risk factors for oral lichen planus. Dermatology. 2001;203(4):303–7.
334. Girardi C, Luz C, Cherubini K, de Figueiredo MAZ, Nunes MLT, Salum FG. Salivary cortisol and dehydroepiandrosterone (DHEA) levels, psychological factors in patients with oral lichen planus. Arch Oral Biol. 2011;56(9):864–8.
335. Delavarian Z, Javadzade-Bolouri A, Dalirsani Z, Arshadi H-R, Toofani-Asl H. The evaluation of psychiatric drug therapy on oral lichen planus patients with psychiatric disorders. Med Oral, Patol Oral Cir Bucal. 2010;15(2):e322–e7.
336. Bagan J, Compilato D, Paderni C, Campisi G, Panzarella V, Picciotti M, et al. Topical therapies for oral lichen planus management and their efficacy: a narrative review. Curr Pharm Des. 2012;18(34):5470–80.
337. Nasr MM, Ebrahim HM, Khattab FM, Marei AM. Bacillus Calmette-Guerin, polysaccharide nucleic acid in the treatment of cutaneous and oral lichen planus. Dermatol Ther. 2018;31(3):e12591.
338. Bascones-Martinez A, Mattila R, Gomez-Font R, Meurman JH. Immunomodulatory drugs: Oral and systemic adverse effects. Med Oral, Patol Oral Cir Bucal. 2014;19(1):e24.
339. Chun Y. BCG-polysaccharide nucleic acid with prednisolone in the treatment of alopecia areata. Pract J Clin Med. 2010;37:78–9.
340. Li N, Cao N, Niu YD, Bai XH, Lu J, Sun Y, et al. Effects of the polysaccharide nucleic acid fraction of bacillus calmette-guérin on the production of interleukin-2 and interleukin-10 in the peripheral blood lymphocytes of patients with chronic idiopathic urticaria. Biomed Rep. 2013;1(5):713–8.
341. Sloot S, Rashid OM, Sarnaik AA, Zager JS. Developments in intralesional therapy for metastatic melanoma. Cancer Control. 2016;23(1):12–20.
342. Zuo C, Huang J, Liao Z, Lu J, Chen J. Effects of BCG-PSN on serum levels of IL-4 and IL-12 in patients with condyloma acuminatum. Zhong Nan Da Xue Xue Bao Yi Xue Ban. 2004;29(6):690–2.
343. Sharquie K, Hayani R. BCG as a new therapeutic and prophylactic agent in patients with severe oral aphthosis. Clin Exp Rheumatol. 2005;23(6):914.
344. Zhan L, Xiong X, Wang L. Treatment of BCG polysaccharide nucleic acid combined with CO2 laser

reduces Th17 cells and their related cytokines in cutaneous lesion of vitiligo patients. Xi bao yu fen zi Mian yi xue za zhi= Chinese journal of. Cell Mol Immunol. 2014;30(12):1300–3.
345. Xiong C, Li Q, Lin M, Li X, Meng W, Wu Y, et al. The efficacy of topical intralesional BCG-PSN injection in the treatment of erosive oral lichen planus: a randomized controlled trial. J Oral Pathol Med. 2009;38(7):551–8.
346. Shaik S, Jyothi PN, Kumar BV, Suman S, Praveen KS, Sravanthi M. Platelet rich plasma a new prospective in treatment of recalcitrant Erosive Lichen Planus.
347. Pietrzak WS, Eppley BL. Platelet rich plasma: biology and new technology. J Craniofac Surg. 2005;16(6):1043–54.
348. Merigo E, Oppici A, Parlatore A, Cella L, Clini F, Fontana M, et al. Platelet-rich plasma (PRP) rinses for the treatment of non-responding oral lichen planus: a case report. Biomedicine. 2018;6(1):15.
349. Loré B, Saraceno R, Poladas G, Fida M, Khoury C, Arcuri C, et al. Oral lichen planus: therapy and phenotype. G Ital Dermatol Venereol. 2016;153(4):459–63.
350. Axéll T, Henriksen BM. Treatment of gingival lichen with free palatal grafts. J Oral Pathol Med. 2007;36(2):105–9.
351. Hovick C, Kalkwarf K. Treatment of localized oral erosive lichen planus lesions with free soft tissue grafts. Periodontal Case Rep. 1987;9(2):21–4.
352. Tamizi M, Moayedi M. Treatment of gingival lichen planus with a free gingival graft: a case report. Quintessence Int. 1992;23(4):249.
353. Katz J, Goultschin J, Benoliel R, Rotstein I, Pisanty S. Lichen planus evoked by periodontal surgery. J Clin Periodontol. 1988;15(4):263–5.
354. Ishida MDCE, Ramos-e-Silva MDP, Marcia. Cryosurgery in oral lesions. Int J Dermatol. 1998;37(4):283–5.
355. Malmström M, Leikomaa H. Experiences with cryotherapy in the treatment of oral lesions. Proc Finn Dent Soc. 1980;76(3):117–23.
356. Pakfetrat A, Falaki F, Ahrari F, Bidad S. Removal of refractory erosive-atrophic lichen planus by the CO2 laser. Oral Health Dent Manag. 2014;13(3):595–9.
357. Van der Hem P, Egges M, Van der Wal J, Roodenburg J. CO2 laser evaporation of oral lichen planus. Int J Oral Maxillofac Surg. 2008;37(7):630–3.
358. Fornaini C, Raybaud H, Augros C, Rocca J-P. New clinical approach for use of Er: YAG laser in the surgical treatment of oral lichen planus: a report of two cases. Photomed Laser Surg. 2012;30(4):234–8.
359. Akbulut N, Kursun ES, Tumer MK, Kamburoglu K, Gulsen U. Is the 810-nm diode laser the best choice in oral soft tissue therapy? Eur J Dent. 2013;7(02):207–11.
360. Aras MH, Göregen M, Güngörmüş M, Akgül HM. Comparison of diode laser and Er: YAG lasers in the treatment of ankyloglossia. Photomed Laser Surg. 2010;28(2):173–7.
361. Akram Z, Abduljabbar T, Vohra F, Javed F. Efficacy of low-level laser therapy compared to steroid therapy in the treatment of oral lichen planus: a systematic review. J Oral Pathol Med. 2018;47(1):11–7.
362. Jajarm HH, Falaki F, Mahdavi O. A comparative pilot study of low intensity laser versus topical corticosteroids in the treatment of erosive-atrophic oral lichen planus. Photomed Laser Surg. 2011;29(6):421–5.
363. Walsh L. The current status of low level laser therapy in dentistry, part 1. Soft tissue applications. Aust Dent J. 1997;42(4):247–54.
364. Conlan MJ, Rapley JW, Cobb CM. Biostimulation of wound healing by low-energy laser irradiation a review. J Clin Periodontol. 1996;23(5):492–6.
365. Karu TI, Pyatibrat LV, Moskvin SV, Andreev S, Letokhov VS. Elementary processes in cells after light absorption do not depend on the degree of polarization: implications for the mechanisms of laser phototherapy. Photomed Laser Surg. 2008;26(2):77–82.
366. Agha-Hosseini F, Moslemi E, Mirzaii-Dizgah I. Comparative evaluation of low-level laser and CO2 laser in treatment of patients with oral lichen planus. Int J Oral Maxillofac Surg. 2012;41(10):1265–9.
367. Elshenawy HM, Eldin AM, Abdelmonem MA. Clinical assessment of the efficiency of low level laser therapy in the treatment of Oral lichen planus. Open Access Maced J Med Sci. 2015;3(4):717–21. https://doi.org/10.3889/oamjms.2015.112.
368. Passeron T, Zakaria W, Ostovari N, Mantoux F, Lacour J, Ortonne J. Treatment of erosive oral lichen planus by the 308 nm excimer laser. Lasers Surg Med. 2004;34(3):205.
369. Köllner K, Wimmershoff M, Landthaler M, Hohenleutner U. Treatment of oral lichen planus with the 308-nm UVB excimer laser—early preliminary results in eight patients. Lasers Surg Med. 2003;33(3):158–60.
370. Trehan M, Taylor CR. Low-dose excimer 308-nm laser for the treatment of oral lichen planus. Arch Dermatol. 2004;140(4):415–20.
371. Fornaini C. LLLT in the symptomatic treatment of oral lichen planus. Laser Therapy. 2012;21(1):51–3.
372. Mahdavi O, Boostani N, Jajarm H, Falaki F, Tabesh A. Use of low level laser therapy for oral lichen planus: report of two cases. J Dent. 2013;14(4):201.
373. Sivolella S, Berengo M, Cernuschi S, Valente M. Diode laser treatment is effective for plaque-like lichen planus of the tongue: a case report. Lasers Med Sci. 2012;27(2):521–4.
374. Cafaro A, Albanese G, Arduino PG, Mario C, Massolini G, Mozzati M, et al. Effect of low-level laser irradiation on unresponsive oral lichen planus: early preliminary results in 13 patients. Photomed Laser Surg. 2010;28(S2):S-99–S-103.
375. Cafaro A, Arduino PG, Massolini G, Romagnoli E, Broccoletti R. Clinical evaluation of the efficiency of low-level laser therapy for oral lichen planus: a prospective case series. Lasers Med Sci. 2014;29(1):185–90.

376. El Shenawy HM, Eldin AM. A comparative evaluation of low-level laser and topical steroid therapies for the treatment of erosive-atrophic lichen planus. Open Access Maced J Med Sci. 2015;3(3):462–6. https://doi.org/10.3889/oamjms.2015.072.
377. Othman N-A, Shaker O-G, Elshenawy H-M, Abd-Elmoniem W, Eldin A-M, Fakhr M-Y. The effect of diode laser and topical steroid on serum level of TNF-alpha in oral lichen planus patients. J Clin Exp Dent. 2016;8(5):e566.
378. Dillenburg CS, Martins MAT, Munerato MC, Marques MM, Carrard VC, Sant'Ana Filho M, et al. Efficacy of laser phototherapy in comparison to topical clobetasol for the treatment of oral lichen planus: a randomized controlled trial. J Biomed Opt. 2014;19(6):068002.
379. Mostafa D, Tarakji B. Photodynamic therapy in treatment of oral lichen planus. J Clin Med Res. 2015;7(6):393.
380. Costa RA, Farah ME, Cardillo JA, Belfort R. Photodynamic therapy with indocyanine green for occult subfoveal choroidal neovascularization caused by age-related macular degeneration. Curr Eye Res. 2001;23(4):271–5.
381. Donnelly RF, McCarron PA, Woolfson D. Drug delivery systems for photodynamic therapy. Recent Pat Drug Deliv Formul. 2009;3(1):1–7.
382. Ochsner M. Photophysical and photobiological processes in the photodynamic therapy of tumours. J Photochem Photobiol B Biol. 1997;39(1):1–18.
383. Moan J, Streckyte G, Bagdonas S, Bech Ø, Berg K. Photobleaching of protoporphyrin IX in cells incubated with 5-aminolevulinic acid. Int J Cancer. 1997;70(1):90–7.
384. Aghahosseini F, Arbabi-Kalati F, Fashtami LA, Fateh M, Djavid GE. Treatment of oral lichen planus with photodynamic therapy mediated methylene blue: a case report. Medicina Oral, Patología Oral y Cirugía Bucal (Internet). 2006;11(2):126–9.
385. Pavlic V, Vujic-Aleksic V. Phototherapy approaches in treatment of oral lichen planus. Photodermatol Photoimmunol Photomed. 2014;30(1):15–24.
386. Korbelik M. PDT-associated host response and its role in the therapy outcome. Laser Surg Med. 2006;38(5):500–8.
387. Sobaniec S, Bernaczyk P, Pietruski J, Cholewa M, Skurska A, Dolińska E, et al. Clinical assessment of the efficacy of photodynamic therapy in the treatment of oral lichen planus. Lasers Med Sci. 2013;28(1):311–6.
388. Aghahosseini F, Arbabi-Kalati F, Fashtami LA, Djavid GE, Fateh M, Beitollahi JM. Methylene blue-mediated photodynamic therapy: a possible alternative treatment for oral lichen planus. Laser Surg Med. 2006;38(1):33–8.
389. Paula LF, Santos RO, Menezes HD, Britto JR, Vieira JB Jr, Gontijo Filho PP, et al. A comparative study of irradiation systems for photoinactivation of microorganisms. J Braz Chem Soc. 2010;21:694–700.
390. Lundquist G, Forsgren H, Gajecki M, Emtestam L. Photochemotherapy of oral lichen planus: a cotrolled study. Oral Surg Oral Med Oral Pathol Oral Radiol Endodontol. 1995;79(5):554–8.
391. Tanew A, Radakovic-Fijan S, Schemper M, Hönigsmann H. Narrowband UV-B phototherapy vs photochemotherapy in the treatment of chronic plaque-type psoriasis: a paired comparison study. Arch Dermatol. 1999;135(5):519–24.
392. Kassem R, Yarom N, Scope A, Babaev M, Trau H, Pavlotzky F. Treatment of erosive oral lichen planus with local ultraviolet B phototherapy. J Am Acad Dermatol. 2012;66(5):761–6.
393. Kunte C, Erlenkeuser-Uebelhoer I, Michelsen S, Scheerer-Dhungel K, Plewig G. Treatment of therapy-resistant erosive oral lichen planus with extracorporeal photopheresis (ECP). Journal der Deutschen Dermatologischen Gesellschaft= Journal of the German Society of Dermatology: JDDG. 2005;3(11):889–94.
394. Guyot A, Farhi D, Ingen-Housz-Oro S, Bussel A, Parquet N, Rabian C, et al. Treatment of refractory erosive oral lichen planus with extracorporeal photochemotherapy: 12 cases. Br J Dermatol. 2007;156(3):553–6.
395. Marchesseau-Merlin A, Perea R, Kanold J, Demeocq F, Souteyrand P, D'Incan M. Photopheresis: an alternative therapeutic approach in corticoresistant erosive oral lichen planus. Ann Dermatol Venereol. 2008;135:209–12.
396. Biasotto M, Campisi G, Lodi G, Lo Muzio L, Mignogna MD, Montebugnolie L, Sardella A. Patologia e Medicina Orale - SIPMO. Edra, 1° Edition, 2022.
397. Del Gaizo C, Panzarella V, Giannatempo G, Lo Russo L, Canepa F, Mauceri R, ... & DI FEDE O. Oral Lichen Planus: a new experimental therapeutic protocol by means of oxygen-ozone mixture injection. J. Osseointegration. 2019;11(2):413–414.
398. Adamo D, Mignogna MD, Pecoraro G, Aria M, Fortuna G. Management of reticular oral lichen planus patients with burning mouth syndrome-like oral symptoms: a pilot study. J Dermatolog Treat. 2018;29(6):623–29.

Batch number: 10732801

Printed by Printforce, the Netherlands